Springer Texts in Education

Springer Texts in Education delivers high-quality instructional content for graduates and advanced graduates in all areas of Education and Educational Research. The textbook series is comprised of self-contained books with a broad and comprehensive coverage that are suitable for class as well as for individual self-study. All texts are authored by established experts in their fields and offer a solid methodological background, accompanied by pedagogical materials to serve students such as practical examples, exercises, case studies etc. Textbooks published in the Springer Texts in Education series are addressed to graduate and advanced graduate students, but also to researchers as important resources for their education, knowledge and teaching. Please contact Natalie Rieborn at textbooks.education@springer.com for queries or to submit your book proposal.

More information about this series at http://www.springer.com/series/13812

Jimmie Leppink

The Art of Modelling the Learning Process

Uniting Educational Research and Practice

Springer

Jimmie Leppink
Hull York Medical School
University of York
York, UK

ISSN 2366-7672 ISSN 2366-7680 (electronic)
Springer Texts in Education
ISBN 978-3-030-43081-8 ISBN 978-3-030-43082-5 (eBook)
https://doi.org/10.1007/978-3-030-43082-5

This Springer imprint is published by the registered company Springer Nature Switzerland AG
The registered company address is: Gewerbestrasse 11, 6330 Cham, Switzerland

I dedicate this book to my wife

Patricia Pérez Fuster

Just when I thought I would never say 'no'
To a great opportunity to continue my career
on another continent
Life happened, we met—totally
unexpected—and everything changed

That 'no' to the other continent
Has been one of the best decisions
In my life thus far

Thank you for always being by my side

Preface

Eighteen years ago, I decided to study Psychology, because I thought I wanted to become a clinical psychologist. However, I soon developed a passion for research methods as a way to do good research and to provide an evidence base for clinical practice. I learned about heuristics and biases in human reasoning and slowly but steadily learned that the Leitmotiv question that fascinates me is: *What is evidence?* I had not lost my interest in Clinical Psychology but realised that there was a field where my interest in Clinical Psychology and my interest in the evidence question would fit in very well: Forensic Psychology. I wanted to become an eyewitness expert and advise judges, lawyers, and juries on the reliability and validity of eyewitness testimonies and about the strength of evidence available in a criminal case, and so I decided to continue my studies in that direction.

At the same time, as a tutor in Statistics during my Bachelor's and Master's studies in Psychology, I also developed a keen interest in how to make Statistics Education better, to make it more accessible for students in Psychology, Health Sciences, Medicine, Law, and other domains. An unexpected opportunity to do a Ph.D. in exactly that topic emerged, and I decided to go for it and leave forensics as an option for after my Ph.D. Instead of eventually returning to Forensics, I decided to stay in Education and expand my work from Statistics Education to Language Education, Medical Education, and related fields. The key question since the start of my Ph.D. in September 2008 has been how we can establish evidence for what works in Education for what type of learners and under what circumstances. Looking back at my research over the years, especially during and the first years after my Ph.D., I would have done many things differently, but that change in perspective is—and, in my view, should be—part of a researcher's journey.

What I would *not* have done differently is to be trained in different domains and fields. A Latin proverb goes: *Non scholae, sed vitae discimus*, or: we learn not for school but for life. The world around us is changing rapidly, and although we have to make choices in how much time we devote to different things, a background in different domains and fields allows for more flexibility in learning new things, for preparing for the jobs of tomorrow, and for developing a broader and more diverse perspective on complex phenomena such as human learning. Although I would have done quite a few things differently if I was about to start my Postdoc now—and all positions have their pros, cons, and challenges—looking back, being a

Postdoc for five years has been one of the best things that could happen. I spent time at institutes in Australia, Canada, Spain, Germany, and the Netherlands, before eventually moving to the United Kingdom, and slowly but steadily developed my own perspective on learning and the evidence question. For the three books (including this one) that I have written thus far, most of the ideas were born while travelling during that five-year Postdoc time.

In this book, I discuss a variety of ways to model learning processes from the perspectives of the different domains and fields I passed over the eighteen years since I decided to study Psychology, using a variety of methods and both commercial and zero-cost Open Source software packages.

York, UK Jimmie Leppink

Acknowledgements

After *Instructional Design Principles for High-Stakes Problem-Solving Environments*, written in collaboration with my colleagues from Western Sydney University Dr. Chwee Beng Lee and Dr. José Hanham, and *Statistical Methods for Experimental Research in Education and Psychology*, this text on modelling the learning process is my third book. Even though this book, like my second book, is a monograph, many people have had their impact on its content. Through studies, conferences, visiting researcher trips, and other opportunities, I have been fortunate to learn from many people at a variety of sites across the world. At **Maastricht University**, I learned from quite a few people but above all from my mentor the late Dr. Arno Muijtjens. At the **Catholic University of Leuven**, I found great teachers in among others: Emeritus Prof. Dr. Jacques Tacq; Prof. Dr. Geert Molenberghs; Prof. Dr. Kelvyn Jones; and the late Emeritus Prof. Dr. Allan McCutcheon. I am proud to be a Maastricht University and Catholic University of Leuven graduate!

Since my postdoctoral visit to Australia in 2015, I have been greatly inspired by Dr. Paul Ginns (**University of Sydney**), Dr. José Hanham (**Western Sydney University**), and Prof. Dr. Martin Veysey (**University of Newcastle**, and later as colleague at **Hull York Medical School**). During my trips to Canada in December 2015 and April 2016, I learned from a variety of great scholars, including Dr. Kulamakan (Mahan) Kulasegaram (**University of Toronto**), Dr. Saad Chahine (**Western University**, later **University of Ottawa**), and Dr. Adam Szulewski (**Queen's University**).

The first of a series of research visits to the **Universitat de València** (University of Valencia, Spain) was the single best thing in my life thus far, not in the last place because this is where I met my wife, Dr. Patricia Pérez Fuster, who has been by my side since that first visit and with whom I have published several papers on methodological and statistical topics. During my several stays at the University of Valencia, I also learned a great deal from several great Educational Psychologists, including Dr. Ladislao Salmeron, Emeritus Prof. Dr. Eduardo Vidal Abarca, and Dr. Raquel Cerdán.

Technology has made it very easy to learn from people who are stationed far away and whom you may only meet occasionally, for instance at a conference. Through collaboration or through dialogue in online platforms that aim to unite scientists across the globe, I have learned from many people, and above all from

Dr. Shane Tutwiler (**Harvard University**, later **University of Rhode Island**, thank you for reviewing the previous version of this book), Prof. Dr. Patricia O'Sullivan (**University of California**, **San Francisco**), and Dr. Kalman Winston (**University of Liverpool Online** and **Cambridge University**).

With my move to **Hull York Medical School**, **University of York**, I found many great new colleagues, including Mrs. Joanna Micklethwaite, Dr. Steven Oliver, and Dr. Kit Fan. It is exciting to be part of a team of many enthusiasts with great ideas who each in their own way contribute to the collective effort to make bold steps in the expansion and development of a medical school.

All the people mentioned here, and many more, including the reviewers of the proposal with which this book started—Dr. Shane Tutwiler and Prof. Dr. Bart Rienties—have had their impact on the content of this book; for all this, I am very grateful.

York, UK Jimmie Leppink

Contact

For a quick tour through the book and data files, syntax, and worked examples of studies discussed in this book, please visit: https://wordpress.com/view/research489962293.wordpress.com (this website is also used for my previous book *Statistical Methods for Experimental Research in Education and Psychology*). The website also has a contact form, which allows you to send emails to me. For any questions, comments, or suggestions—which I will consider for an eventual next edition—please use the contact form on the website or get in touch with me directly via j.leppink@gmail.com (Gmail) or hyjl17@hyms.ac.uk (my Outlook email address at Hull York Medical School).

Contents

About the Author

Jimmie Leppink (28 April 1983) obtained degrees in Psychology (M.Sc., Cum Laude), Law (LLM), and Statistics Education (Ph.D.) from Maastricht University, the Netherlands, and obtained a degree in Statistics (M.Sc., Magna Cum Laude) from the Catholic University of Leuven, Belgium. He was a Postdoc in Education and Assistant Professor of Methodology and Statistics at Maastricht University's School of Health Professions Education. In January 2019, he moved to the University of York, where he has been working as Senior Lecturer in Medical Education (since January 2019), as Deputy Chair of Board of Studies (since June 2019), and as Academic Lead and Director of Assessment (since September 2019) at Hull York Medical School. His research, teaching, and consulting activities revolve around applications of research methods in Education, Psychology, and a broader Social Science context as well as the use of learning analytics for the design of learning environments, instruction, and assessment in Medical Education and the broader Education.

Symbols and Abbreviations

α	Statistical significance level in some cases, Cronbach's alpha in other cases
θ	Ability
λ	Constant factor in HF, also standardised item (-factor) loadings in factor analysis
μ	Population mean
π	Population proportion
ρ	Reliability in some examples, Spearman's correlation coefficient in other examples
σ	Population *SD*, and in squared form the population variance
σ_M	σ of *M*
φ	Coefficient φ, a measure of the strength of association for categorical variables that, when all variables involved are dichotomous, yields the same point estimate as r, ρ, τ, and V
χ^2	Chi-square, a test statistic
τ	Kendall's τ
τ_b	Kendall's τ-b, a Kendall's τ-coefficient included in most statistical software packages
τ^2	Heterogeneity in effect of interest across studies (e.g., in a meta-analysis)
ω	McDonald's omega
–2LL, –2RLL	The minus two log likelihood aka deviance of a model using FIML (–2LL; fixed effects) or using REML (–2RLL; random effects): LL stands for log likelihood
1PL, 2PL, 3PL	One-, two-, and three-parameter logistic model
A, B	In the context of randomised controlled experiments used to refer to treatment factors, and in the context of SCEDs sometimes used to denote baseline (A) and treatment (B), and in some examples used to denote different scenarios
AB	Example of a baseline (A)-treatment (B) phase design in the context of SCED
AD1	First-order ante-dependence residual covariance structure

AI	Artificial Intelligence
AIC	Akaike's information criterion
AICc	Corrected AIC, a variant of AIC that has a slightly lower tendency towards more complex models than AIC, though the difference between AIC and AICc reduces with increasing sample size
AIG	Automatic item generation
ALS	Applied life sciences
AR1	First-order autoregressive residual covariance structure
AR1H	Extension of AR1 structure that accounts for varying V_{RES}
ARIMA	Autoregressive integrated moving average
ARIMA(0,0,0)	Mean (*M*) model
ARIMA(0,0,1)	MA1 model
ARIMA(0,1,0)	Random walk model
ARIMA(1,0,0)	AR1 model
ARIMA(1,0,1)	ARMA(1,1) residual covariance structure that combines AR1 and MA1
ATD	Alternating treatments design
B, *b*	Regression coefficient
B_0	Fixed intercept
BF	Bayes factor
BF_{01}	Bayes factor for $\boldsymbol{H_0}$ verses $\boldsymbol{H_1}$
BF_{10}	Bayes factor for $\boldsymbol{H_1}$ verses $\boldsymbol{H_0}$
BIC	Schwarz' Bayesian information criterion
C%	Percentage of CI, often 95% although in this book I also hold a plea for 90%
CAIC	An extension of AIC that, somewhat like BIC, provides a stricter penalty for adding more parameters and as such reduces the likelihood of too complex models being selected when many parameters can be estimated
CAT	Computerised adaptive testing
CI	Frequentist confidence interval
CRI	Credible interval aka posterior interval, a Bayesian alternative to the Frequentist confidence interval
CS	Compound symmetry
CSH	CS heterogenous (i.e., allowing V_{RES} to vary)
CSI	Crime Scene Investigation
d	Cohen's *d*, a measure of effect size which expresses the differences between two *M*s in *SD*s instead of in actual scale (e.g., points or minutes) units
DC	Degree centrality
df	Degrees of freedom
DI	Diagonal covariance structure, which assumes independence of residuals but varying V_{RES}
DIF	Differential item functioning

DRF	Deviance reduction factor, also known as R^2_{McF} in fixed-effects categorical outcome variable models, and for any comparison of fixed-effects solutions in fixed-effects and mixed-effects models in studies involving categorical or quantitative outcome variables, a straightforward indicator of the reduction in –2LL or deviance by a more complex model relative to a simpler (i.e., special case) variant of that more complex model (e.g., Model 1 vs. Model 0, or a main-effects plus interaction model vs. a main-effects model)
E	In some cases evidence, in some cases the number of edges that can be estimated in a network analysis
e	Exponent
EBIC	Extended BIC
EBICglasso	The combination of EBIC and LASSO
EDM	Educational Data Mining
E_E	The number of non-zero (i.e., estimated) edges in a network analysis
EMM	Estimated marginal means
ESEM	Exploratory structural equation modelling
E_x	Piece of evidence
FA1	First-order factor-analytic covariance structure
FA1H	A variant of FA1 in which V_{RES} is allowed to vary
FIML	Full Informed Maximum Likelihood, used for the estimation of fixed effects, sometimes also referred to simply as ML (Maximum Likelihood)
FOST	Four one-sided testing
GPS	Global Positioning System
GR	Ganz Rasch, a software package used for this book, version 1.0
$\boldsymbol{H_0}$	Null hypothesis
$\boldsymbol{H_{0.1}}$, $\boldsymbol{H_{0.2}}$, $\boldsymbol{H_{0.3}}$, $\boldsymbol{H_{0.4}}$	The coherent set of four H_0s tested in FOST, the first two of which are also used in TOST
$\boldsymbol{H_1}$	Alternative hypothesis
H(1:1), H(1:2)	(Some of the) hidden layers in an artificial neural network
HF	Huynh-Feldt residual covariance structure
H&S	Health and society
i	Lowest level in multilevel (i.e., mixed-effects) model
ICC	Intraclass correlation
ID	Independence residual covariance structure, basically a linear regression model assuming independence of residuals and assuming a constant V_{RES}
IGLS	Iterative generalised least squares
i.i.d.	Independently and identically distributed
IRT	Item response theory

j	Second-lowest level in multilevel (i.e., mixed-effects) model (e.g., upper level in two-level model)
Jamovi	In other sources sometimes denoted with small J as *jamovi*, a statistical software package used in this book, version 1.1.5.0
JASP	A statistical software package used in this book, version 0.11.1.0
JZS	Jeffrey-Zellner-Siow, used to refer to a set of common prior distributions (e.g., for *M*, difference in *M*, and *r*) in Bayesian analysis
k	Number of items (and in the context of AR1 and AR1H, the number of items in between a given pair of two items, for instance for adjacent items $k = 0$); in some cases, *k* refers to the third-lowest level in a multilevel (i.e., mixed-effects) model (e.g., upper level in a three-level model)
LA	Learning Analytics
LASSO	Least absolute shrinkage and selection operator
LB	Lower bound
$ln(OR)$	Logit
LR	Likelihood Ratio
LR_E	LR of E
LR_x	LR of E_x
M	(Arithmetic) mean in a sample, group, or condition
MA	Moving average
MA1	First-order moving average
MAR	Missing at random
MAR1	In repeated-measures and longitudinal studies, MAR depending on the previous response
MAR2	In repeated-measures and longitudinal studies, MAR depending on the previous two responses
MBBS	Bachelor of Medicine Bachelor of Surgery
MCAR	Missing completely at random
M_d	Mean difference
MI	Multiple imputation
MLwiN	A statistical software package used in this book, version 3.02
M_N	A factor by which to multiply *N* based on $ICC = 0$ to account for $ICC > 0$
MNAR	Missing not at random
Model 0	Null model ($\boldsymbol{H_0}$ or simplest of models under comparisons)

Model 1	Alternative model ($\boldsymbol{H_1}$), a more complex version of the null model, and when there are several alternatives to Model 0, together with Model 0 among several competing models in model comparison/selection (e.g., also Models 2–4 when we deal with possible main and interaction effects of two factors)
MOOC	Massive open online course
Mplus	A statistical software package used in this book, version 8
N, n	Total sample size (N) and size of condition or group within total sample size (n)
NHST	Null hypothesis significance testing
n_{TEST}	Sample size (n) of a testing sample
n_{TRAIN}	Sample size (n) of a training sample
OR	Odds ratio
OSCE	Objective structured clinical examination
P, p	Probability
PAND	Percentage of all non-overlapping data, generally a better alternative to PND
PAND-B	Bayesian Binomial alternative to PAND, which yields a point estimate slightly less extreme than PAND and, contrary to PAND, comes with a 95% CRI
PAND-BC	PAND-B corrected for correlated residuals
PASTE	Pragmatic approach to statistical testing and estimation, a core approach in this book, which is about combining different methods of testing and estimation to make informed decisions
PND	Percentage of non-overlapping data
PND-B	Bayesian Binomial alternative to PND, which yields a point estimate slightly less extreme than PND and, contrary to PND, comes with a 95% CRI
PND-BC	PND-B corrected for correlated residuals
Q	Ljung-Box Q-statistic to test for independence of residuals in time series
r	Pearson's correlation coefficient
R^2, R^2 adjusted	Proportion of variance explained in fixed-effects models for quantitative outcome variables, with a penalty for model complexity in the case of the adjusted variant
R^2_{CS}	R-squared statistic attributed to Cox and Snell, potentially useful for categorical outcome variable models though its upper bound is (well) below 1
R^2_{M}, R^2_{R}, R^2_{C}	R^2 of fixed (M), random (R), and fixed and random (C) effects
R^2_{McF}	R-squared statistic attributed to McFadden, my recommended default R-squared statistic for categorical outcome variable models

R^2_N	*R*-squared statistic attributed to Nagelkerke, potentially useful for categorical outcome variable models
R^2_T	*R*-squared statistic attributed to Tjur, potentially useful for categorical outcome variable models though its upper bound is (well) below 1
REML	Restricted Maximum Likelihood, used for the estimation of random effects
REVC	Rescaled eigenvector centrality
RI	Random intercept
RIC	Rescaled information centrality
RIGLS	Restricted iterative generalised least squares
r_M	Square root of R^2_M
ROPE	Region of practical equivalence, a Bayesian concept similar to the region of relative equivalence in TOST, and part of the TOST-ROPE uniting FOST
r_{RES}	Residual correlation
RS	Random slope
S	Sparsity
SABIC	Sample-size adjusted BIC
SCED	Single-case experimental design, sometimes referred to as single-subject experimental design (SSED)
SD	Standard deviation in a sample, group, or condition
SE	Standard error
SEM	Standard error of measurement
SocNetV	Stands for Social Network Visualizer, and is a statistical package used in this book, version 2.5
SOST	Sequential one-sided testing
SPSS	Stands for Statistical Package for the Social Sciences, and is a statistical package used in this book, version 25
Stata	A statistical package used in this book, version 15.1
t	Probability distribution and test statistic, slightly wider than the standard Normal distribution *z* though the difference between *t* and *z* converges to zero as sample size goes to infinity; squaring *t*, we obtain *F* for $df_{groups} = 1$ or $df_{effect} = 1$. In some cases, *t* refers to time point or occasion *t*
t_c	Critical *t*-value
TIF	Test information function
TOST	Two one-sided tests, an approach to (relative) equivalence testing
TP	Toeplitz residual covariance structure
TPH	Extension of TP that accounts for varying V_{RES}

Type I error	Traditionally, seeing a difference (in the sample) where there is none; in FOST, concluding sufficient evidence against relative equivalence while actually relative equivalence holds
Type II error	Traditionally, failing to see a difference (in the sample) where there is one; in FOST, concluding sufficient evidence in favour of relative equivalence while actually relative equivalence does not hold
Type M error	(Substantial) misestimation of an effect of interest in magnitude
Type S error	Seeing a negative effect that is actually positive or vice versa
UB	Upper bound
UN	Unstructured residual covariance structure
V	Cramér's V
VAS	Visual analogue scale
V_{FIXED}	Variance of fixed effects
V_{RANDOM}	Variance of random effects
V_{RES}	Residual variance
V_{RI}	RI variance
X_1–X_3	Set of items in some cases, set of repeated measurements in other cases
X, Y, Z	Commonly used to refer to variables (e.g., X being main predictor or factor, Y being response variable, and Z being a background variable that moderates, mediates or confounds the relation between X and Y)
Y_1–Y_3	Set of items in some cases, set of repeated measurements in other cases
z	Probability distribution (i.e., standard Normal distribution) and test statistic; squaring z yields χ^2_1

Part I
Common Questions

Learning Processes 1

Abstract

This is the first of four chapters of Part I of this book. The focus of Part I lies on different types of research questions as well as practice-driven questions that may refer to groups or to individual learners. In this first chapter, several contemporary theories of learning and assessment are discussed and compared in terms of their relative pros and cons. From this comparison, a working definition of 'learning processes' for this book is formulated along with a series of research- and practice-oriented questions, several of which are revisited in later chapters in this book. Finally, this chapter provides a drone view of subsequent chapters in this first part of the book and of the in total thirteen chapters that follow in the other parts of the book.

1.1 Introduction

Learning is by definition a longitudinal phenomenon; it is largely about dynamic, nonlinear processes that require longitudinal studies with carefully planned measurements and statistical methods that allow to appropriately account for questions of interest, the study design, and key features of the data at hand. Questions of interest may result from theory, data or practical experience, and the outcomes of our research can help to advance existing theory or develop new theory about learning in a particular context. In this chapter, contemporary questions from educational research and practice are discussed in the light of a variety of theories of learning and assessment. These theories are discussed in terms of their relative pros and cons, largely in terms of the types of studies that have been used to develop and inform these theories and in terms of the actual evidence available. Several questions discussed in this chapter, and some of the theories behind these questions, are revisited in later chapters in this book. A working definition of learning processes is

J. Leppink, *The Art of Modelling the Learning Process*, Springer Texts in Education,
https://doi.org/10.1007/978-3-030-43082-5_1

provided that serves as a red thread throughout the book and allows for an early introduction of a longitudinal approach that can help us to acquire a better understanding of learning processes, can inform both future learning and the revision of educational content and formats, and may help to foster self-regulated learning skills (Bjork, Dunlosky, & Kornell, 2013) and adaptive expertise (i.e., the ability to adapt to new territory and to new types of problems and challenges: Ellström, 2001; Hanham & Leppink, 2019; Hatano & Inagaki, 1986; Holyoak, 1991).

1.2 A Helicopter Tour Through the Theories

Going through the immense and rapidly growing body of literature on theories of learning and assessment, one can find dozens if not hundreds of different theories, which—in terms of the paradigms they are based on and in terms of their orientation—have more or less in common with other theories out there. The goal of this chapter, or of this book for that matter, is *not* to discuss any of these theories in detail let alone to provide a full-blown review of all the similarities and differences between all these theories; this chapter provides a helicopter view of the confusing world of Education with what seems a wild-growth of theories and models based on these theories, and how they may or may not inform educational research and/or practice.

1.2.1 Stimulus, Processing, and Response

Some theories of learning have been strongly influenced by *behaviourism* (Pavlov & Anrep, 1928; Skinner, 1974; Watson, 1928), the central tenet of which is that behaviour is a response to external stimuli and learning is a *change* in *observable* behaviour due to reinforcement and/or punishment. Although this seemingly *objective* focus has its attractiveness and may provide straightforward explanations for a range of behaviours where reinforcement and/or punishment is applied, its ignorance of internal influences such as motivation and emotion has constituted a common source of critique.

Behaviourism precedes cognitivism (e.g., Cooper, 1993; Ertmer & Newby, 1993), which argues that we must 'open' and understand the *black box* of the human mind. A theory that is commonly considered to be a bridge between behaviourism and cognitivism is Bandura's *social learning theory* (Bandura, 1969, 1973, 1977, 1986; Bandura & Walters, 1963), which revolves around the idea of continuous interaction between cognitive, behavioural, and environmental factors. Social learning theory is largely about learning behaviour through *modelling* or observing and imitating others (e.g., examples or role models), and attention, memory, and motivation are all considered in this process. This theory is intuitively appealing and is sometimes used to explain aggressive behaviour and homicide rates in some countries or states where people are allowed to possess guns for their own defence and aggressive video games are common. However, it fails to explain why in some other countries where the possession of guns is legal and aggressive video games are common aggressive behaviour and homicide are considerably less common.

Two fairly influential cognitive theories in which learning is about limited-capacity processing, organising, and integrating information into cognitive schemas are *cognitive theory of multimedia learning* (Mayer, 1997, 2002; Mayer & Moreno, 2003) and *cognitive load theory* (Leppink & Hanham, 2019; Sweller, Van Merriënboer, & Paas, 1998, 2019). These two theories have provided support for robust phenomena such as the *multimedia effect* or novices in a topic learning more from combinations of verbal and visual information than from verbal or visual information alone. A strength of these two theories is that they have been built on a tradition of carefully designed randomised controlled experiments. However, the vast majority of these experiments are based on fairly small samples under conditions the practical relevance of which is rather questionable (e.g., Lee, Hanham, & Leppink, 2019; Leppink, 2019). For example, participants come to a lab to study for 15–20 min a particular content that for most of them has no relevance outside the lab, and undergo a small-size post-test to measure learning outcomes immediately after that study period. Students attending a 15–20 min lecture on for them meaningless content to regurgitate that content in an exam straight after the lecture (and to not forget it right away once the exam is over) is not particularly an example of how learning happens in the real world. Moreover, both theories largely treat the learner as an *individual* and do not really consider the social context in which learning takes place. This may partly explain why experiments informed by (one of) these two theories appear to provide clear support in favour of *fading* instructional guidance from worked examples (through completion problems) to autonomous problem solving but fail to explain why under some conditions (e.g., working in small groups) initial struggle and failure can be productive (i.e., *productive failure*; Kalyuga & Singh, 2016; Kapur, 2008, 2011, 2014; Kapur & Rummel, 2012; Lee, Leppink, & Hanham, 2019).

Another theory that has been influential is *deliberate practice theory* (Ericsson, Krampe, & Tesch-Römer, 1993). In this theory, expertise can be explained in terms of extensive and long-term deliberate practice, and apart from height in sports such as basketball, individual differences in physical features or talent are not really considered. Much of the evidence that appears to support this idea has come from studies that compare experts with non-experts retrospectively, while people who quit practice at some point (i.e., dropouts) are not really considered. The latter is problematic, because it does not help to rule out beyond reasonable doubt the possibility that deliberate practice works for a select group (i.e., those who eventually become expert) but not for a particular other group of people (i.e., the dropouts). There is little research on the effect of general intelligence or innate talent on expertise development, and some of the research that has been done in that area appears to provide evidence in favour of this effect and thus against the idea that deliberate practice—and not intelligence or innate talent—explains the development of expertise (e.g., De Bruin, Kok, Leppink, & Camp, 2014). Finally, deliberate practice theory appears largely focussed on *routine* expertise (i.e., expertise in a particular set of tasks or with particular methods or tools in a specific context or territory), and it remains unclear how it can explain the development of *adaptive* expertise.

1.2.2 Information Constructor

Theories such as cognitive theory of multimedia learning and cognitive load theory have resulted in guidelines for how to design instruction, including the fading of instructional guidance and the gradual increase in task complexity as learners advance such as in the *four-component instructional design* (4C/ID) model (e.g., Van Merriënboer & Kirschner, 2017). However, scholars of constructivism (e.g., Cooper, 1993; Ertmer & Newby, 1993) oppose that learning is about *constructing* subjective representations of information using personal experience and our perspectives on the environment. An important theory in this area is Vygotsky's *social development theory* (Vygotsky, 1978), which states that learning takes place in a *zone of proximal development*: the zone between what one can understand and do by oneself (i.e., without support) and what one can learn through social interaction with one or several more knowledgeable others. Interestingly, although several cognitive load theorists have consistently rejected the constructivist perspective and findings that can be explained from that perspective (e.g., findings inspired by the previously mentioned *productive failure* framework), some of these cognitive load theorists do refer to Vygotsky's concept of zone of proximal development in an attempt to explain cognitive load and learning outcomes in their experiments.

With the advent of technology and online learning, we have also seen a rise of *connectivism* (Downes, 2010; Siemens, 2005): with the ever-increasing variety of media, we have plenty new opportunities for online learning and co-creation of new education. Examples included *massive open online courses* (MOOCs; Kop, 2011), online special interest group discussion platforms on social media like *LinkedIn*, *Facebook*, and *YouTube*. These and other initiatives can also provide very powerful tools for the study of social networks from small to very large.

Although not all learning takes place in interaction, this certainly appears to be the case for most of our learning, and constructivist theories such as social development theory and connectivism take this interaction element into account. Examples of educational approaches inspired by constructivism are *problem-based learning* (Schmidt, 1983) and *research-based learning* (Bastiaens, Van Tilburg, & Van Merriënboer, 2017).

1.2.3 Intelligent Motivation

Another collection of theories is rooted in the philosophical paradigm called *humanism* (e.g., DeCarvalho, 1991), which considers learning to be a personal act to fulfil one's potential. Within this collection, one group of theories identifies motivation as a key factor of learning. Influential examples in this group are *self-determination theory* (Gagné & Deci, 2005; Ryan & Deci, 2000) and *flow theory* (Csikszentmihalyi, 2008). Self-determination theory predicts that people will perform and learn optimally if three innate psychological needs are met: self-perceived competence, relatedness, and autonomy. Similarly, flow theory predicts optimal performance and learning when we are engaged in activities that match our current skill level and stimulate immersion and concentration. These and other motivation theories can be very useful in settings where substantial differences in motivation can be encountered (e.g., high school settings) but are less useful in setting where the range in motivation is more limited (e.g., Year 5 in Medical School).

A second group of theories in the humanist collection is found in theories that focus on or are linked to notions of so-called *learning styles*, including *experiential learning theory* (Kolb, 1984), *multiple intelligences theory* (e.g., Gardner, 1983), and *adult learning theory* (Blondy, 2007; Palis & Quiros, 2014). One of the problems with these theories is that notions of multiple intelligences and learning styles are not backed by any serious empirical evidence. If tailoring education to someone's preferred learning style was to result in better learning outcomes, we should be able to establish that phenomenon in randomised controlled experiments that compare a condition where that tailoring is done (i.e., treatment condition) and a condition where that is not done (i.e., control condition). We have failed to find such evidence, and for this and other reasons we should conclude that the notion of tailoring education to preferred learning styles resulting in better learning outcomes should be placed in the genre of *science fiction* (e.g., Kirschner & Van Merriënboer, 2013; Leppink, 2017, 2019; Pashler, McDaniel, Rohrer, & Bjork 2008). Theories such as cognitive theory of multimedia learning, cognitive load theory, and several constructivist theories can explain why some of the core assertions from learning style theorists fly in the face of consistent evidence of what works under what conditions.

1.2.4 Learning and Assessment

Some educational theories and approaches recognise assessment as an inherent part of a solid instructional design. For example, *programmatic assessment* (Schuwirth & Van der Vleuten, 2012; Van der Vleuten & Schuwirth, 2005) is about "*assessing learners longitudinally with a variety of methods that are embedded in the educational process, and that afford both assessment of learning and assessment for learning*" (Uijtdehaage & Schuwirth, 2018, p. 350). Programmatic assessment recognises that learning is a longitudinal process, that performance of the moment is part of a bigger growth picture, and that different methods can shed light on somewhat different aspects of competence and learning. This and other longitudinal approaches to assessment also fit well with theory around the development of metacognition and self-regulated learning skills (e.g., Bjork et al., 2013). Skills like accurate self-assessment and appropriate learning task selection do not come naturally; they need to be explicitly taught and stimulated through carefully placed, repeated measurements with meaningful feedback. Knowing what we know is easier than knowing what we do not know; as we become more familiar with new content, we become more aware of how much is out there that we do not know.

Traditionally, educational practitioners and researchers have frequently averaged scores from repeated measurements to a single score, and by doing so we tend to lose a lot of information about variation in performance within the individual assessed. Besides, although different assessment methods tend to shed light on different aspects of performance or learning, they may share some variance. For example, in a medical context, performance on a clinical exam of a patient's shoulder is likely correlated with performance on an example of MCQs about shoulder anatomy; although these two exams measure somewhat different skills, without a critical degree of knowledge of the shoulder one is rather unlikely to perform well on a carefully designed MCQ exam or on a clinical exam of a patient's shoulder. Therefore, in programmatic assessment, "*information about a student's strengths and weaknesses is collected across different assessment methods rather than within*" (Uijtdehaage & Schuwirth, 2018, p. 350). However, this choice is largely a response to the traditional practice of averaging repeated measurements from the same method (i.e., within method), while—as this book demonstrates—true longitudinal analysis has *nothing* to do with averaging repeated measurements. True longitudinal analysis, which includes longitudinal assessment, is about using *the same methods repeatedly* and using *within-individual variance* in an outcome of interest assessed with that method instead of 'erasing' that variance by averaging scores. At the same time, the type of triangulation as in programmatic assessment (e.g., MCQ performance and clinical exam performance sharing some variance) is very meaningful and frequently not considered in other longitudinal assessment approaches. Therefore, starting point of this book is that *both within-method and between-methods* comparisons matter.

1.3 A Pragmatic Working Definition of Learning Processes

There are many more theories out there, but they often share concepts with the theories discussed thus far in this chapter, and even in some of the theories discussed we have seen some movement towards each other. For instance, some cognitive load theorists have attempted to incorporate a *collaborative* component (e.g., Kirschner, Sweller, Kirschner, & Zambrano, 2018). Perhaps, research inspired by this *collaborative cognitive load theory* can help to explain apparent contradictions between cognitive load theory, which postulates that optimal learning is achieved by fading instructional guidance from worked examples to autonomous problem solving (eventually through completion problems), and the productive failure framework, which can explain why under some conditions initial struggle resulting from the absence of a particular type of support can actually benefit learning. Either way, common research questions in this area include: effects of presence or absence of *instructional support* at different stages in a learning trajectory, effects of *collaboration* or *peer support* at different stages in a learning trajectory, and effects of variation in (different types of) learning task *complexity* at different stages in a learning trajectory.

1.3.1 Testing Effects

Productive failure and programmatic assessment also fit well with another robust finding from human learning research, the *testing effect*: taking a memory test not only assesses what we know, but also enhances retention (e.g., Karpicke & Aue, 2015; Roediger & Karpicke, 2006a, 2006b). This is not to say that test performance increases linearly over time; rather, with time, the effect of repeated testing may level off. Besides, some learners will profit more from testing than others. For example, Fig. 1.1 (SPSS version 25; IBM Corporation, 2017) presents the performance of each of 25 students on a series of 10 MCQ tests (i.e., 0–9 on the horizontal axis) on probability calculus (test score: 0–50).

Each of the 10 tests is composed by a random sample of 50 items, without replacement (i.e., items in one test are not appearing in any of the other tests), from an item bank that holds over 10,000 MCQs (items) with five response options (choices) each. Given little variation in difficulty level of the questions, different tests of random samples of 50 items can be interpreted as very similar in difficulty

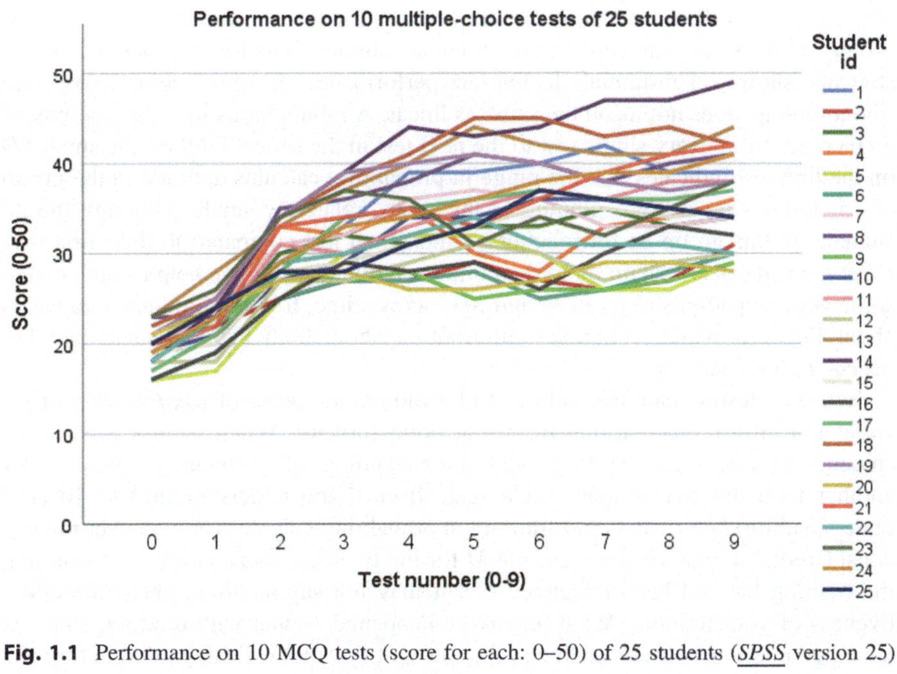

Fig. 1.1 Performance on 10 MCQ tests (score for each: 0–50) of 25 students (SPSS version 25)

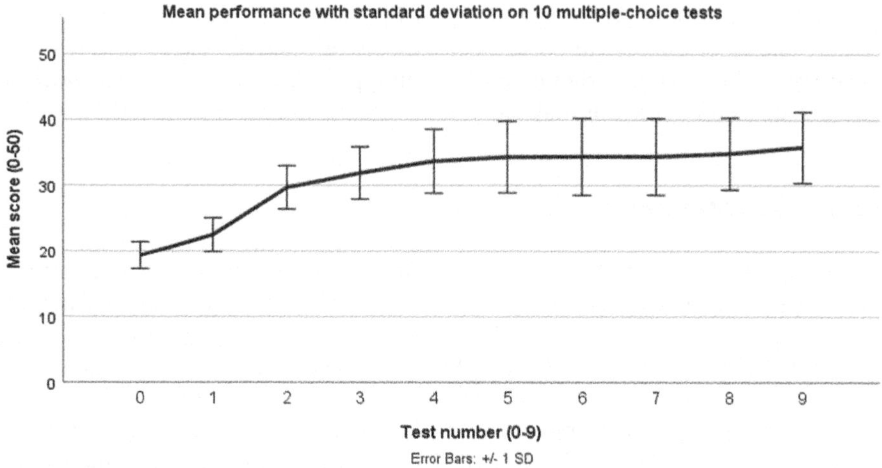

Fig. 1.2 M and SD of 10 MCQ tests for the group of 25 students (*SPSS* version 25)

and increases in scores can be interpreted as learning. Figure 1.2 (*SPSS* version 25) indicates the mean performance (*M*) and standard deviation (*SD*) around that mean performance of the group of 25 candidates for each of the 10 tests.

As becomes clear from Fig. 1.2, *M* increases quite substantially in the early rounds but then levels off, and *SD* increases somewhat across tests. Figure 1.1 illustrates the different performance trajectories for the 25 students that form the group; while some students demonstrate an almost monotonous increase, other students show a substantial decline in performance at some point. Note that 'monotonous' does not mean the same as linear. A monotonous increase just means an increase from every single test to the next test in the series. Further, the small *SD* on the first test indicates that the range in probability calculus aptitude in the group of 25 students is, at the beginning of the series, relatively small. Although the 25 students in this group perform better on their final test compared to their first test, some students clearly learn more than others. While Fig. 1.2 can help us understand some general patterns (e.g., in *M* and *SD*) across time, true longitudinal analysis is about Fig. 1.1, which comprises information about both *within-student* and *between-students* variance.

Repeated testing can also help us to become more aware of *what we do not yet know* and inform our learning from that point forward. When we ask a group of students to rate their self-perceived understanding of probability calculus—or another topic for that matter—on a scale from 0 (no understanding) to 10 (full understanding) *before* and *after* training in probability calculus (or whatever topic is considered), we may obtain the same *M* for the two occasions. Does this mean that the training has not been effective? No, it may not say anything about the effectiveness of your training. What has likely happened, is that with training, students have become more aware of things they do not (yet) know, things that before the training they did perhaps not even know they existed. With that, we have a recalibration of our response scale, due to which at least some of the options in the scale no longer have the same meaning. This is one of the fundamental problems with self-report measures that is often ignored. For instance, researchers may ask learners to self-rate variables like how much mental effort they invested in a task or how difficult or complex a given task was and interpret differences between repeated measurements as differences in effort, difficulty or complexity, while the very meaning of these scales may change from task to task due to learning.

Our self-assessment of competence in a particular domain is likely to change while we learn. Figure 1.3 (*SPSS* version 25) presents the deviation in self-assessed performance on a task from the assessment provided by a teacher for each of 30 students who form a cohort. After each of a series of six tasks (0–5), the teacher and individual student X independently rate student X's performance on a scale from 0 (minimum) to 50 (maximum). Positive differences indicate that the student's self-assessment was higher than the teacher's assessment, while negative differences indicate self-assessments lower than the teacher's assessment.

Figure 1.3 indicates that the majority of students initially rated their own performance higher than the teacher did, then had a phase in which they rated their own performance slightly lower than the teacher, and then moved to a zone around zero difference. An explanation for this pattern could be that an initial blindness for all that is out there to be learned resulted in a tendency towards overestimation, which was slowly replaced by a tendency towards underestimation in response to

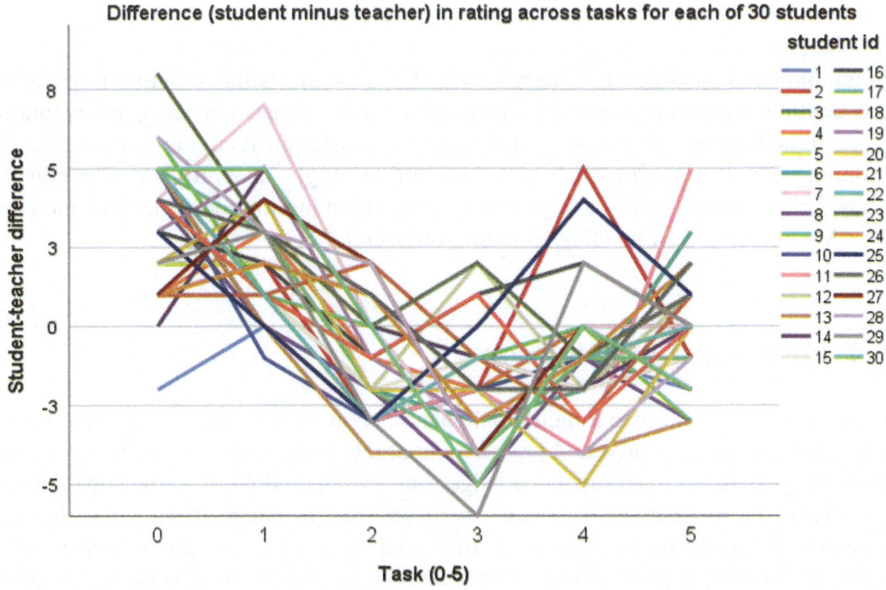

Fig. 1.3 Self-assessed minus teacher's rating on 6 tasks for each of 30 students (*SPSS* version 25)

becoming more aware of that world out there to be explored, and with time students became more aware of the assessment criteria and of what is good and bad performance, resulting in differences closer to zero.

Whether we deal with performance (Figs. 1.1 and 1.2), with self-assessments (Fig. 1.3) or other learning-relevant variables that are monitored longitudinally, averaging across measurements to obtain a single score for each student comes with a tremendous loss of information: all within-subject variance is erased, and we learn nothing about how initial performance, self-assessment, or the like, changes with practice and/or other factors. Figures 1.1 and 1.3 help us to shed light on research questions like how performance and self-assessment change over time and which variables may influence or at least to a certain degree explain that change.

1.3.2 Intercorrelation

From the previous, it becomes clear that two types of processes of interest in the context of learning are *within-individual* change and *between-individuals* differences in that change over time: why do some individuals learn more or faster than other individuals, and how can we help learners to grow and develop further? Second, this *within-individual* change and these *between-individuals* differences in that change, in combination with features of the methods or instruments used to measure variables of interest (e.g., the type of test and what knowledge or skill[s] they capture), create an *intercorrelation structure* which defines how repeated measurements with the same method or instrument are correlated with one another (i.e., needed for true longitudinal analysis) as well as how measurements from different methods or instruments are correlated with one another (cf. triangulation in programmatic assessment). Understanding this intercorrelation structure is vital for the continuous development of educational programmes, for early intervention (e.g., remediation) for learners who stagnate or decline (and may be at risk of dropping out of a programme), and for justifying high-stakes decisions in educational programmes such as a Psychology student having to redo a block or module or a Medicine student needing to redo a clerkship.

1.4 Remainder of This Book

Learning is by definition a longitudinal phenomenon. Nevertheless, the methods we use in educational research and practice are largely cross-sectional: performance of a given type (e.g., anatomy knowledge, survey methodology knowledge, interviewing skills) is assessed at a single point in time. In much of our research, that assessment usually takes place right after a study or practice period, and in educational practice, that assessment often takes place weeks or in some cases even months after study or practice. By uniting key concepts and methods from Education, Psychology, Econometrics, Medicine, Language, and Forensic Science, this book provides an interdisciplinary methodological approach to study human learning longitudinally. This longitudinal approach can help us to acquire a better understanding of learning processes, can inform both future learning and the revision of educational content and formats, and may help to foster self-regulated learning skills.

1.4.1 Part I: Common Questions (Chaps. 1–4)

This book consists of four parts of four chapters each and a seventeenth, concluding chapter. Part I (*Common Questions*) focusses on different types of research questions as well as practice-driven questions that may refer to groups or to individual learners. This first chapter constitutes the first chapter of this first part. Chapter 2 (*Study Designs*) explains how questions—theory-driven, data-driven or emerging from practical experience—can inform our methodological approach in a given context. Key questions such as the availability or sampling of participants, the planning of measurements (e.g., assessments), and pros and cons of different types of measures are discussed in this second chapter as well. Chapter 3 (*Statistical Learning*) provides a pragmatic approach to statistical testing and estimation for large samples as well as for studies involving small samples or individual cases. Finally, Chap. 4 (*Anchoring Narratives*) focusses on different types of quality criteria (e.g., reliability and validity) and provides a framework for combining different types of evidence into a validity argument in favour of a particular hypothesis about what is going on or about what works in a given context, relative to several competing hypotheses. This framework attempts to unite contemporary validity frameworks such as the ones from Messick (1989) and Kane (2006), as well as similar approaches from forensic science such as the theory of anchored narratives discussed by Wagenaar, Van Koppen, and Crombag (1993) as a framework for thinking about evidence in a criminal case.

The first part lays the foundation for the rest of the book: key theories on what seems to (not) work in for different types of learners, moving from a punishment culture to a growth mindset by moving away from the current largely cross-sectional to an increasingly longitudinal dynamic approach to assessment, facilitating the development of metacognition and self-regulated learning skills, and theory informing and being informed by research. Further, since different assessment methods may shed light on somewhat different aspects of learning, the key message from this book is: *multi-time* (or, where possible, continuous) and *multi-method* assessment.

1.4.2 Part II: Variable Types (Chaps. 5–8)

Part II (*Variable Types*) focusses on different types of outcome variables in educational research and practice: pass/fail and other dichotomies (Chap. 5), multi-category nominal choices (Chap. 6), ordered performance categories (Chap. 7; e.g., good, sufficient, poor; excellent, pass, borderline, fail), and different types of quantifiable (i.e., interval or ratio level of measurement) variables (Chap. 8). For each of these types of outcome variables, single-measurement and repeated-measurements scenarios are discussed with examples. This approach serves three purposes. First, there is a habit among both researchers and practitioners to reduce quantitative information into two or three categories (e.g., above vs. below average; good, medium, poor); this habit usually comes at the cost of a substantial loss of information and is, in the light of the wide variety of methods available, unnecessary. Second, it is common practice to compute Cronbach's alpha and other statistics of limited use in situations where these statistics provide inadequate outcomes but where more viable alternatives, which are readily available, perform well. Third, covering the concept of repeated measurements in a series of fairly basic chapters allows for a smooth introduction to the novel concepts and methods discussed in the next part, in such a way that we do not lose readers who may have a somewhat limited background in Methodology and Statistics but who are keen to learn in this area.

1.4.3 Part III: Variable Networks (Chaps. 9–12)

Part III (*Variable Networks*) focusses on cross-sectional and longitudinal interdependence of learning-related variables through emerging network-analytic methods. In Chap. 9 (*Instrument Structures*), network analysis is discussed as an approach to the study of the features of the psychometric instruments we used, and this approach is compared with common latent variable methods in terms of relative pros and cons. In Chap. 10 (*Cross-Instrument Communication*), the network-analytic approach discussed in Chap. 9 is extended to the study of interrelations of measures derived from a series of instruments. Where Chaps. 9 and 10 leave out the longitudinal component for the sake of simplicity, Chap. 11 (*Temporal Structures*) discusses the network-analytic approach introduced in these two previous chapters in a context of longitudinal measurement and analysis. This allows for consolidation and practice with concepts and methods discussed in Chaps. 5–10 and creates useful visuals for some of the key concepts in Chaps. 12–16. Chapter 12 (*Longitudinal Assessment Networks*) constitutes the final chapter in this third part and demonstrates how a network-analytic approach can enhance our understanding of the interdependence of different assessment components in for example a Bachelor's or Master's programme.

1.4.4 Part IV: Time Series (Chaps. 13–16)

In Part IV (*Time Series*), we apply the concepts learned in Chaps. 5–12 to different types of studies involving time series. First, Chap. 13 (*Randomised Controlled Experiments*) uses a straightforward context of randomised controlled experiments that involve either a series of measurements after treatment or some combination of one or several measurements prior to treatment and one or several measurements after treatment. Chapter 14 (*Static and Dynamic Group Structures*) demonstrates a variety of ways in which the analysis of group structures—including through social network analysis—can help us to account for why some learners may (have) become more similar in their knowledge or skill, or in their perspectives on particular questions, and why some individuals may learn more than others in a given context. Where Chaps. 13 and 14 focus on somewhat smaller series of repeated measurements (i.e., 5–7 measurements), Chap. 15 (*Progress Testing in Larger Cohorts*) discusses a longstanding tradition in medical schools in among others the Netherlands and the United Kingdom called *progress testing*. Succinctly put, progress testing involves series of 15–24 knowledge tests (i.e., the exact number depends on country or medical school) intended to measure growth in knowledge over time. Placing this chapter after Chaps. 13 and 14 and before Chap. 16 (*Studies with Small Samples or Individuals*) provides a natural extension of core concepts discussed in the earlier chapters at present and to inform subsequent learning. Chapter 16 discusses some contemporary settings where longitudinal assessment is already practiced to some extent, or at least considered for the time forward, but where numbers of learners are very small (e.g., 1–20 students). In this chapter, the reader learns about individual and small-group time series models as a means to model change in performance (or learning outcomes otherwise) with time and to estimate changes in that change with time-specific events like training.

1.4.5 Part V: Conclusion (Chap. 17)

Finally, Part V (*Conclusion*) provides some general guidelines for (a united) educational research and practice, for groups large and small as well as for the study of the individual, for the time ahead (Chap. 17).

1.4.6 A Note on Data and Software Used Throughout This Book

The goal of this book is neither to cover all possible methods out there nor to use all possible software packages or focus on a single software package. For a recent overview of excellent textbooks on statistical methods already available, see for instance Leppink (2019). The data used in this book are not from actual research or educational settings, but are simulated such that they represent examples of different types of data—that fairly well or clearly do not meet certain assumptions—and allow to discuss different types of approaches to data analysis for different types of variables and situations. As far as software is concerned, both commercial and zero-cost Open Source packages are used in this book. Commercial packages used in this book are *Mplus* version 8.1 (Muthén & Muthén, 2017), *Stata* 15.1 (StataCorp, 2017), *SPSS* version 25 (IBM Corporation, 2017), and *MLwiN* version 3.02 (Charlton, Rasbash, Browne, et al., 2019). Zero-cost Open Source packages used throughout this book are *JASP* version 0.11.1.0 (Love, Selker, Marsman, et al., 2018), *Jamovi* version 1.1.5.0 (Jamovi project, 2019), *Ganz Rasch* (*GR*) 1.0 (Alexandrowicz, 2012), and *SocNetV* version 2.5 (Kalamaras, 2018). In the remainder of this book, I just use the *italic underlined* terms to refer to the versions and references here.

References

Alexandrowicz, R. W. (2012). "GANZ RASCH": A free software for categorical data analysis. *Social Science Computer Review, 30,* 369–379. https://doi.org/10.1177/0894439311417222.

Bandura, A. (1969). *Principles of behavior modification*. New York: Holt, Rinehart & Winston.

Bandura, A. (1973). *Aggression: A social learning analysis*. Englewood Cliffs, NJ: Prentice-Hall.

Bandura, A. (1977). *Social learning theory*. New York: General Learning Press.

Bandura, A. (1986). *Social foundations of thought and action*. Englewood Cliffs, NJ: Prentice-Hall.

Bandura, A., & Walters, R. (1963). *Social learning and personality development*. New York: Holt, Rinehart & Winston.

Bastiaens, E., Van Tilburg, J., & Van Merriënboer, J. J. G. (2017). *Research-based learning: Case studies from Maastricht University*. Cham: Springer. https://doi.org/10.1007/978-3-319-50993-8.

Bjork, R. A., Dunlosky, J., & Kornell, N. (2013). Self-regulated learning: Beliefs, techniques, and illusions. *Annual Review of Psychology, 64,* 417–444. https://doi.org/10.1146/annurev-psych-113011-143823.

Blondy, L. C. (2007). Evaluation and application of andragogical assumptions to the adult online learning environment. *Journal of Interactive Online Learning, 6*(2), 116–130.

Charlton, C., Rasbash, J., Browne, W. J., Healy, M., & Cameron, B. (2019). *MLwiN Version 3.02*. Centre for Multilevel Modelling, University of Bristol. http://www.bristol.ac.uk/cmm/software/mlwin/refs.html.

Cooper, P. A. (1993). Paradigm shifts in designed instruction: From behaviorism to cognitivism to constructivism. *Educational Technology, 33*(5), 12–19. https://www.jstor.org/stable/44428049.

Csikszentmihalyi, M. (2008). *Flow: The psychology of optimal experience*. New York: Harper Perennial Modern Classics.

De Bruin, A. B. H., Kok, E. M., Leppink, J., & Camp, G. (2014). Practice, intelligence, and enjoyment in novice chess players: A prospective study at the earliest stage of a chess career. *Intelligence, 45,* 18–25. https://doi.org/10.1016/j.intell.2013.07.004.

DeCarvalho, R. (1991). The humanistic paradigm in education. *The Humanistic Psychologist, 19* (1), 88–104. https://doi.org/10.1080/08873267.1991.9986754.

Downes, S. (2010). New technology supporting informal learning. *Journal of Emerging Technologies in Web Intelligence, 2*(1), 27–33.

Ellström, P. (2001). Integrating learning and work: Problems and prospects. *Human Resource Development Quarterly, 12,* 421. https://doi.org/10.1002/hrdq.1006.

Ericsson, K. A., Krampe, R. Th., & Tesch-Römer, C. (1993). The role of deliberate practice in the acquisition of expert performance. *Psychology Review, 100*(3), 363-406. https://doi.org/10.1037/0033-295X.100.3.363.

Ertmer, P. A., & Newby, T. J. (1993). Behaviorism, cognitivism, constructivism: Comparing critical features from an instructional design perspective. *Performance Improvement Quarterly, 6*(4), 50–72. https://doi.org/10.1111/j.1937-8327.1993.tb00605.x.

Gagné, M., & Deci, E. L. (2005). Self-determination theory and work motivation. *Journal of Organizational Behavior, 26*(4), 331–362. https://doi.org/10.1002/job.322.

Gardner, H. (1983). *Frames of mind: The theory of multiple intelligences*. New York: Basic Books.

Hanham, J., & Leppink, J. (2019). Expertise and problem solving in high-stakes environments. In C. B. Lee, J. Hanham, & J. Leppink (Eds.), *Instructional design principles for high-stakes problem-solving environments*. Singapore: Springer. https://doi.org/10.1007/978-981-13-2808-4_3.

Hatano, G., & Inagaki, K. (1986). Two courses of expertise. In H. Stevenson, H. Azuma, & K. Hakuta (Eds.), *Child development and education in Japan* (pp. 262–272). New York: Freeman.

Holyoak, K. J. (1991). In K. A. Ericsson & J. Smith (Eds.), *Toward a general theory of expertise: Prospects and limits of symbolic connectionism: Toward third-generation theories of expertise* (pp. 301–335). Cambridge, UK: Cambridge University Press.

IBM Corporation (2017). SPSS version 25. Retrieved Feb 1, 2020, from https://www-01.ibm.com/support/docview.wss?uid=swg24043678.

Jamovi project (2019). Jamovi version 1.1.5.0. Retrieved Feb 1, 2020, from https://www.jamovi.org/.

Kalamaras, D. V. (2018). Social network visualizer version 2.5. Retrieved Feb 1, 2020, from http://socnetv.org/.

Kalyuga, S., & Singh, A. M. (2016). Rethinking the boundaries of cognitive load theory in complex learning. *Educational Psychology Review, 28*(4), 831–852. https://doi.org/10.1007/s10648-015-9352-0.

Kane, M. T. (2006). Validation. In R. L. Brennan (Ed.), *Educational measurement* (4th ed., pp. 17–64). Westport: Praeager.

Kapur, M. (2008). Productive failure. *Cognition and Instruction, 26,* 379–424. https://doi.org/10.1080/07370000802212669.

Kapur, M. (2011). A further study of productive failure in mathematical problem solving: Unpacking the design components. *Instructional Science, 39,* 561–579. https://doi.org/10.1007/s11251-010-9144-3.

Kapur, M. (2014). Productive failure in learning math. *Cognitive Science, 38,* 1008–1022. https://doi.org/10.1111/cogs.12107.

Kapur, M., & Rummel, N. (2012). Productive failure in learning from generation and invention activities. *Instructional Science, 40,* 645–650. https://doi.org/10.1007/s11251-012-9235-4.

Karpicke, J. D., & Aue, W. R. (2015). The testing effect is alive and well with complex materials. *Educational Psychology Review, 27*(2), 317–326. https://doi.org/10.1007/s10648-015-9309-3.

Kirschner, P. A., Sweller, J., Kirschner, F., & Zambrano, J. R. (2018). From cognitive load theory to collaborative cognitive load theory. *International Journal of Computer-Supported Collaborative Learning, 13*(2), 213–233. https://doi.org/10.1007/s11412-018-9277-y.

Kirschner, P. A., & Van Merriënboer, J. J. G. (2013). Do learners really know best? *Urban legends in education. Educational Psychologist, 48*(3), 169–183. https://doi.org/10.1080/00461520.2013.804395.

Kolb, D. A. (1984). *Experiential learning: Experience as the source of learning and development*. Englewood Cliffs, NJ: Prentice-Hall.

Kop, R. (2011). The challenges to connectivist learning in open online networks: Learning experiences during a massive open online course. *The International Review of Research in Open and Distributed Learning, 12*(3), 19–38. https://doi.org/10.19173/irrodl.v12i3.882.

Lee, C. B., Hanham, J., & Leppink, J. (2019a). *Instructional design principles for high-stakes problem-solving environments*. Singapore: Springer. https://doi.org/10.1007/978-981-13-2808-4.

Lee, C. B., Leppink, J., & Hanham, J. (2019b). On the design of instruction and assessment. In: C. B. Lee, J. Hanham, & J. Leppink (Eds.), *Instructional design principles for high-stakes problem-solving environments*. Singapore: Springer. https://doi.org/10.1007/978-981-13-2808-4_11.

Leppink, J. (2017). Science fiction in medical education: The case of learning styles. *Journal of Graduate Medical Education, 9*(3), 394. https://doi.org/10.4300/JGME-D-16-00637.1.
Leppink, J. (2019). *Statistical methods for experimental research in education and psychology*. Cham: Springer. https://doi.org/10.1007/978-3-030-21241-4.
Leppink, J., & Hanham, J. (2019). Human cognitive architecture through the lens of cognitive load theory. In: C. B. Lee, J. Hanham, & J. Leppink (Eds.), *Instructional design principles for high-stakes problem-solving environments*. Singapore: Springer. https://doi.org/10.1007/978-981-13-2808-4_2.
Love, J., Selker, R., Marsman, M., et al. (2018). JASP version 0.11.1.0. Retrieved Feb 1, 2020, from https://jasp-stats.org/.
Mayer, R. E. (1997). Multimedia learning: Are we asking the right questions? *Educational Psychologist, 32*(1), 1–19. https://doi.org/10.1207/s15326985ep3201_1.
Mayer, R. E. (2002). Multimedia learning. *Psychology of Learning and Motivation, 41,* 85–139. https://doi.org/10.1016/S0079-7421(02)80005-6.
Mayer, R. E., & Moreno, R. (2003). Nine ways to reduce cognitive load in multimedia learning. *Educational Psychologist, 38*(1), 43–52. https://doi.org/10.1207/S15326985EP3801_6.
Messick, S. (1989). Validity. In R. L. Linn (Ed.), *Educational measurement* (3rd ed., pp. 13–103). New York: Macmillan.
Muthén, L. K., & Muthén, B. (2017). Mplus user's guide, version 8. Retrieved Feb 1, 2020, from https://statmodel.com.
Palis, A. G., & Quiros, P. A. (2014). Adult learning principles and presentation pearls. *Middle East African Journal of Ophthalmology, 21*(2), 114–122. https://doi.org/10.4103/0974-9233.129748.
Pashler, H., McDaniel, M., Rohrer, D., & Bjork, R. (2008). Learning styles: Concepts and evidence. *Psychological Science in the Public Interest, 9,* 105–119. https://doi.org/10.1111/j.1539-6053.2009.01038.x.
Pavlov, I. P., & Anrep, G. V. (1928). Conditioned reflexes. *Journal of Philosophical Studies, 3* (11), 380–383.
Roediger, H. L., & Karpicke, J. D. (2006a). Test-enhanced learning: Taking memory tests improves long-term retention. *Psychological Science, 17*(3), 249–255. https://doi.org/10.1111/j.1467-9280.2006.01693.x.
Roediger, H. L., & Karpicke, J. D. (2006b). The power of testing memory: Basic research and implications for educational practice. *Perspectives on Psychological Science, 1*(3), 181–210. https://doi.org/10.1111/j.1745-6916.2006.00012.x.
Ryan, R. M., & Deci, E. L. (2000). Self-determination theory and the facilitation of intrinsic motivation, social development, and well-being. *American Psychologist, 55*(1), 68–78.
Schmidt, H. G. (1983). Problem-based learning: Rationale and description. *Medical Education, 17,* 11–16. https://doi.org/10.1111/j.1365-2923.1983.tb01086.x.
Schuwirth, L. W. T., & Van der Vleuten, C. P. M. (2012). Programmatic assessment and Kane's validity perspective. *Medical Education, 46*(1), 38–48. https://doi.org/10.1111/j.1365-2923.2011.04098.x.
Siemens, G. (2005). Connectivism: A learning theory for the digital age. *International Journal of Instructional Technology and Distance Learning, 2*(1), 3–10.
Skinner, B. F. (1974). *About behaviorism*. Oxford, UK: Alfred A. Knopf.
StataCorp (2017). Stata statistical software: Release 15.1. College Station, TX: StataCorp LLC. Retrieved Feb 1, 2020, from https://www.stata.com.
Sweller, J., Van Merriënboer, J. J. G., & Paas, F. (1998). Cognitive architecture and instructional design. *Educational Psychology Review, 10*(3), 251–296. https://doi.org/10.1023/A:1022193728205.
Sweller, J., Van Merriënboer, J. J. G., & Paas, F. (2019). Cognitive architecture and instructional design: 20 years later. *Educational Psychology Review, 31*(2), 261–292. https://doi.org/10.1007/s10648-019-09465-5.

Uijtdehaage, S., & Schuwirth, L. W. T. (2018). Assuring the quality of programmatic assessment: Moving beyond psychometrics. *Perspectives on Medical Education, 7*(6), 350–351. https://doi.org/10.1007/s40037-018-0485-y.

Van der Vleuten, C. P. M., & Schuwirth, L. W. T. (2005). Assessing professional competence: From methods to programmes. *Medical Education, 39*(3), 309–317. https://doi.org/10.1111/j.1365-2929.2005.02094.x.

Van Merriënboer, J. J. G., & Kirschner, P. A. (2017). *Ten steps to complex learning: A systematic approach to four-component instructional design* (3rd ed.). New York: Routledge. https://doi.org/10.4324/9781315113210.

Vygotsky, L. S. (1978). *Mind in society: The development of higher psychological processes*. Cambridge, MA: Harvard University Press.

Wagenaar, W. A., Van Koppen, P. J., & Crombag, H. F. M. (1993). *Anchored narratives: The psychology of criminal evidence*. Hertfordshire, UK: Harvester Wheatsheaf.

Watson, J. B. (1928). *The ways of behaviourism*. Oxford, UK: Harper.

Study Designs 2

Abstract

There is a bridge connecting questions of interest, study designs, and analytic methods used to make sense of data collected. Whether questions are based on theory, on research data observed earlier on, or from practical experience, questions inform our methodological approach for a new study; they may have implications for the sampling of participants, the planning of measurements, and choice of measures used in the study. Some questions may call for a randomised controlled experiment, whereas other questions may call for other types of studies. In this chapter, a variety of study types are discussed, including randomised controlled experiments and quasi-experimental studies, cohort studies, individual growth studies, and other study designs used in later chapters in this book. It is explained how a multi-time (or, where possible, continuous) and multi-method approach to assessment can help us to shed light on somewhat different aspects of learning, can help us to get a better grip on complex, dynamic learning processes, and—from a practical point of view—can help us to move from a punishment (i.e., pass/fail) culture to more of a growth mindset culture, where performance of the moment is a fraction of a bigger growth picture.

2.1 Introduction

Different types of questions call for different types of designs or different choices within a given type of design, and the questions we ask and the design we choose also influence what kind of conclusions can be drawn. In the domain of Education, some types of questions concern the effectiveness of study, teaching, practice or assessment methods on learning outcomes or other learning-relevant variables (e.g., effort, motivation) in a given context. Examples include the effect of a particular

J. Leppink, *The Art of Modelling the Learning Process*, Springer Texts in Education,
https://doi.org/10.1007/978-3-030-43082-5_2

type of instructional support in Mathematics Education in high school and the effect of checklists on the development of self-regulated learning skills among undergraduates in an online degree programme. This kind of questions generally calls for some form of randomised controlled experiment, where we randomly sample students from our target population and randomly assign them to different conditions (e.g., Bloom, 2008; Leppink, 2019).

In other cases, we may be interested in differences between pre-existing groups in some outcome variables of interest. Examples include differences in performance on a particular type of computer task between novices and experts in a particular topic and differences in English proficiency among high-school graduates from a number of non-English speaking countries in the European Union. Although we may well have to leave causality in the middle in this second type of questions, both types of questions have in common that they are best addressed by sufficiently large random samples from the target population(s) of interest. Using smaller and/or non-random samples does not mean that our studies are useless, but the more we move away from sufficiently large and random samples, the more our interpretations and generalisations of findings may be questioned, unless we can demonstrate that differences between individuals in an outcome variable of interest are much smaller than usual and/or—as far as sample size is concerned—the effect of an intervention under study is considerably larger than common in educational research. Besides, as becomes clear later on in this chapter and is repeated in later chapters in this book, a somewhat smaller sample size may, under some circumstances, to some degree be compensated by taking repeated measurements from the same individuals sampled on the same outcome variable of interest.

Finally, there are questions in Education for which random sampling is not needed or even does not make sense. This includes common questions in everyday educational practice, such as if there are substantial differences between subsequent cohorts in a Psychology undergraduate programme at University A in a given block or module exam or if Learner M demonstrates growth on subsequent occasions of a progress test (e.g., see Chap. 1). These questions are so specific that generalisation to a broader population is neither asked nor makes sense. For the cohort type of question, we can simply compare exam performance of the cohorts who completed the exam, and for the individual type of question, we need a testing practice as described in Chaps. 1 and 16 to draw a meaningful conclusion.

2.2 Types of Comparisons

Whenever the interest lies in generalising beyond a sample, as in among others randomised controlled experiments and quasi-experiments, random sampling constitutes a way to eliminate sampling *bias*, because only the laws of probability determine which individuals are sampled. Even though given population *SD* (σ) > 0, *M* in a sample of size *N* is virtually always at least somewhat different from *M* in the population (μ) randomly sampled from, and *M* varies across possible samples of N, no bias means that the average of M across all possible samples of size N drawn from the same population equals M of the population of interest. The *SD* of *M*s across possible samples of N decreases with increasing sample size N. Dealing with single samples of size N to estimate μ, given σ, the *SD* of *M*s across all possible samples of size N drawn from the population of interest (σ_M) equals:

$$\sigma_M = \sigma/\sqrt{N}.$$

This quantity, σ_M, is also referred to as *standard error* (*SE*). In research practice, we rarely know σ, but we use *SD* to estimate it. The resulting *SE* is then:

$$SE = SD/\sqrt{N}.$$

As for M, there is less sample-to-sample fluctuation in *SD* across larger than across smaller samples, meaning less fluctuation in *SE* from sample to sample as well. Where the laws of probability apply (i.e., in the case of random sampling), the formula of and reasoning behind *SE* make sense, and *confidence intervals* (CIs) and statistical significance tests can account for the uncertainty due to sample-to-sample fluctuation. Given M and *SE*, the 95% CI is:

$$95\%\ \text{CI} = M \pm t_c * SE.$$

In this formula, t_c is the critical t-value at the given degrees of freedom (*df*) and statistical significance level (α, in the case of the 95% CI: 0.05, tested two-sided), which is slightly larger than the critical z-value at that α (at $\alpha = 0.05$, the critical z-value is about 1.96) but gradually approaches that critical z-value with increasing N. The same holds for other α levels (e.g., for the 90% CI, the critical z-value is about 1.645, and t_c is slightly larger than that but approaches 1.645 with increasing N). The C% CI should include the population parameter of interest (here: μ) in C% of all possible samples of the same size N drawn from the same population.

In studies where the population of interest is available, for instance in cohort studies in a very specific setting or in individual assessment like the progress testing example, thinking in terms of random sampling from a larger population or generalising beyond the individual(s) studied to a larger population is pointless and using CIs and statistical significance tests—which are based on *SE*s that work in the case of random sampling from a larger population—no longer make sense.

2.2.1 Randomised Controlled Experiments

In the case of a randomised controlled experiment, there is not only random sampling from a population of interest but random allocation to conditions of interest as well. In the case of random allocation, "*the short-term and long-term future experiences of the control group provide valid estimates of what these experiences would have been for the treatment group had it not been offered the* *treatment*" (Bloom, 2008, p. 128). It is important to note that random sampling from a population of interest should not be expected to compensate for non-random allocation to conditions, and that random allocation to conditions does not justify convenience sampling or purposeful sampling from the population of interest. Besides, deviations from random sampling and/or random allocation may substantially decrease the replicability of findings from one experiment in future experiments (Hedges, 2018; Ioannidis, 2005a, 2005b; Tipton, Hallberg, Hedges, & Chan, 2017). Finally, another factor that impacts the likelihood of findings being replicated is found in the sample size of our experiments. We have already seen that, randomly sampling from populations of interest, *SE*s decrease with increasing *N*. In the case of small samples, different experiments may yield quite different outcomes even if the population sampled from is the same and the phenomenon of interest remains unchanged. Therefore, it is important to do required sample size calculations for an aimed statistical power and precision (e.g., Buchner, Erdfelder, Faul, & Lang, 2009; Dong & Maynard, 2013; Dong, Kelcey, & Spybrook, 2017; Dong, Kelcey, Spybrook, & Maynard, 2016; Kelcey, Dong, Spybrook, & Cox, 2017; Kelcey, Dong, Spybrook, & Shen, 2017; Spybrook, Kelcey, & Dong, 2016). Limited statistical power is a bigger problem than one might think at first. With a statistical power of 0.7, for example, there is a 70% chance of obtaining a statistically significant finding for an effect of interest. However, with two independent experiments of a power of 0.7 each, the chance of obtaining a statistically significant finding in *both* experiments is 0.7 * 0.7 = 0.49 (i.e., 49%), and when we add a third independent experiment with a power of 0.7, the chance that all three experiments yield a statistically significant finding for that phenomenon of interest is 0.7 * 0.7 * 0.7 = 0.343 meaning 34.3% (e.g., Leppink, 2019a).

In not so few experiments, there are either two (or in some cases, three) experimental treatment factors or there is one treatment factor yet one or two pre-existing grouping variables play a role as well. An example of an experiment with two treatment factors (i.e., two-way experiment) is found in presenting a self-use checklist during study or not presenting it to participants (i.e., treatment factor A) and providing instructor feedback during study or not providing it to participants (i.e., treatment factor B). An extension to a three-way experiment, to study the *testing effect* discussed in Chap. 1, could be achieved by adding a third factor: immediate and delayed post-test or delayed post-test only. In line with the *testing effect*, one would expect the group of participants taking a post-test immediately after study (i.e., immediate post-test) to on average perform better on a post-test sometime after study (i.e., delayed post-test) than participants who were not offered the immediate post-test. Either way, two factors or three, statistical power and precision will usually be optimal if all cells (i.e., combinations of A and B, or of A, B, and C) have the same *n* (i.e., *N* is the overall sample size, and *n* is the size per condition). In other words, random allocation would be done such that equal proportions of *N* fill the different cells in the design.

An example of an experiment with one treatment factor and a pre-existing grouping variable is autonomous problem solving versus studying worked examples of problems (i.e., treatment factor) for novices versus advanced learners in the topic at hand (i.e., pre-existing grouping variable). In such cases, *stratified random sampling* (e.g., Kish, 1965), meaning that random sampling is applied among novices and advanced learners (i.e., the strata) in such a way that the proportions of novices and advanced learners are the same across conditions, will normally result in more precision and power than simple random sampling; in the latter, some imbalance (i.e., slightly different novice-advanced ratios across conditions) is likely, and that imbalance comes at the cost of a loss of precision and power.

In some experiments, one or more quantitative *covariates* are included, the role of which partly depends on whether these covariates are measured prior to or after the start of treatment; covariates measured *after* the start of treatment are commonly better treated as *mediators* or intermediate variables in a causal chain that are affected by the treatment and in their turn predict one or more outcome variables of interest (e.g., Leppink, 2019a).

Finally, there are experiments where interaction between participants, repeated measurements, or some combination thereof (e.g., Leppink, 2019a; Snijders & Bosker, 2012; Tan, 2010), creates a so-called *intraclass correlation* (*ICC*) that reduces the effective sample size and hence needs to be accounted for in required sample size calculations and data analysis. For example, in learning groups of size *n* in which group discussion constitutes part of participants' study, the multiplication factor for the required sample size needed (M_N) to account for $ICC > 0$ is:

$$M_N = 1 + [(n-1) * ICC].$$

In cases where we deal with *dyads* ($n = 2$) instead of groups ($n > 2$), this formula comes down to:

$$M_N = 1 + ICC.$$

The larger *ICC*, the larger M_N needed to account for *ICC*. These considerations of *ICC* and M_N also apply to quasi-experimental studies and other studies that do use random sampling but not random allocation to conditions.

2.2.2 Quasi-experiments

Although quasi-experimental research (e.g., Class A in School J happening to be the control condition and Class B in School K the treatment condition; Leppink, 2019a) certainly has its use and is not necessarily inferior to experimental research, causal inference is a lot more difficult in quasi-experimental than in experimental research (e.g., Cook & Campbell, 1979; Cook & Wong, 2008; Hedges, 2018; Huitema, 2011; Stuart & Rubin, 2010). In the case of random allocation to conditions, differences between participants in key variables are randomised. Although this will rarely result in conditions that are *exactly* the same in these key variables in a given experiment, and there will be experiment-to-experiment variation, over large series of experiments the average difference between conditions in these key variables should be about zero (i.e., with infinite numbers of experiments, which would include all possible samples of the same size from the same population, the difference would be zero). However, in the absence of random allocation to conditions, conditions may start off substantially different on several key variables, and these differences may persist across replications of the study. Accounting for these differences in data analysis is not always possible, but even if it is possible it will require a number of steps (e.g., Cook & Wong, 2008; Hedges, 2018; Stuart & Rubin, 2010). Besides, causal inference is not always of interest in quasi-experimental studies; the question of interest is often whether groups *differ* in one or more outcome variables of interest, and we can estimate differences while leaving causality in the middle.

2.2.3 Cohort Studies

In some studies, the interest is not in generalising beyond individuals observed, and it does not make much sense to view the individuals observed as a random sample of possible individuals that could have been observed. For example, being enrolled in a degree programme is rarely if ever a completely random event; it is not that universities send out random invitations to possible students to sign up for Programme X and these students then enrol. Rather, students make a choice for a particular programme and may or may not be accepted to the programme for one or several, often institution-specific or programme-specific, reasons. Nevertheless, we are sometimes interested in studying differences between cohorts in for instance exam performance.

Consider five subsequent cohorts in Medical School A, the sizes of which vary from 179 to 222 students. In Year 1 of the Bachelor of Medicine, students complete a variety of exams including an end-of-year 100-item MCQ exam on topics covered during the first year and an objective structured clinical examination (OSCE: e.g., Khan, Gaunt, Ramachandran, & Pushkar, 2013; Khan, Ramachandran, Gaunt, & Pushkar, 2013). Both result in a score ranging from 0 (minimum) to 100 (maximum). We are interested in cohort differences in performance on the two exams and in the correlation between the two exams. Figure 2.1 presents the distribution of MCQ exam performance across cohorts, Fig. 2.2 presents the distribution of OSCE performance across cohorts, and Fig. 2.3 presents the scatterplot of the joint distribution of the two exams for each of the cohorts (*Jamovi*).

Figures 2.1, 2.2 and 2.3 indicate some differences between cohorts. Table 2.1 presents *M* and *SD* per exam and Pearson's correlation (*r*; Pearson, 1900) of the two exams for the five cohorts (*Jamovi*).

The correlations between the two exams reported in Table 2.1 are not unusual; in practical educational settings, correlations between MCQ exams and OSCEs in the 0.3–0.5 range are common. Squaring *r*, we learn how much of the variance in one exam is explained by performance on the other exam. Thus, the proportion of variance explained varies from about 0.095 (9.5%, Cohort 3) to about 0.171 (17.1%, Cohort 2). When we evaluate the mean difference (M_d) for the different

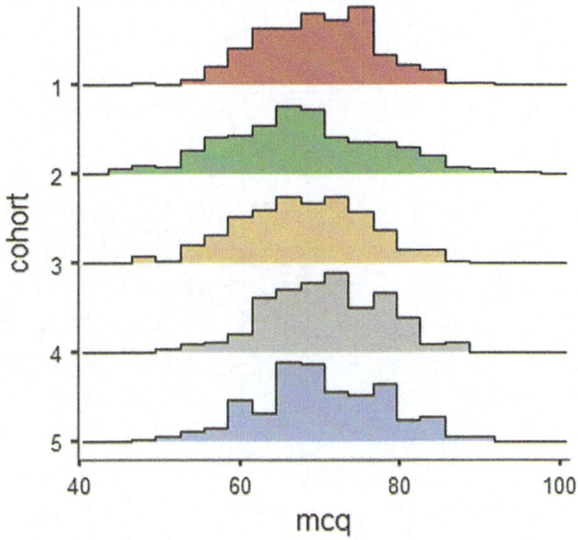

Fig. 2.1 Distribution of MCQ exam performance in the five cohorts (1–5) (*Jamovi*)

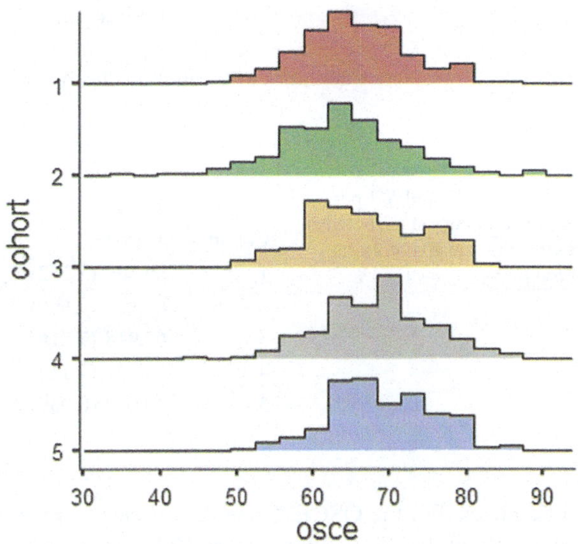

Fig. 2.2 Distribution of OSCE exam performance in the five cohorts (1–5) (*Jamovi*)

pairs of cohorts, we see slightly larger differences on the OSCE than on the MCQ exam, and the same holds when we evaluate these M_ds relative to the *SD*s of these cohorts, as for instance with Cohen's *d* (i.e., M_d divided by the pooled *SD* of the two groups compared; Cohen, 1988). For the MCQ exam, Cohen's *d* varies from about 0.008 (Cohort 2 vs. Cohort 3) to about 0.392 (Cohorts 3 vs. Cohort 4). Although the meaning of numbers in educational settings always depends on the context, most would agree that *d*-values in this range represent fairly small

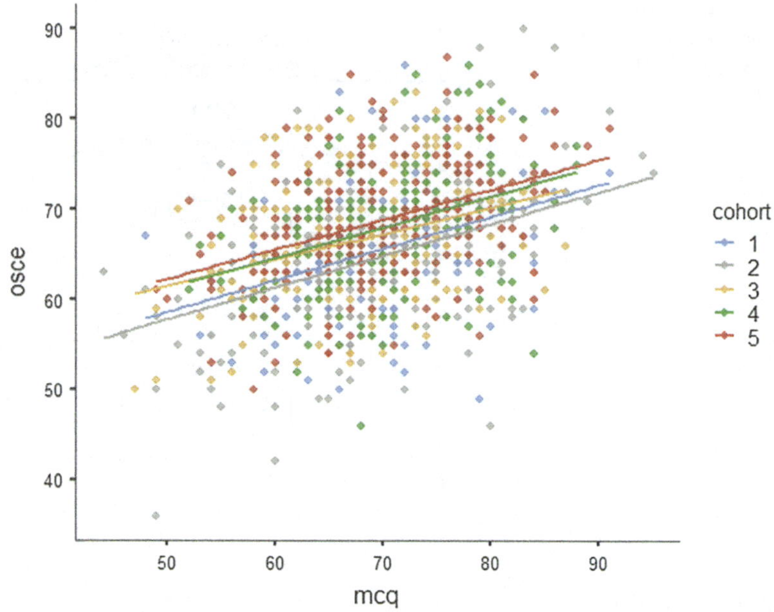

Fig. 2.3 Scatterplot of the joint distribution of the two exams for each of the cohorts (1–5) (Jamovi)

Table 2.1 *M* and *SD* per exam and Pearson's *r* between exams for the five cohorts (Jamovi)

Exam	MCQ	OSCE	MCQ-OSCE
Cohort	*M (SD)*	*M (SD)*	*Pearson's r*
1	69.603 (7.252)	65.536 (7.252)	0.354
2	67.847 (9.669)	64.099 (8.253)	0.414
3	67.918 (7.716)	66.712 (7.213)	0.309
4	70.838 (7.114)	68.335 (7.000)	0.348
5	70.099 (8.039)	68.932 (6.806)	0.393

differences. For the OSCE, Cohen's *d* varies from about 0.087 (Cohort 4 vs. Cohort 5) to about 0.642 (Cohort 2 vs. Cohort 5); *d*-values in the 0.5–0.8 range are commonly interpreted as medium-size difference, so the difference between Cohort 2 and Cohort 5 would probably be interpreted as such (and the same goes for the difference between Cohort 2 and Cohort 4, where $d = 0.552$).

Note that none of these differences can be interpreted as one cohort being smarter, more motivated or whatever; a multitude of observed and unobserved variables may contribute to cohort differences in performance, and among these variables is that exams for different cohorts are rarely exactly the same (here: different MCQ exams and different stations in an OSCE for different cohorts).

Adding CIs or *p*-values is not meaningful in this kind of setting either, since the cohorts are not random samples from larger populations of interest and our interest does not lie in any kind of generalisation beyond the students in these cohorts anyway. Combinations of graphs and descriptive statistics provide all the information we need in response to our questions on cohort differences in average performance on the two exams and the correlation between the exams. Some may wonder if some of the observations are not actually outliers that influence some of our statistics, and such questions can be studied by computing the statistics of interest *with* and *without* these potential outliers. For the data at hand, that exercise would not result in any meaningful differences in outcomes.

2.2.4 Individual Trajectories

As with the cohort example, everyday educational practice questions concerning the learning of particular individuals in a programme do not call for CIs or significance tests; the individual under study was not randomly sampled from a population of interest, and there is no interest in generalising an individual's exam performance to other individuals either. The progress testing example discussed in Chap. 1 and mentioned earlier in this chapter is an example of that. However, there is an increasing interest in some fields in Education in so-called *single-case experimental designs* (SCEDs, sometimes also referred to as *single-subject experimental designs* or SSEDs) for the evaluation of treatments and interventions in individuals (e.g., Michiels & Onghena, 2018; Michiels, Heyvaert, Meulders, & Onghena, 2017; Tanious, De, & Onghena, 2019) or fairly small populations which may be difficult to study for a variety of reasons and therefore often result in researchers having to resort to small samples (e.g., Pérez-Fuster, 2017; Pérez-Fuster, Sevilla, & Herrera, 2019). Although there are different types of SCEDs, key feature of these different designs is that we have time series of measurements on the same outcome variable (s) of interest from the same individual(s). Although the individuals under study do not necessarily constitute a random sample from a broader population of interest and the interest does not necessarily lie in generalising beyond the individuals studied (e.g., the effect of a treatment or intervention for a given individual), randomisation can be found in the exact sequence of *baseline* (A) and *treatment* (B) within this series, and the scores observed from each individual may be considered a random sample from a 'population' or 'universe' of possible scores from that individual under A and B, respectively.

The deliberate baseline-treatment manipulation is one of the features in which SCEDs can be distinguished from nonexperimental research. Simultaneously, contrary to traditional experimental designs where different individuals are allocated to different conditions (e.g., control vs. treatment), the interest in SCEDs lies *not* in comparing groups but in estimating *within-individual* differences using repeated measurements from these individuals. Michiels and Onghena (2018) provide a comprehensive SCED typology based on the *type of design*, the use of *replication*, and the use of *random assignment*.

Two main types of designs, which can be combined, are *phase* designs and *alternation* designs (Heyvaert & Onghena, 2014; Onghena & Edgington, 2005; Rvachew & Matthews, 2017). While phase designs divide the full series or sequence of measurements into separate phases for baseline and treatment, alternation designs involve rapid alternation of these conditions throughout the series. Perhaps the simplest example of a phase design is the AB or *interrupted time series design* (e.g., Michiels & Onghena, 2018), in which a sequence of As (i.e., baseline measurements) is followed by a series of Bs (i.e., treatment measurements), while common examples of alternation designs are the *completely randomised design*, the *randomised block design*, and the *alternating treatments design* (ATD; Onghena, 2005).

Baseline-treatment decisions may constitute a random variable. For example, in the aforementioned AB design, given a multitude of measurements, the start of treatment can be randomised. If we have five, ten or fifteen individuals and ten measurements, we could create for example five possible sequences and randomly assign individuals to these five sequences:

AAA BBBBBBB
AAAA BBBBBB
AAAAA BBBBB
AAAAAA BBBB
AAAAAAA BBB

This way, we would have for each individual at least three baseline and at least three treatment measurements. Michiels and Onghena (2018) provide several examples of how to apply randomisation with other types of designs.

Finally, replication can greatly enhance the internal validity of an SCED (e.g., Kratochwill et al., 2010) and can be done in two ways: *simultaneously* or *sequentially* (e.g., Onghena & Edgington, 2005). While simultaneous replication is about using multiple alternation or phase designs simultaneously (e.g., the *multiple baseline across participants design*), sequential replication comes down to carrying out individual series sequentially in an attempt to test the generalisability of findings to other individuals, settings or outcomes (e.g., Harris & Jenson, 1985; Mansell, 1982; Michiels & Onghena, 2018).

2.3 Types of Information

Of course, SCEDs are not the only designs that can include repeated measurements; any of the other types of studies discussed in this chapter can incorporate a component of repeated measurements. In randomised controlled experiments, where random samples of individuals are randomly assigned to different (orders of) conditions, series of measurements may take place after the start of treatment or partially before partially after the start of treatment. The same may sometimes happen in quasi-experimental studies and even cohort studies, although the statistical treatment of measurements prior to treatment will likely be different from that in randomised controlled experiments (e.g., Leppink, 2019a; Twisk et al., 2018; Van Breukelen, 2006; Van Breukelen & Van Dijk, 2007). Studies including repeated measurements allow us to separate within-individual variance from between-individuals variance and can help us to study not only how particular variables of interest can explain performance of the moment but change in that performance as well. Performance of the moment is part of a bigger growth picture, and that performance may change in response to several factors. For a variety of reasons discussed in later chapters in this book, treatment effects estimated through changes within (groups of) individuals may be quite different from the same effects estimated through differences between (groups of) individuals.

The cohort study example discussed earlier in this chapter illustrates how MCQ exams and OSCEs may measure different types of knowledge or skill but do share some variance. In an assessment programme where we have multiple measurements for each—within a year, a two-year phase or a Bachelor stage—we will likely see both substantial within-instrument between-occasions correlations and between-instruments correlations within and between measurements. Even though we may better not speak in terms of causal inference, if early-stage performance on MCQ exams and OSCEs can to some extent help to predict performance on MCQ exams and OSCEs at a later stage, we can use early-stage poor performance to recommend and inform remediation instead of send students to re-sit exams without any remediation (i.e., growth mindset instead of punishment practice).

How many repeated measurements are needed depends on several factors, including what kind of effect or trend we expect and in how much detail we want to go. In cases where an effect or trend of interest is (expected to be) linear, having two time points may do. Some experiments, for example, include two post-tests: one immediately after study or practice (i.e., immediate post-test) and one sometime later (i.e., delayed post-test). However, if the interest lies in a nonlinear effect or trend, having only two measurements is problematic because every change appears linear even if it is not. For example, for a quadratic trend, we will need at least three (and ideally: equidistant) measurements and perhaps preferably more than three measurements in order to test for higher-order polynomials (e.g., cubic) that may invalidate quadratic interpretations (e.g., Leppink, 2019a).

Finally, whichever study we find ourselves in, it is good to keep in mind that *methodological control* (i.e., control by *design*) is almost always better than *statistical control* (i.e., control by *analysis*), with more of the latter being needed usually increasing risks of our estimates being inaccurate and our conclusions being incorrect.

References

Bloom, H. S. (2008). In: Alasuutari, P., Bickman, L., & Brannen, J. (Eds.), *The SAGE handbook of social research methods* (Chap. 9, pp. 115–133). London: Sage.

Buchner, A., Erdfelder, E., Faul, F., & Lang, A. G. (2009). G*Power version 3.1.2. Retrieved February 1, 2020, from http://www.gpower.hhu.de/.

Cohen, J. (1988). *Statistical power analysis for the behavioural sciences*. New York: Routledge.

Cook, T. D., & Campbell, D. T. (1979). *Quasi-experimentation: Design and analysis for field settings*. Chicago, IL: Rand McNally.

Cook, T. D., & Wong, V. C. (2008). Better quasi-experimental practice. In P. Alasuutari, L. Bickman, & J. Brannen (Eds.), *The SAGE handbook of social research methods* (Chap. 10, pp. 134–165). London: Sage.

Dong, N., Kelcey, B., & Spybrook, J. (2017). Power analyses of moderator effects in three-level cluster randomized trials. *Journal of Experimental Education, 86*(3), 489–514. https://doi.org/10.1080/00220973.2017.1315714.

Dong, N., Kelcey, B., Spybrook, J., & Maynard, R. A. (2016). Designing and analyzing multilevel experiments and quasi-experiments for causal evaluation (Version 1.07). Retrieved February 1, 2020, from https://www.causalevaluation.org/power-analysis.html.

Dong, N., & Maynard, R. A. (2013). PowerUp!: A tool for calculating minimum detectable effect sizes and minimum required samples sizes for experimental and quasi-experimental design studies. *Journal of Research on Educational Effectiveness, 6*(1), 24–67. https://doi.org/10.1080/19345747.2012.673143.

Harris, F. N., & Jenson, W. R. (1985). Comparisons of multiple-baseline across persons designs and AB designs with replications: Issues and confusions. *Behavioral Assessment, 7,* 121–127.

Hedges, L. V. (2018). Challenges in building usable knowledge in education. *Journal of Research on Educational Effectiveness, 11*(1), 1–21. https://doi.org/10.1080/19345747.2017.1375583.

Heyvaert, M., & Onghena, P. (2014). Analysis of single-case data: Randomisation tests for measures of effect size. *Neuropsychological Rehabilitation, 24,* 507–527. https://doi.org/10.1080/09602011.2013.818564.

Huitema, B. E. (2011). *The analysis of covariance and alternatives: Statistical methods for experiments, quasi-experiments, and single-case studies* (2nd ed., Part VII, pp. 565–617). New York: Wiley.

Ioannidis, J. P. A. (2005a). Contradicted and initially stronger effects in highly cited clinical research. *Journal of the American Medical Association, 294*(2), 218–228. https://doi.org/10.1001/jama.294.2.218.

Ioannidis, J. P. A. (2005b). Why most published research findings are false. *PLoS, Medicine, 2*(8), e124. https://doi.org/10.1371/journal.pmed.0020124.

Kelcey, B., Dong, N., Spybrook, J., & Cox, K. (2017). Statistical power for causally defined indirect effects in group-randomized trials with individual-level mediators. *Journal of Educational and Behavioral Statistics, 42*(5), 499–530. https://doi.org/10.3102/1076998617695506.

Kelcey, B., Dong, N., Spybrook, J., & Shen, Z. (2017). Experimental power for indirect effects in group-randomized studies with group-level mediators. *Multivariate Behavioral Research, 52*(6), 699–719. https://doi.org/10.1080/00273171.2017.1356212.

Khan, K. Z., Gaunt, K., Ramachandran, S., & Pushkar, P. (2013). The objective structured clinical examination (OSCE): AMEE guide no. 81. Part II: Organisation & administration. *Medical Teacher, 35*(9), e1447–e1463. https://doi.org/10.3109/0142159X.2013.818635.

Khan, K. Z., Ramachandran, S., Gaunt, K., & Pushkar, P. (2013). The objective structured clinical examination (OSCE): AMEE guide no. 81. Part I: An historical and theoretical perspective. *Medical Teacher, 35*(9), e1437–e1446. https://doi.org/10.3109/0142159X.2013.818634.

Kish, L. (1965). *Survey sampling*. New York: Wiley. https://doi.org/10.1002/bimj.19680100122.

Kratochwill, T. R., Hitchcock, J., Horner, R. H., Levin, J. R., Odom, S. L., Rindskopf, D. M., & Shadish, W. R. (2010). Single-case designs technical documentation. Retrieved February 1, 2020, from https://files.eric.ed.gov/fulltext/ED510743.pdf.

Leppink, J. (2019). *Statistical methods for experimental research in education and psychology*. Cham: Springer. https://doi.org/10.1007/978-3-030-21241-4.

Mansell, J. (1982). Repeated direct replication of AB designs. *Journal of Behavior Therapy and Experimental Psychiatry, 13*(3), 261–262. https://doi.org/10.1016/0005-7916(82)90017-9.

Michiels, B., Heyvaert, M., Meulders, A., & Onghena, P. (2017). Confidence intervals for single-case effect size measures based on randomization test inversion. *Behavior Research Methods, 49*(1), 363–381. https://doi.org/10.3758/s13428-016-0714-4.

Michiels, B., & Onghena, P. (2018). Randomized single-case AB phase designs: Prospects and pitfalls. *Behavior Research Methods*. https://doi.org/10.3758/s13428-018-1084-x.

Onghena, P. (2005). Single-case designs. In B. Everitt & D. Howell (Eds.), *Encyclopedia of statistics in behavioral science* (Vol. 4, pp. 1850–1854). Chichester, UK: Wiley.

Onghena, P., & Edgington, E. S. (2005). Customization of pain treatments: Single-case design and analysis. *The Clinical Journal of Pain, 21*(1), 56–68.

Pearson, K. (1900). On the criterion that a given system of deviations from the probable in the case of a correlated system of variables is such that it can be reasonably supposed to have arisen from random sampling. *Philosophical Magazine, 50*(5), 157–175. https://doi.org/10.1080/14786440009463897.

Pérez-Fuster, P. (2017). *Enhancing skills in individuals with autism spectrum disorder through technology-mediated interventions*. Valencia, Spain: Universitat de València. https://dialnet.unirioja.es/servlet/dctes?codigo=137925.

Pérez-Fuster, P., Sevilla, J., & Herrera, G. (2019). Enhancing daily living skills in four adults with autism spectrum disorder through an embodied digital technology-mediated intervention. *Research in Autism Spectrum Disorders, 58,* 54–67. https://doi.org/10.1016/j.rasd.2018.08.006.

Rvachew, S., & Matthews, T. (2017). Demonstrating treatment efficacy using the single subject randomization design: A tutorial and demonstration. *Journal of Communication Disorders, 67,* 1–13. https://doi.org/10.1016/j.jcomdis.2017.04.003.

Snijders, T. A. B., & Bosker, R. J. (2012). *Multilevel analysis: An introduction to basic and advanced multilevel modelling* (2nd ed.). London: Sage.

Spybrook, J., Kelcey, B., & Dong, N. (2016). Power for detecting treatment by moderator effects in two and three-level cluster randomized trials. *Journal of Educational and Behavioral Statistics, 41*(6), 605–627. https://doi.org/10.3102/1076998616655442.

Stuart, E. A., & Rubin, D. B. (2010). Best practices in quasi-experimental designs: Matching methods for causal inference. In: J. W. Osborne (Ed.), *Best practices in quantitative methods* (Chap. 11, pp. 155–176). London: Sage.

Tan, F. E. S. (2010). Best practices in analysis of longitudinal data: A multilevel approach. In J. W. Osborne (Ed.), *Best practices in quantitative methods* (Chap. 30, pp. 451–470). London: Sage.

Tanious, R., De, T. K., & Onghena, P. (2019). A multiple randomization testing procedure for level, trend, variability, overlap, immediacy, and consistency in single-case phase designs. *Behaviour Research and Therapy, 119,* 103414. https://doi.org/10.1016/j.brat.2019.103414.

Tipton, E., Hallberg, K., Hedges, L. V., & Chan, W. (2017). Implications of small samples for generalization: Adjustments and rules of thumb. *Evaluation Review, 41*(59), 472–505. https://doi.org/10.1177/0193841X6655665.

Twisk, J. W. R., Bosman, L., Hoekstra, T., Rijnhart, J., Welten, M., & Heymans, M. (2018). Different ways to estimate treatment effects in randomised controlled trials. *Contemporary Clinical Trials Communications, 10,* 80–85. https://doi.org/10.1016/j.conctc.2018.03.008.

Van Breukelen, G. J. P. (2006). ANCOVA versus change from baseline: More power in randomized studies, more bias in nonrandomized studies. *Journal of Clinical Epidemiology, 59* (9), 920–925. https://doi.org/10.1016/j.jclinepi.2006.02.007.
Van Breukelen, G. J. P., & Van Dijk, K. R. A. (2007). Use of covariates in randomized controlled trials. *Journal of the International Neuropsychological Society, 13*(5), 903–904. https://doi.org/10.1017/S1355617707071147.

Statistical Learning

3

Abstract

Where Chaps. 1 and 2 provide the foundation for types of questions and study designs, respectively, this third chapter provides a pragmatic approach to statistical testing and estimation (PASTE). This approach is an extension of PASTE introduced in my recent Springer Texts in Education Series book entitled "Statistical Methods for Experimental Research in Education and Psychology" in two ways: moving beyond experimental research and including small samples as well. Both extensions require specific modifications in the pragmatic approach for larger-sample experimental research as introduced in the aforementioned book, including in criteria used for statistical testing and in terms of causal inference. However, like in the approach presented in my book on experimental research, the approach discussed in this chapter is about uniting traditional and emerging approaches to statistical testing and estimation: Frequentist CIs and equivalence testing, Bayesian posterior intervals and the region of practical equivalence, Likelihood ratio testing, and information criteria that are—through the use of Likelihoods—related to the other methods but provide testing outcomes under slightly different assumptions. Concepts of Big Data, Artificial Intelligence, Machine Learning, Educational Data Mining, and Learning Analytics are introduced in this chapter, with examples that are revisited in later chapters in this book. Finally, PASTE as introduced in this chapter incorporates a decision-making framework for dealing with different types of missing data as well.

J. Leppink, *The Art of Modelling the Learning Process*, Springer Texts in Education,
https://doi.org/10.1007/978-3-030-43082-5_3

3.1 Introduction

There is a bridge between (research) *questions* (and, where available, hypotheses), *design* (i.e., study design and methods used for data collection), and data *analysis* (e.g., Leppink, 2019). Besides, apart from the questions and design, the nature of the data collected should also inform our analytic choices. Graphs and descriptive statistics together provide a very good way to get a grip on the data. Given these different sources of information for analytic decision making—questions, design, and the type of data at hand—different teams of researchers may well make different choices and consequently end up with different findings and conclusions for the same data (e.g., Leppink & Pérez-Fuster, 2019; Silberzahn et al., 2018; Twisk, Hoogendijk, Zwijsen, & De Boer, 2016; Twisk et al., 2018). It is therefore of paramount importance to be fully transparent about all choices made at any point in the analytic stage, and the same holds for the design and data collection stage. In the words of Van der Zee and Reich (2018, p. 3): "*For both qualitative and quantitative research, interpretation of results depends on understanding what stances researchers adopted before an investigation, what constraints researchers placed around their analytic plan, and what analytic decisions were responsive to new findings. Transparency in that analytic process is critical for determining how seriously practitioners or policymakers should consider a result.*" Finally, we should bear in mind that even if two teams independently carry out the same experiment, with exactly the same design and materials and procedure and for simplicity assuming no measurement error in our instruments (i.e., perfect reliability, which is usually not the case), given different samples for each experiment and variation between people in learning and similar outcome variables of interest, the two teams will obtain somewhat different results even if the phenomenon of interest in the population of interest is exactly the same (cf. the notion of *SE* discussed in Chap. 2). Consider the following example.

3.2 Series of Experiments

In a team of Educational Psychologists, there is an interest in the effectiveness of a particular type of instructional support on learning inferential statistics among undergraduate Psychology students. The psychologists carry out an experiment in which they randomly allocate $N = 50$ participants to an instructional support (i.e., treatment) condition ($n = 25$) or a no instructional support (i.e., control) condition ($n = 25$). Although some of their colleagues from the Medical Education department criticise this experiment because they see no point in trying to prove that 'something works better than nothing', the psychologists justify their choice by pointing at the seas of literature on effects of instructional support that demonstrate that support may have positive as well as negative effects, or no effect at all, and that for the type of support at hand the literature does not provide any clear reason to expect a positive effect on learning beforehand. Besides, the psychologists argue that most of their colleagues in the field of Educational Psychology would say that even though the effect of a particular type of support may not be exactly zero it may be so small that we may as well call the two options—presence or absence of this type of instructional support—*relatively* or *practically equivalent* (Kruschke, 2013, 2014, 2018; Kruschke & Liddell, 2017; Lakens, 2017; Leppink, 2019). More precisely, they specify the interval of $-0.3 < d < 0.3$ as region of relative or practical equivalence. They carry out their experiment and publish the results (henceforth: Experiment 1).

3.2.1 Replication

Reading the article reporting on Experiment 1, seven other teams of Educational Psychologists independently decide to replicate the experiment (from this point forward: Experiments 2–8), using the same design, materials, and procedure as in the original experiment. The outcome variable in these experiments is a 100-item MCQ test score on a scale from 0 (minimum, all incorrect) to 100 (maximum, all correct). Students in the experiments participate individually throughout the study, without interaction with peers. Since Experiment 1 does not provide substantial evidence in favour of a positive or negative effect of instructional support, no one-sided hypothesis with regard to the direction of any possible treatment effect is formulated in any of Experiments 2–8 either. The only thing that differs across experiments is the sample size. Table 3.1 presents *n*, *M*, and *SD* per condition and the 90% CI of *d* for the difference between conditions in each of Experiments 1–8.

You may wonder why the researchers in each of the experiments computed 90% CIs and not 95% CIs, although they had no one-sided hypothesis about a positive or negative treatment effect. The reason is that the approach chosen by the researchers is *four one-sided testing* (FOST; Leppink, 2019). As the name indicates, in FOST, four one-sided tests are performed in response to a set of four null hypotheses:

Table 3.1 Sample size, *M*, and *SD* per condition and 90% CI of *d* for the difference between conditions in each of Experiments 1–8 (*JASP*)

Experiment	*n* (*N*)	*M* (*SD*) control	*M* (*SD*) treat	90% CI of *d*
1	25 (50)	55.200 (4.761)	57.400 (4.646)	[−0.006; 0.937]
2	65 (130)	54.780 (5.727)	56.030 (5.598)	[−0.070; 0.509]
3	20 (40)	51.850 (5.641)	55.700 (4.835)	[0.190; 1.266]
4	39 (78)	56.080 (4.349)	53.490 (4.994)	[−0.931; −0.172]
5	31 (62)	56.810 (4.736)	53.940 (4.312)	[−1.060; −0.203]
6	35 (70)	55.340 (5.280)	55.370 (4.741)	[−0.388; 0.399]
7	27 (54)	55.700 (5.105)	56.260 (4.662)	[−0.335; 0.561]
8	115 (230)	55.940 (4.867)	55.670 (5.162)	[−0.271; 0.163]

Table 3.2 FOST in a nutshell with six examples of 90% CIs of d

H_0 is rejected					
90% CI of d	$H_{0.1}$	$H_{0.2}$	$H_{0.3}$	$H_{0.4}$	Interpretation
I: [−0.731; −0.367]	No	Yes	Yes	No	Evidence for substantial negative effect
II: [0.327; 1.007]	Yes	No	No	Yes	Evidence for substantial positive effect
III: [−0.257; 0.156]	Yes	Yes	No	No	Evidence for relative equivalence
IV: [−0.458; −0.104]	No	Yes	No	No	Inconclusive
V: [−0.057; 0.543]	Yes	No	No	No	Inconclusive
VI: [−0.359; 0.455]	No	No	No	No	Inconclusive

$$\begin{gathered}\boldsymbol{H_{0.1}} : d < -0.3 \text{ (i.e., more negative treatment effect);} \\ \boldsymbol{H_{0.2}} : d > 0.3 \text{ (i.e., more positive treatment effect);} \\ \boldsymbol{H_{0.3}} : d > -0.3 \text{ (i.e., either a less negative or a positive treatment effect);} \\ \boldsymbol{H_{0.4}} : d < 0.3 \text{ (i.e., either a less positive or a negative treatment effect).}\end{gathered}$$

The first two null hypotheses, $\boldsymbol{H_{0.1}}$ and $\boldsymbol{H_{0.2}}$, are also used in *two one-sided tests equivalence testing* (TOST; Lakens, 2017, 2018). Table 3.2 summarises the rationale behind FOST with six examples of 90% CIs of d.

The first two (I and II) represent the two possible scenarios where researchers find sufficient evidence *against* relative (or practical) equivalence, because in none of these two cases the 90% CI has any overlap with the [−0.3; 0.3] interval that represents the interval of relative (or practical) equivalence. To conclude sufficient evidence *in favour* of relative equivalence, we need a situation like in the third scenario (III): the 90% CI lies fully within the [−0.3; 0.3] interval. Therefore, in the other three scenarios (IV, V, and VI), we can conclude *neither* sufficient evidence against *nor* sufficient evidence in favour of relative equivalence. Note that in none of the scenarios we can be 'conclusive' as in absolute evidence; it is just that in three scenarios we have evidence *beyond reasonable doubt* against (scenarios I and II) or in favour of (scenario III) relative equivalence. Comparing Tables 3.1 and 3.2, we learn that in Experiments 1–7 in Table 3.1 we remain inconclusive, and that in Experiment 8 we have a case of sufficient evidence in favour of relative equivalence. The conclusion drawn from Experiments 1–7 is to be expected given the sample sizes in each of these experiments. With a sample size like the one in Experiment 8, we already have somewhat more chance to find sufficient evidence against or in favour of relative equivalence, although even there, chances are not that high. There are plenty of examples in educational research of studies where a statistically non-significant p-value from $\boldsymbol{H_0}$: 'no difference' against $\boldsymbol{H_1}$: 'difference' is interpreted as evidence in favour of $\boldsymbol{H_0}$ while the 90% CI is something like in scenario IV, V or VI in Table 3.2, or where a statistically significant p-value from

$\boldsymbol{H_0}$: 'no difference' against $\boldsymbol{H_1}$: 'difference' is interpreted as evidence against $\boldsymbol{H_0}$ while the 90% CI is still very wide and partly overlaps with the [−0.3; 0.3] interval.

3.2.2 Meta-analysis

In our series of Experiments 1–8, Experiments 3 (p = 0.026), 4 (p = 0.017), and 5 (p = 0.015) yield a statistically significant p-value at α = 0.05 (tested two-sided) testing $\boldsymbol{H_0}$: 'no difference' against $\boldsymbol{H_1}$: 'difference'. Still, across the series of experiments, the picture looks different. To establish sufficient evidence against or in favour of relative equivalence, we will often need series of studies on the same phenomenon, but Statistics is not about drawing bold conclusions based on single studies anyway.

Table 3.3 presents the 90% CI of the standardised mean difference of a meta-analysis based on Experiments 1–8, with *Jamovi*, under different assumptions.

The differences between *homoscedastic* (i.e., equal) and *heteroscedastic* (i.e., unequal) variances are not noticeable on the second decimals, because as indicated in Table 3.1 differences in *SD*s are small. However, the different estimators do give somewhat different outcomes because they are based on somewhat different assumptions.

The *fixed effect* estimator (Hedges & Vevea, 1998) can be used if the goal of the meta-analysis is to estimate the true effect in Experiments 1–8, and there is no interest in generalising beyond this *fixed* set of experiments. In practice, this is rarely the case; rather, as in the separate experiments, the interest usually lies in generalising beyond the individuals and studies at hand. Using the fixed effect estimator when the interest lies in generalising beyond the studies tends to result in too narrow CIs for the effect or phenomenon of interest. The other estimators in Table 3.3 treat Experiments 1–8 as a random sample from a population of possible studies and allow for generalising beyond Experiments 1–8, which is of interest in the current context.

Table 3.3 The 90% CI of the standardised mean difference based on Experiments 1−8 (*Jamovi*)

Model estimator	Population variances	
	Homoscedastic	Heteroscedastic
DerSimonian-Laird	[−0.22; 0.24]	[−0.22; 0.24]
Hedges-Olkin	[−0.25; 0.28]	[−0.25; 0.28]
Hunter-Schmidt	[−0.20; 0.22]	[−0.20; 0.22]
Sidik-Jonkman	[−0.25; 0.28]	[−0.25; 0.28]
Maximum Likelihood (FIML)	[−0.21; 0.23]	[−0.21; 0.23]
Restricted Maximum Likelihood (REML)	[−0.23; 0.26]	[−0.23; 0.26]
Empirical Bayes	[−0.24; 0.27]	[−0.24; 0.27]
Paule-Mandel	[−0.24; 0.27]	[−0.24; 0.27]
Fixed Effect	[−0.13; 0.12]	[−0.13; 0.12]

For a variety of reasons, there may be some *heterogeneity* in the effect of interest from setting to setting (τ^2). In the case of the fixed effects indicator, τ^2 is assumed to be zero, whereas in the other estimates it is not zero and it varies across estimators. The DerSimonian-Laird estimator (DerSimonian & Laird, 1986; George & Aban, 2016; Raudenbush, 2009) tends to perform well when τ^2 is small, while the Hedges-Olkin estimator (Hedges & Olkin, 1985; Raudenbush, 2009) tends to perform well when τ^2 is more substantial. However, both DerSimonian-Laird and Hedges-Olkin are better when the number of studies is larger than what we are dealing with in the current context, and even then, the Hedges-Olkin estimator may overestimate τ^2 when it is small (i.e., the DerSimonian-Laird estimator will probably be better). The Hunter-Schmidt estimator (Hunter & Schmidt, 2004) is a more efficient estimator than the DerSimonian-Laird and Hedges-Olkin estimators but is associated with substantial negative bias (e.g., Viechtbauer, 2005). The Sidik-Jonkman estimator (Sidik & Jonkman, 2005a, 2005b) tends to be substantially biased for small τ^2-values but is less biased for large τ^2-values than the DerSimonian-Laird estimator.

The (Full Informed) Maximum Likelihood (FIML, sometimes also referred to as ML) estimator and Restricted Maximum Likelihood (REML) estimator (Raudenbush, 2009; Viechtbauer, 2005) serve different functions. Whenever the interest lies in obtaining a CI for an effect size of interest, FIML tends to underestimate τ^2 and more so as τ^2 increases, and this is less the case with REML. However, when testing *moderator variables*—variables that change across larger series of experiments and moderate the treatment effect of interest (e.g., the benefit of blended learning over face-to-face or online-only learning depends on whether formative quizzes are part of the learning programme)—FIML is commonly more appropriate than REML, because these moderator effects are usually to be treated as *fixed* rather than as *random* effects (e.g., the difference between presence or absence of quizzes is not a random sample of a universe of possible outcomes to be generalised to). That said, REML is generally less efficient than FIML or Hunter-Schmidt but is—when estimating τ^2—often a reasonable default estimator that is approximately unbiased and relatively efficient (e.g., Viechtbauer, 2005).

The Paule-Mandel estimator (Paule & Mandel, 1982) provides a better estimator of τ^2 than the DerSimonian-Laird estimator, especially for larger τ^2-values, and if the residuals of scores in the experiments included do not deviate much from a Normal distribution the Paule-Mandel estimator tends to provide a CI of the effect size of interest similar to REML and the last estimator not yet discussed: the empirical Bayes estimator (Berkey, Hoaglin, Mosteller, & Colditz, 1995; Morris, 1983). We get back to Bayesian estimation in a bit.

When in doubt about which estimator to choose, it is always an option to provide the outcomes obtained with a series of estimators (e.g., like in Table 3.3) along with the input used for estimation (i.e., Table 3.1) and leave it to the reader to decide which estimator(s) to prefer. In the example context, with regard to our original question of interest, all estimators provide an interval within the [−0.3, 0.3] interval, indicating that it is reasonable to conclude sufficient evidence for relative equivalence. Based on the evidence available (i.e., Experiments 1–8 with meta-analysis), the effect of interest may or may not be exactly zero but is likely in the prespecified region of differences too small to practically matter (i.e., relative or practical equivalence).

3.3 Bigger and Better Data

While dealing with large volumes of data was a challenge and terms like Big Data, Artificial Intelligence (AI), Machine Learning, Educational Data Mining (EDM), and Learning Analytics (LA) appeared quite futuristic concepts decades ago, with advancements in science and technology, things gradually changed. These days, companies are handling and analysing massive datasets, and this practice is also referred to as *Big Data*. Although many different traits have been attributed to Big Data, careful research of Big Data definitions and analysis of ontological characteristics of varieties of datasets appears to reveal that key definitional boundary markers of Big Data are that entire systems or populations (i.e., *exhaustivity*) are captured real-time (i.e., *velocity*), in contrast to 'small data' where samples are captured in fragments (Kitchin & McArdle, 2016). One example from daily life that we are probably all familiar with is *Global Positioning System* (GPS) data (e.g., Hofmann-Wellenhof, Lichtenegger, & Collins, 2012); we can easily find locations, how to get there, and through our mobile devices we can share our current location and movement with others. Another example that many of us are well familiar with comes from Facebook and other social media that provide platforms for the processing of billions of messages and other communication on a daily basis (e.g., Kitchin & McArdle, 2016). This kind of data creates both challenges and opportunities for data analysis and decision making, and provides one or many examples of why so-called quantitative-qualitative 'divides' may be in the interest of some who have made a career as 'quantitative' or 'qualitative' researcher but are not realistic for or in the interest of the practice of science.

3.3.1 The Nonsense of Quantitative-Qualitative Divides

Discourse in some fields of Education is rife of attempts to pretend that qualitative and quantitative research are very different. Statisticians who comment on the methodological setup of a focus group study are laughed away because they are perceived as weird 'quant nerds' who have no clue of qualitative research, even if these statisticians have considerable experience with focus group research from previous workplaces (and should you wonder, yes, I am one of these statisticians who used to receive comments in that direction every time I raised a question about anything 'qualitative' in certain audiences, despite prior experience with focus-group research). Likewise, given the composition of the Editorial Boards and the kind of reviews that authors of submitted manuscripts receive, some journals managed to build and maintain a reputation of being 'too qualitative' or 'too quantitative'. Besides, it is fairly easy these days to find comments on social media like this one from Twitter recently: "*closing the communication gap between clinicians and academics: the hugely different views clinicians & medical educators have on what constitutes 'evidence'. Is it linear causal quantitative research or does it include qualitative complexity research*" (source not mentioned here, should the poster want to remove it at some point).

This comment was made by a scholar who is quite influential in the field of Medical Education and who had been provided with examples and literature by a variety of people—on Twitter and in meetings—demonstrating why this kind of view and all the reasons and so-called 'philosophy' behind it are wrong. Both among clinicians and among medical educators, there is considerable diversity in views on what constitutes evidence. Besides, 'quantitative' neither equates 'linear' nor 'causal', and 'qualitative' does not equate 'complex' either. Similar comments that rightly spiked criticism from others on Twitter included that 'quantitative' research is about causality while 'qualitative' research is not, quantitative research is confirmatory while qualitative research is exploratory, being a 'qualitative' researcher equals being a 'constructivist' while being a 'quantitative' researcher equals being a 'positivist' or 'post-positivist', that 'quantitative' research is free of bias (or: bias is not recognised) and needs software while 'qualitative' research is done 'by hand' and it is okay to 'bring your own bias', that 'qualitative' methods can help us to study 'how' and 'why' questions while 'quantitative' methods cannot, that randomised controlled experiments are useless because they focus on linear relations (and therefore: they can never be meaningful for 'real life'), that replication research is meaningless in Education because there are no single causal linear relations and therefore we need 'qualitative' methods, and that for complex questions we need 'qualitative' not 'quantitative' research. All this is a bit like stating that water is not H_2O but sometimes H_2 and sometimes O.

Causality can be a question to be left in the middle regardless of whether research is 'quantitative' or 'qualitative', and most so-called 'quantitative' research is *not* about causality or at least should not be interpreted as such. Some fields are rife of examples of confirmatory 'qualitative' research and there are tons of exploratory 'quantitative' methods out there as well. Interviews are typically labelled 'qualitative' but can easily yield quantitative data as well. For experiments, many nonlinear methods are available, provided we ask the right questions and design our experiments appropriately. Replication is not all about single causal linear relations; it is about systematic attempts to investigate the generalisability or transferability of findings in different settings, and this may concern differences, correlations, linear or nonlinear patterns, and we may well leave causality in the middle (which in most of our research we should do anyway). Which methods to use ought to depend on our questions, but both 'qualitative' and 'quantitative' methods can help to study complex questions.

No matter how 'qualitative' or 'quantitative', our research is commonly about describing, explaining and/or predicting phenomena of interest. In this endeavour, so-called 'quantitative' differences are nothing more than 'qualitative' differences that have been measured, and seemingly 'qualitative' differences can be conceived as 'quantitative' differences that have been categorised either because we do not have good measures of these differences or because we have collected our data in a particular way. This includes variables like 'attitude', 'meaning', and 'identity', which according to some 'qualitativists' are not measurable while much of the work done by sociologists, psychologists, and neuroscientists indicates otherwise.

Another common quantitative-qualitative divide already referred to partially is found in the false dichotomy that replication only matters in quantitative research. Replication is often associated with the idea of two or more studies coming up with the same finding, but replication is about redoing a *study*. What we need for that is a careful description of exactly what we have done; without that description, replication research becomes impossible. Replication research is important because the aim of our research is usually to establish evidence for what works under what conditions beyond the random setting studied. Educational research papers do not focus on what works in Programme A at University X but can be used by other researchers in their settings as well. While non-replicable research has its use for exploration and idea generation, no matter how 'qualitative' or 'quantitative' our research, if we really want to understand the usefulness of theoretical concepts and statements, we need to be able to replicate the studies that are supposed to provide support for these concepts and statements.

3.3.2 Artificial Intelligence and Machine Learning

Regardless of what 'qualitative' or 'quantitative' instruments we use, the very process of collecting and processing data can be conceived as a form of measurement. In the Big Data era, the nature of that measurement has been changing, and AI machines have started to make decisions that in former times were only made by humans, by feeding these machines large amounts of data from which they can learn patterns that are needed to solve specific tasks (e.g., self-driving cars). Statisticians are interested in how AI can help to effectively train complex models with ever-increasing volumes of data, neuroscientists are interested in how AI can help to design operational models of the brain, and computer scientists focus on how to improve these AI systems. In these and other questions, Machine Learning is a subset of AI; the latter is about helping machines make decisions that have traditionally been made by humans, while Machine Learning is about using statistical methods to enable machines to improve that process with increasing experience (i.e., more data coming in). In other words, although Machine Learning is not the same as AI, it is *the basis* of AI (e.g., Samuel, 1959; Tiffin & Paton, 2018).

With some methods, such as *linear regression* (e.g., Howell, 2017) and *logistic regression* (e.g., Agresti, 2002), full information about outcome variables of interest is available, while with other methods, such as *principal component analysis* or *exploratory factor analysis* (e.g., Field, 2018), no such information is available; this distinction is also referred to as *supervised* (full information available) versus *unsupervised* (no information available) learning, and methods where partial information about the outcome variables of interest is available are called *semi-supervised* learning methods (e.g., Tiffin & Paton, 2018).

A subfield of Machine Learning, which is inspired by the functionality of human brain neurons and gave rise to the concept of *artificial neural network*, is called *deep learning* (e.g., LeCun, Bengio, & Hinton, 2015). This form of learning is used a lot with large volumes of text, pictures, and videos. For example, a square is a figure that has four equally large sides that are connected with each other as two sets of parallel lines that are perpendicular to each other. Once we understand these simple concepts (i.e., simple tasks) and how they can help us to recognise a square (i.e., a slightly more complex task), we can start to distinguish squares from shapes that do not meet all the criteria for being called a square. As in human learning, this process can be repeated at ever-increasing levels of complexity. For example, we may feed machines large series of x-rays of human lungs to help machines learn to detect the presence of different pathologies. These pictures go through an *input layer*, are then processed through one or more *hidden layers* in which 'neurons' in the artificial neural network are activated, to then reach an *output layer* where predicted outcomes are provided. In the meta-analytic example earlier on in this chapter, if instead of being divided over eight experiments we had a single experiment with $N = 714$ students, Fig. 3.1 could be the resulting artificial neural network.

In this network, the input layer (*left*) includes the two treatment conditions and a 'Bias' element created by the machine, there is a single hidden layer with elements H(1:1), H(1:2), and 'Bias', and the output layer is the score. As we do have full information on the outcome variable of interest (i.e., score), this is a form of supervised learning. Most software programmes, including SPSS which we are using for this example, enable to save the predicted scores. Doing so for this example, we find that Pearson's r between the predicted scores and observed scores

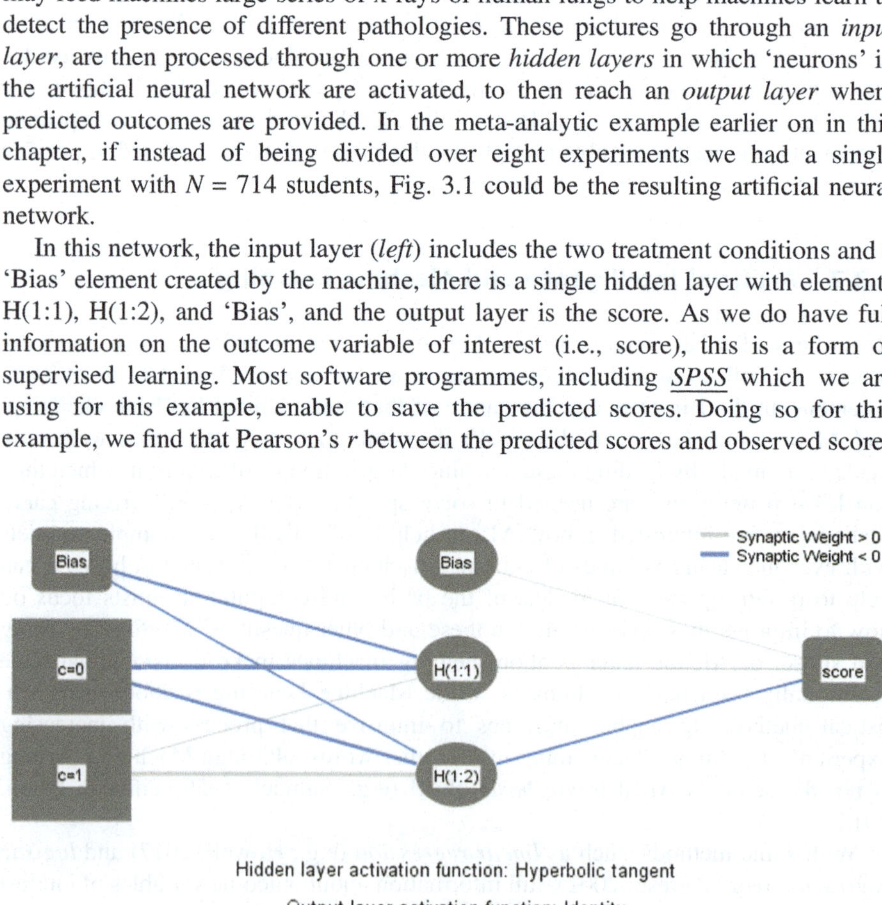

Fig. 3.1 Artificial neural network of the effect of instructional support (treatment: $c = 0$ is control, $c = 1$ is treatment) on learning outcomes (score) (perceptron network in SPSS)

equals $r = 0.002$, which is the same as Pearson's r for the correlation between condition (i.e., treatment vs. control) and observed scores, and for the correlation between condition and network-predicted scores we find: $r = 1$. Thus, we have basically found a complex 'black box' way to estimate a treatment effect which yields the same outcome as a simple linear correlation or standardised regression coefficient.

The term 'black box' is used because contrary to the aforementioned methods used in Machine Learning—linear regression, logistic regression, and principal component analysis—we do not really understand what algorithms are used by the machine to learn from the data. The machine does pick up signals we put in and estimates their importance, but we do not really know what neurons are activated for what reason and what the different elements in the network that we did not put in ourselves (here: Bias and the two H-elements) actually mean. This is why for the volumes of data that educational researchers and practitioners commonly (still) work with, common Machine Learning methods like the regression and component analysis methods just mentioned and other statistical methods where we fully understand the algorithms remain to be preferred. However, for much larger amounts of data, these common methods may become increasingly hard to use and deep learning methods appear to perform well. In the context of x-rays, for example, recent work suggests that deep learning approaches have been able to achieve expert-level performance in medical image interpretation tasks (Rajpurkar et al., 2018). For 'qualitativists' who claim that 'qualitative' is to be done 'by hand' (e.g., thematic coding with sticky notes) instead of with software or machines: a recent article in *Nature* presents an example of how artificial neural networks could have learned *unsupervised*—that is: without any human labelling or supervision—and without any form of prior knowledge otherwise, from abstracts from research published at different points in the past to classify materials as 'thermoelectric' years before that was actually discovered by humans (Tshitoyan et al., 2019). Examples like these are why deep learning is increasingly considered the 'next generation' Machine Learning.

3.3.3 Cross-Validation

An important component of Machine Learning, which has been used in statistical approaches for decades, and works well in the case of sufficiently large samples, is *cross-validation* (Geisser, 1975; Kurtz, 1948; Mosier, 1951; Osborne, 2010; Stone, 1974; Yu, 2010). In studies where the sample size is in the 100 s or larger, cross-validation can help to reduce the risk of *overfitting* (i.e., ending up with more complex models than needed; Osborne, 2010). In its most basic form, we randomly divide our total sample (N) into a *training* sample and a *testing* or *evaluation* sample. A common rule of thumb for this division is 70% of N for the training sample and the remaining 30% for the evaluation sample, although in larger samples the training sample can take up a higher percentage (e.g., up to 80%) while in smaller samples the training sample may include only about 65% of the total sample. The training sample is used to determine the best model, and the testing sample is then used to test that model.

The basic idea behind cross-validation is that if a phenomenon of interest as demonstrated in one sufficiently large random sample actually exists in the population sampled from, it should be found in other sufficiently large samples as well. In small samples, however, this concept does not really work because of increasing sample-to-sample fluctuation of findings with increasingly smaller sample size. Let us look at an example to illustrate this. Suppose, we have a random sample of size N in which two variables X and Y are more or less symmetrically and unimodally distributed with $M = 0$ and $SD = 1$, and their correlation is about 0, in three scenarios. In Scenario A, we randomly divide $N = 40$ into a training set of $n_{\text{TRAIN}} = 20$ and a testing set of $n_{\text{TEST}} = 20$. In Scenario B, we randomly divide $N = 1000$ into a training set of $n_{\text{TRAIN}} = 500$ and a testing set of $n_{\text{TEST}} = 500$. Finally, in Scenario C, we randomly divide $N = 360$ into a training set of $n_{\text{TRAIN}} = 240$ and a testing set of $n_{\text{TEST}} = 120$. Table 3.4 presents Cohen's d for the difference between the training and testing sample in X and Y for twenty trials in each scenario; values closer to 0 are better.

Table 3.4 Cohen's *d* for *X* and *Y* for twenty trials in each scenario (*JASP*)

	Scenario A: $N = 40$		Scenario B: $N = 1000$		Scenario C: $N = 360$	
Trial	$d\,X$	$d\,Y$	$d\,X$	$d\,Y$	$d\,X$	$d\,Y$
1	−0.394	−0.281	0.034	0.020	−0.037	−0.040
2	0.670	0.512	0.083	0.046	0.025	0.192
3	−0.059	0.125	0.017	0.037	0.060	0.204
4	0.242	−0.298	0.092	0.006	−0.161	−0.018
5	−0.438	−0.122	0.027	−0.107	−0.082	−0.050
6	0.330	0.511	−0.008	−0.124	0.068	0.077
7	0.225	−0.290	0.025	−0.026	0.095	−0.255
8	−0.540	0.177	0.022	−0.029	−0.214	−0.206
9	0.186	−0.423	−0.061	−0.033	0.196	0.071
10	0.214	−0.174	0.015	0.026	0.007	0.163
11	−0.309	0.590	0.020	0.042	−0.132	−0.038
12	−0.368	−0.187	0.063	−0.015	−0.172	0.039
13	−0.542	0.037	0.020	−0.091	0.030	−0.096
14	0.015	0.445	−0.004	0.024	−0.153	−0.111
15	−0.205	0.046	−0.025	−0.024	0.090	0.039
16	0.232	−1.082	0.060	0.046	−0.041	0.193
17	−0.017	−0.293	0.001	0.010	0.091	−0.038
18	−0.540	−0.250	−0.055	0.002	−0.114	−0.047
19	0.112	0.362	0.042	0.032	0.179	0.065
20	−0.066	0.530	−0.002	0.029	0.118	−0.006

In line with the concept of *SE* discussed earlier, Scenario A is characterised by considerable sample-to-sample variation in *d*, meaning considerable differences in estimated *M* from μ. If we reported *M* and *SD* instead of *d*, we would see considerable fluctuation from sample to sample in *SD* as well. In Scenario B, nearly all *d*-values are in the [−0.1; 0.1] range, indicating small to very small differences. Although, as to be expected in line with the concept of *SE*, Scenario C finds itself somewhere in between Scenario A and Scenario B in terms of sample-to-sample fluctuation, the vast majority of *d*-values are still in the [−0.2; 0.2] range, indicating small differences.

Table 3.5 presents Pearson's *r* for the correlation between *X* and *Y* in the training and testing sample for twenty trials in each scenario; values closer to 0 are better.

Again, we see considerable fluctuation in Scenario A, little fluctuation in Scenario B, and in most cases also little fluctuation in Scenario C.

Table 3.5 Pearson's *r* for *X*-*Y* correlation in the training and testing sample for twenty trials in each scenario (*JASP*)

Trial	Scenario A: $N = 40$		Scenario B: $N = 1000$		Scenario C: $N = 360$	
	r X-*Y* train	*r X*-*Y* test	*r X*-*Y* train	*r X*-*Y* test	*r X*-*Y* train	*r X*-*Y* test
1	0.191	−0.159	−0.001	0.001	0.068	−0.032
2	0.188	−0.351	0.006	−0.008	−0.108	0.064
3	−0.153	0.270	0.025	−0.025	−0.113	0.049
4	0.153	−0.154	−0.019	0.020	−0.083	0.035
5	−0.154	0.118	0.059	−0.054	0.025	−0.011
6	−0.091	0.031	0.028	−0.028	−0.060	0.033
7	−0.178	0.167	0.025	−0.023	−0.041	0.033
8	−0.233	0.240	0.000	0.001	−0.060	0.011
9	0.174	−0.194	−0.007	0.006	0.153	−0.072
10	−0.041	0.041	−0.040	0.038	0.073	−0.029
11	0.059	0.035	0.035	−0.031	−0.048	0.024
12	0.010	−0.046	0.065	−0.067	−0.093	0.054
13	−0.203	0.242	−0.037	0.042	−0.001	0.003
14	0.007	−0.013	0.016	−0.014	0.041	−0.027
15	−0.059	0.054	0.026	−0.025	0.037	−0.017
16	0.278	−0.098	−0.052	0.055	−0.071	0.039
17	−0.049	0.051	−0.014	0.013	0.037	−0.011
18	−0.103	0.017	0.007	−0.006	−0.017	0.007
19	−0.079	0.045	−0.040	0.041	0.127	−0.061
20	0.156	−0.159	0.046	−0.049	0.070	−0.033

3.3.4 Educational Data Mining and Learning Analytics

The process of discovering patterns in large data sets using database systems, statistics, and Machine Learning is also known as *data mining* (Alani, Tawfik, Saeed, & Anya, 2018) or, in the context of education, EDM (Aldowah, Al-Samarraie, & Fauzy, 2019; Baker, 2019; Bakhshinategh, Zaiane, ElAtia, & Ipperciel, 2018; Bogarín, Cerezo, & Romero, 2018; Hussain, Dahan, Ba-Alwib, & Ribata, 2018; Rodrigues, Isotani, & Zárate, 2018; Santos, Menezes, De Carvalho, & Montesco, 2019). Besides, an emerging subfield of EDM, which focusses on logs, audit trails, log files or processes alike, is also called *process mining* (Bogarín et al., 2018). Big Data in educational context is sometimes also referred to as *Big Educational Data* (e.g., Aldowah et al., 2019), and EDM is about discovering patterns even where theory is absent (i.e., data-driven), in order to evaluate educational and training programmes and to improve educational and learning processes. EDM and LA have somewhat different origins. In the words of Ray and Saeed (2018, p. 137), "*LA has an origin in Semantic Web, intelligent curriculum, and systematic interventions, while EDM has origin in educational software, student modeling, and predicting course outcomes*" and therefore classification, clustering, and prediction methods are very important in EDM (e.g., Hussain et al., 2018; Santos et al., 2019) whereas LA is often perceived to be of a more descriptive nature, which is not to say that classification, clustering, and prediction methods have no importance in LA. Or, as others put it, EDM is more oriented towards processing large amounts of data, while LA is more about the relationship between the learner and the learning environment and how the learner can function better in or make better use of that environment (e.g., Viberg, Hatakka, Bälter, & Mavroudi, 2018; Vieira, Parsons, & Byrd, 2018). Nevertheless, EDM and LA have a lot of common ground in terms of objectives and goals, such as modelling student behaviour, predicting performance, increasing reflection and (self-)awareness, predicting dropout, facilitating and improving assessment and feedback, facilitating social interactions in learning environments, understanding students' mood, and recommending resources (e.g., Aldowah et al., 2019; Ray & Saeed, 2018; Schumacher & Ifenthaler, 2018; Vieira et al., 2018). In short, the overall purpose of both LA and EDM is to understand how students learn (Viberg et al., 2018), and the methods used in EDM can support LA.

3.4 Missing Data

An important topic that many researchers do not really know how to deal with is *missing data*. Missing data is a problem, because it comes with a loss of information and a loss of statistical power and precision with it, can create complications in data management and analysis, and can increase the risk of biased estimation and testing outcomes (Barnard & Meng, 1999; Cole, 2010). How to best deal with missing data depends on a number of factors, including on the variable of interest being measured once or repeatedly (e.g., De Rooij, 2018), variables where missing occurs being outcome variables or predictor variables (covariates; Horowitz & Manski, 2000; Janssen et al., 2010; White & Carlin, 2010), and the type of missingness: *missing completely at random* (MCAR), *missing at random* (MAR), or *missing not at random* (MNAR) (Rubin, 1976).

3.4.1 Types of Missingness

Under MCAR, the missingness is completely *unsystematic*, for example due to random issues in a server in online research (Abraham & Russell, 2004); the subsample of participants with *complete data* is a random sample of all participants in the experiment (e.g., Cole, 2010), and in complete data the subsample and full sample should not differ significantly (e.g., Little, 1988). In the case of MAR, the probability of missingness on variable Y is related to one or more other observed variables in the dataset but not to the value of Y itself (e.g., Acock, 2005) or—in research that involves repeated measurements—it depends on the *previous response* (MAR1) or on the *previous two responses* (MAR2) (De Rooij, 2018; Rubin, 1976). An example of MAR can be found in some participants not being able to respond to all items of a questionnaire due to a lack of time. While Little's MCAR test (Little, 1988) provides researchers with a tool to test $\boldsymbol{H_0}$: 'MCAR' against $\boldsymbol{H_1}$: 'not MCAR', there is no formal MAR test, because there is no way to verify that the probability of missing data on Y is related only to observed variables and not to unobserved variables as well (Leppink, 2019). Some of the observed variables that may correlate with the occurrence of missingness of Y may be used as explanatory or *auxiliary variables* (i.e., variables that are correlated with the variable that needs imputation or with the probability of missing response on that variable; Collins, Schafer, & Kam, 2001) to estimate correlates of missingness to decide on how to deal with the missing data.

While there is no formal MAR test, treating MAR data as MCAR or vice versa often has minor effects on estimation and testing outcomes (Cole, 2010; Collins et al., 2001) and, contrary to MNAR, there is no need to model the mechanism of missingness: MCAR and MAR data are *ignorable* (Cole, 2010). In MNAR, we need to model the mechanism of missingness, because the probability of missingness on Y depends on the actual value of the non-responding participant(s) on Y, even after controlling for other observed variables. For this kind of *nonignorable* missing data (Cole, 2010), we need sophisticated methods to model the missingness mechanism (e.g., De Rooij, 2018; Molenberghs & Verbeke, 2005). In well-controlled and carefully managed experiments, MCAR and MAR are generally more likely than MNAR (Leppink, 2019), but in less controlled studies MNAR may more often than not be the most likely candidate.

3.4.2 Missing Data Methods

Commonly encountered fairly simple methods for imputing missing data have been *mean imputation* (i.e., imputing missing values with the mean of Y from complete data on Y or, in a two-way variant, it is a function of both the mean of Y and the mean of the participant's scores on observed variables; Van Ginkel, Sijtsma, Van der Ark, & Vermunt, 2010), *listwise* or casewise deletion (i.e., all participants with any missing data are removed from the analysis, even if they have complete data on some variables; Abraham & Russell, 2004; Acock, 2005; Cole, 2010), *pairwise* or available-case analysis (i.e., missingness on X but complete data on Y and Z results in dropping that participant for X-Y and X-Z but not for Y-Z relations; Cole, 2010), and—in studies with repeated measurements—*last observation carried forward* (i.e., imputing a missing value on Y at time point t with the observed value on Y at time point 't minus 1'; Peto et al., 1977). Although simple in use, these approaches have their problems unless we have a study with only a few percent of missingness of the MCAR type. Mean imputation comes at the cost of underestimated *SD*s and biased estimation and testing outcomes (Eekhout et al., 2014; Haitovsky, 1968). Listwise deletion comes at the cost of unnecessary loss of statistical power and precision even under MCAR, unless we are dealing with small percentages of missing in large samples (Cole, 2010; Leppink, 2019), and under MAR and MNAR it tends to result in biased estimation and testing outcomes (Enders, 2010). Pairwise deletion suffers from both loss in statistical power and inconsistency in *SE*s and other statistics across comparisons (e.g., Little & Rubin, 2002; Schafer & Graham, 2002) and, like listwise deletion, it tends to come with biased estimation and testing outcomes under MAR and MNAR (Baraldi & Enders, 2010). Finally, carrying the last observation forward only makes sense in studies with repeated measurements where change does not occur frequently or where changes are generally small (Leppink, 2019), which is unrealistic in many cases (Wood, White, & Thompson, 2004) and therefore can normally be expected to result in underestimated *SD*s and biased estimation and testing outcomes with it.

Two slightly more robust approaches to missing data imputation are *matching* or *hot-deck imputation* (i.e., non-responding participants are matched to similar participants to obtain imputations; Fox-Wasylyshyn & El-Masri, 2005; Little & Rubin, 2002; Roth, 1994) and *regression imputation* (i.e., using regression models to predict imputations for missing data; Allison, 2002; Cole, 2010). However, risks of underestimated *SE*s remain in both matching (Roth, 1994) and regression imputation (Enders, 2010). An approach that attempts to resolve this and other problems of the missing data methods discussed thus far is found in *multiple imputation* (MI; Azur, Stuart, Frangakis, & Leaf, 2011; Horton & Lipsitz, 2001; Luo, Szolovits, Dighe, & Baron, 2017; Rubin, 1987; Schafer, 1997; Van Buuren, 2012; Van Buuren & Groothuis-Oudshoorn, 2011). In this three-stage process, different versions of the dataset (e.g., 5–10) are created in which the imputed values differ according to an iterative regression approach (*imputation stage*), which are then analysed with statistical methods we would normally use (*analysis stage*) and pooled to parameter estimates and *SE*s to obtain outcomes that respect the distributions of all variables involved (*pooling stage*). This can be expected to produce unbiased estimates under MAR and MCAR (e.g., Eekhout et al., 2014), and in the case of MNAR, like in the matching and the regression approach, the robustness of estimates can be studied with auxiliary variables (Collins et al., 2001). With the advent of Machine Learning, we will likely see new developments in missing data handling in near future, especially building forth on the regression imputation and MI approach.

While in missing data methods discussed thus far some form of imputation takes place, in the FIML approach there is no imputation at all; instead, all information is used without pairwise deletion. FIML is a common and often recommendable approach to missing data in multilevel analysis, factor analysis, and structural equation and latent growth modelling (Leppink, 2019). Evidence with regard to which of MI and FIML performs better is somewhat mixed. Although some studies provide some evidence in favour of MI (e.g., Graham & Schafer, 1999; Schafer & Graham, 2002), others recommend to have at least ten times as many participants as variables for MI (e.g., Cole, 2010), and recent work suggests that both MI and FIML may result in biased outcomes in small samples (Yuan, Yang-Wallentin, & Bentler, 2012) but MI more so (Hayes & McArdle, 2017).

3.4.3 A Pragmatic Approach for Missing Data Handling

Apart from the type of missingness, how to best deal with missing data depends on whether the missingness occurs on predictor variables or outcome variables and whether the variables where missing occurs are measured once or repeatedly (Leppink, 2019). Generally speaking, not imputing missingness is less of a concern with outcome variables than with predictor variables, because it is the latter that creates inconsistencies (e.g., in *SE*s) in model comparison. Therefore, missingness in predictor variables is probably better approached with MI than with FIML, or—when missingness is MCAR and only a small percentage (e.g., 5%, preferably not more than 10%) of missingness—listwise deletion can be used. With missingness in the outcome variable, FIML should be fine under MAR and MCAR, although under MNAR we will probably be better off with MI. Where missingness occurs in multi-item questionnaires, MI can be done at item level (i.e., imputing item scores) unless the majority of items in a scale have missing data; in the latter, it is probably better to apply MI on the scale score. Both MI (under MCAR, MAR, and MNAR) and FIML (under MCAR and MAR) may provide decent solutions with levels of missingness of say 20% or 30%, especially when samples are large, but when missingness exceeds 50% things do become more difficult and one may wonder if analysing the data any further at all is meaningful, unless we have repeated measurements. In the latter case, larger proportions of missing data are not only more likely—especially in less tightly controlled studies—but can also be dealt with more easily, since trajectories of previous observations often do have some predictive power for current and in some cases near-future observations. That said, if we reach a point where over 80% of participants have missing data on the same variables at several occasions, and the effective sample size due to missingness becomes too small to reasonably deal with missing data, we may want to refrain from drawing any conclusions from the data altogether. Luckily, such levels of missingness do not occur in many settings.

3.5 Testing and Estimation

For statistical testing and estimation, and decisions such as which of a series of competing models is to be preferred, there are many options to choose from depending on the features of our variables of interest and whether we treat effects as fixed or random. Although in many statistical textbooks written for students and researchers in Education and Psychology either only one option is presented or two options are presented as if they were very different and are not really compatible, there are ways to combine different options into a multi-method approach for a more informed decision making. For examples and practical applications in the context of experimental research in Education and Psychology, see Leppink (2019). The remainder of this chapter provides a helicopter view of options and how to combine them in different settings, experimental and other, where the interest lies in human learning.

Suppose, we are in a study where a total of $N = 750$ first-year bachelor students are asked to self-rate six items on a visual analogue scale (VAS) with 0 (neutral) as midpoint and −4 (completely disagree) to +4 (completely agree). We have evidence from previous research on this instrument that the six items can be grouped together in two sets of three items, which for the sake of simplicity we call X_1–X_3 and Y_1–Y_3, are in our sample all distributed around $M = 0$ with $SD = 1$ and with skewness and kurtosis values all in the [−0.4; 0.4] range, with no outliers or other severe departures from Normality. Table 3.6 presents Pearson's r for each pair of variables.

This correlation pattern is well in line with what we would expect whenever there are two sets of items that can be grouped together: substantial correlations within set (i.e., among X_1–X_3 and among Y_1–Y_3) but clearly weaker correlations between items from different sets (i.e., between any X item with any Y item). Now,

Table 3.6 Bivariate correlation per item pair (*Jamovi*)

	X_1	X_2	X_3	Y_1	Y_2	Y_3
X_1						
X_2	0.731					
X_3	0.609	0.802				
Y_1	0.020	−0.004	0.002			
Y_2	0.022	0.018	0.015	0.731		
Y_3	−0.017	−0.028	−0.032	0.598	0.827	

there are several possible ways how to proceed depending on strong the evidence from previous research is.

On the one hand, if there was no previous research on the interrelations between items in settings similar to the one in the study at hand, we could do an *exploratory factor analysis* (e.g., Osborne, Costello, & Kellow, 2010) on the full dataset of $N = 750$ students. On the other hand, if previous research provided a lot of evidence on the structure, we might as well do a *confirmatory factor analysis* (e.g., Hoyle, 2000) on the full dataset of $N = 750$ students. However, these relative 'extremes' are not the only options we have. One possible middle-way option is found in *exploratory structural equation modelling* (ESEM; e.g., Marsh, Morin, Parker, et al., 2014): this method combines features of exploratory and confirmatory factor analysis, for instance by specifying a predetermined number of factors (i.e., as in confirmatory factor analysis) but allowing loadings of items to be estimated for more than one factor (i.e., cross-loadings, which are estimated by default in exploratory factor analysis but are normally fixed to 0 in confirmatory factor analysis). This may help to reduce a tendency towards *over-dimensionalisation* (i.e., distinguishing more factors than should be distinguished), which is especially a risk with categorical rating scale data and above all in exploratory factor analysis (Van der Eijk & Rose, 2015). Another option is to use exploratory factor analysis on a *training* sample and confirmatory factor analysis on a *testing* sample (cf. cross-validation and Machine Learning; Mulaik, 1987; Yu, 2010) or, in line with the recent developments around ESEM, to use ESEM on a training sample and confirmatory factor analysis on a testing sample. In the study at hand, if for example previous studies are consistent in their evidence of two factors but provide inconsistent outcomes with regard to which items can be grouped together, ESEM could be done on the training sample with two factors. Another option could be that some previous studies indicate a preference towards a one-factor solution whereas other studies indicate a preference towards a two-factor solution. In that case, the training sample could be used to compare one-factor and two-factor solutions, and the best model would then be used for the testing sample. Let us apply this final option to the study at hand.

We randomly divide the total sample ($N = 750$) into a training sample ($n_{\mathrm{TRAIN}} = 500$) and a testing sample ($n_{\mathrm{TEST}} = 250$) and run two models: (1) a confirmatory one-factor model, in which all six items are grouped together as indicators of a single factor or latent variable; and (2) a confirmatory two-factor model, in which items X_1–X_3 are indicators of one factor and Y_1–Y_3 are indicators of another factor. In the second model, the factors are allowed to correlate. These models can be run with a variety of software packages, including *Jamovi*, *JASP*, *Stata*, and *Mplus*.

3.5.1 Testing Criteria

Table 3.7 presents outcomes for model comparison: the *deviance* (−2 * log Likelihood, −2LL; Wilks, 1938), *Akaike's information criterion* (AIC; Akaike, 1973,

1992), *Schwarz' Bayesian information criterion* (BIC; Schwarz, 1978), and the *sample-size adjusted BIC* (SABIC; Enders & Tofighi, 2008; Tofighi & Enders, 2007).

For two models that have all features in common except for one feature or a set of features that is present in one model (i.e., the more complex model) but not in the other model (i.e., the simpler model, which is nested within or a special case of the more complex model), the difference in *deviance* (i.e., the difference in -2LL) between the two models converges to a χ^2-distribution as the sample size goes to infinity, if $\boldsymbol{H_0}$ is true. $\boldsymbol{H_0}$ is rejected if that difference in −2LL exceeds the critical χ^2-value at $\alpha = 0.05$ for df = the difference in number of parameters between the two models. The simpler model *always* has a −2LL at least as large as and virtually always larger than the more complex model. However, the χ^2-test, which is also referred to as Likelihood Ratio (LR) test (for the philosophy behind Likelihood and LR, see: Hacking, 1965; Leppink, 2019; Royall, 1997, 2004), is about the question whether in the population sampled from these extra parameters are different from zero; if so, that should, in a sufficiently large sample, result in a statistically significant drop in −2LL when accounting for these parameters through the more complex model. For the comparison at hand, the difference between models is only *one* parameter: the *correlation* between the two latent variables. The number of parameters used for item loadings is the same for the two models: 6 loadings on a single factor in the (simple) one-factor model, and 2 sets of 3 loadings in the (more complex) two-factor model. Thus, the difference in −2LL is to be tested with a χ^2-distribution of $df = 1$ (i.e., χ^2_1, which is a squared z-distribution). The critical χ^2-value at $\alpha = 0.05$ for $df = 1$ is 3.84; the difference in −2LL exceeds that critical value, and thus $\boldsymbol{H_0}$ is rejected.

Although the aforementioned χ^2-test (i.e., LR test) can be used with nested models like the ones just compared, it cannot be used in a straightforward manner for non-nested models, for instance two-factor models that differ in which items load on which of the two factors. However, it *can* be used in another comparison where item loadings are the same: a two-factor model as presented in Table 3.7 versus a two-factor model in which the correlation between factors is fixed to 0. We cannot use the LR test to compare the one-factor model with a two-factor model in which the correlation between factors is fixed to 0, because the difference in numbers of parameters used is 0 and there is no such a thing as a χ^2-distribution with $df = 0$. Yet, for the two variants of the two-factor model, the one in which the correlation between factors is fixed to 0 counts as a nested (i.e., simpler) version of the two-factor model in Table 3.7, with $df = 1$ (i.e., the correlation is either fixed to

Table 3.7 Model comparison outcomes in the training sample (*Mplus*)

	One factor	Two factors: X_1–X_3, Y_1–Y_3
−2LL	7617.101	6698.778
AIC	7653.101	6736.778
BIC	7728.964	6816.856
SABIC	7671.831	6756.549

0 or estimated). For this simpler two-factor model, we find: −2LL = 6700.259; AIC = 6736.259; BIC = 6812.122; and SABIC = 6754.989. For the difference between the two variants of the two-factor model, the LR test yields: $\chi_1^2 = 1.481$, $p = 0.224$. This is not statistically significant at the $\alpha = 0.05$ level, so we have insufficient evidence to reject H_0: 'factors are uncorrelated'. Note that a statistically non-significant p-value is *not* the same as evidence in favour of 'no correlation': p is the probability of the observed χ_1^2-value or more extreme, under the condition that H_0 is true, so p itself cannot be interpreted as evidence for H_0, which is its very condition in the first place.

For fixed effects like differences in M, correlations, and item-factor loadings, the LR test can be used whenever two models under comparison are nested, and the other three criteria can be used regardless of whether the two models under comparison are nested (see Leppink, 2019 for a variety of examples of model selection in experimental studies). For each of AIC, BIC, and SABIC, the model with the lowest value is to be preferred. AIC, BIC, and SABIC are functions of −2LL but differ in the penalty they apply for more parameters being added and are therefore positioned somewhat differently on the simple-complex model preference dimension. Of the four criteria discussed, AIC is most easily 'convinced' of a more complex model; it may indicate a preference for adding a parameter where the LR test yields a p-value somewhere in the [0.05; 0.11] range (e.g., Forster, 2000; Leppink, 2019), and that tendency is especially noticeable in small samples (Claeskens & Hjort, 2008; Giraud, 2015; McQuarrie & Tsai, 1998). For smaller samples, adaptations of the AIC such as the corrected AIC (AICc) provide more realistic model comparison outcomes (Burnham & Anderson, 2002, 2004; Cavanaugh, 1997; Hurvich & Tsai, 1989).

The criterion that is most difficult to convince is BIC; it may prefer a simpler model even though the LR test yields a p-value somewhere in the [0.001; 0.05] range. SABIC is positioned somewhere in between AIC and BIC, because it applies a stricter penalty for added parameters than AIC but not as strict as BIC. In the example at hand, AIC, BIC, and SABIC all prefer the *no correlation* two-factor model over the other models. Although none of this ought to be interpreted in terms of absolute evidence, all criteria indicate a preference for the *no correlation* two-factor model over the model in which the two factors are correlated. This model can then be used to obtain model fit criteria with the test sample (e.g., Hoyle, 2000).

It has been known for a while that differences in AIC, BIC, and criteria alike can be used to compute ratios that behave like Bayes factors (BFs), but under different prior distributions (Burnham & Anderson, 2002, 2004; Leppink, 2019). The term *prior distribution* is a Bayesian concept: it is the probability of a population parameter of interest *before* seeing the data from Study S. With that data coming in, we obtain a *posterior distribution* (i.e., the probability distribution of the same parameter of interest but *after* seeing the data from Study S) which may serve as a prior distribution for next studies. This is just like life: our prior beliefs are updated as new data come in; as a metaphor, life itself could be viewed as a high-dimensional posterior distribution that is continuously updated with all kinds of internal and external stimuli.

A prior distribution commonly used in for example Bayesian *t*-tests (i.e., Jeffrey-Zellner-Siow, JZS; Rouder, Speckman, Sun, Morey, & Iverson, 2012) is something in between the 'AIC prior' and the 'BIC prior', meaning that the AIC prior most easily results in a Bayes factor in favour of more complexity (e.g., $\boldsymbol{H_1}$ preferred over $\boldsymbol{H_0}$, hence $BF_{10} > 1$ and BF_{01} [=1 / BF_{10}] < 1) while the BIC prior most easily results in a Bayes factor in favour of less complexity (e.g., $\boldsymbol{H_0}$ preferred over $\boldsymbol{H_1}$, hence $BF_{10} < 1$ and $BF_{01} > 1$).

Advantages of the information-criteria-and-Bayes-factors approach over the traditional *null hypothesis significance testing* (NHST) approach are that (1) direct comparison of non-nested models is enabled and fairly easy to do, (2) larger numbers of models can be tested simultaneously (e.g., no series of *p*-values from one model to the next), and (3) contrary to *p*-values differences in AIC, BIC, SABIC, and criteria alike for competing models can actually provide evidence in favour of a simpler model (e.g., $\boldsymbol{H_0}$) relative to a more complex model (e.g., $\boldsymbol{H_1}$). That said, when the interest lies not in whether a given parameter is 0 or not zero but rather in the concept of *relative* or *practical equivalence* discussed earlier in this chapter, we need CIs or their Bayesian equivalents called *credible intervals* (CRIs) and also known as *posterior intervals* (e.g., Kruschke, 2014; Kruschke & Liddell, 2017). Besides, AIC, BIC, BF, and related criteria are mainly useful when dealing with sufficiently large samples; in small samples, these criteria tend to behave oddly.

3.5.2 Estimation Methods

We might agree that correlations in the [−0.15; 0.15] (i.e., proportion of variance explained in the 0–2.25% range) are too small to really matter. The 90% CI of *r* for the correlation between the two factors is [−0.019; 0.128] for the training sample and [−0.153; 0.061] for the testing sample. These intervals are not much different, and while for testing purposes splitting the total sample into a training and testing sample can help to reduce the risk of overfitting, for interval estimation we can use the full sample, which yields a 90% CI of [−0.040; 0.082].

Given its fixed [−1; 1] range of possible values, the default prior distribution for correlation coefficients is a Uniform prior distribution: prior to seeing the data, all *r*-values within the [−1; 1] range are equally likely. With this prior, the Bayesian 90% CRI of *r* for the correlation between the two factors in our study is about the same as the 90% CI, and the Bayesian 95% CRI is about the same as the 95% CI. For differences in *M*s, such as treatment effects in experiments and quasi-experiments, the default prior is usually a Cauchy distribution (e.g., Rouder et al., 2012), which is effectively a distribution like the Normal distribution but wider (i.e., less peaked and with thicker, longer tails); with such priors, the C% CRI tends to be slightly narrower and slightly more pulled towards 0 than the C% CI, although that difference between CI and CRI tends to be small in larger samples and converges to 0 as the sample size goes to infinity. Similar to TOST, the Bayesian *region of practical equivalence* (ROPE) can be used to determine if we have sufficient evidence for practical equivalence: if the 95% CRI is fully within the ROPE (e.g., [−0.3; 0.3] in the case of *d* and [−0.15; 0.15] in the case of *r*), we have sufficient evidence in favour of practical equivalence. Note that, contrary to TOST, ROPE uses the 95% interval, which in the case of Cauchy priors in terms of width usually lies somewhere in between the 90% CI and the 95% CI. In FOST, the 95% CI can be used when slightly more stringent testing is needed, such as in specific multiple-testing situations (Leppink, 2019); otherwise, the 90% CI is more logical given $\alpha = 0.05$ for one-sided testing. The 95% CRI of *r* in the full sample is [−0.052; 0.093], well within the [−0.15; 0.15] range.

In general, when one-sided testing is considered, one-sided *p*-values with 90% CIs and one-sided BFs are generally to be preferred over two-sided *p*-values and 95% CIs or two-sided BFs. Of the other criteria discussed, AIC is probably closest to a one-sided *p*-value; it may indicate a preference over a more complex model while the two-sided *p*-value is somewhere in the [0.05; 0.11] region meaning the one-sided *p*-value in the 'more complex' direction (provided that this is the direction formulated prior to seeing the data) is in the [0.025; 0.055] region. That said, for fixed effects of interest, such as *M*s, differences in *M*s, and correlations, it is always informative to report a 90% (and eventually 95%) CI of that parameter of interest instead of only a *p*-value, and/or to report a 95% CRI of that parameter of interest instead of only a BF. A drawback of *p*-values, BFs, and (differences in) criteria such as AIC, AICc, BIC, and SABIC is that they do not provide us with any point or interval estimates of the parameter of interest. Therefore, these criteria can be reported additional to but should not replace point estimates and CIs and/or CRIs of parameters of interest. Also note that the use of CIs and CRIs in the context of TOST, ROPE, and FOST is not limited to standardised statistics such as *d* or *r*; they are equally useful in the context of percentage points or instrument-specific (i.e., non-standardised) measures. While *d* and *r* provide examples of standardised statistics that facilitate cross-study and cross-setting comparisons, where researchers agree on regions of relative or practical equivalence on other scales (e.g., percentage, points, financial gain in American Dollars), TOST, ROPE, and FOST can also be used with those scales.

When dealing with smaller samples, CIs and CRIs do need to be used with more caution. CIs are commonly forced to be symmetric (e.g., the same *SE* to the right as to the left of *M*); while this is rarely a problem when dealing with large samples, it can be a problem when samples are small (e.g., we are interested in estimating μ using *M* in a sample of $N = 12$ and the distribution of sample scores is very skewed). While CRIs come with more flexibility than CIs (i.e., they may take different kinds of shapes), and are less sensitive to different choices of prior distribution than BFs when sample sizes are on the larger side (e.g., Leppink, 2019), in small samples different prior choices substantially affect both BFs and CRIs. Checking CRIs with a range of prior distributions is therefore recommended, especially when samples are on the smaller side.

3.5.3 Four Types of Error: I, II, S, and M

Traditionally, there has been a strong tendency to think in terms of *Type I* (rejecting $\boldsymbol{H_0}$ where it should not be rejected) and *Type II* (failing to reject $\boldsymbol{H_0}$ where it should be rejected) errors. However, if we take the view that "*in social science everything correlates with everything to some extent, due to complex and obscure causal influences*" (Meehl, 1990, p. 125, on the *crud factor*) and differences are rarely if ever *exactly* zero (e.g., Perneger, 1998), thinking in terms of *Type S* (wrong sign) and *Type M* (incorrect magnitude) (e.g., Gelman & Tuerlinckx, 2000) is perhaps more useful. Three possible outcomes of FOST are: (a) sufficient evidence against relative equivalence (i.e., either a substantial positive or a substantial negative difference or correlation), (b) sufficient evidence in favour of relative equivalence, or (c) inconclusive. In this approach, we can give Type I and II errors somewhat wider definitions as follows.

If we conclude (b) from our sample while it is (a) in the population we sampled from, we are dealing with a Type II error, whereas if we conclude (a) from our sample while it is (b) from the population we sampled from, we are dealing with a Type I error; both cases can be considered Type M errors. However, if we conclude (c) from our sample while it is either (a) or (b) in the population we sampled from, a (substantial) Type M error is unlikely. Finally, Type S error may occur in all these cases.

In this approach, Type I and II errors relate to the region of relative or practical equivalence instead of to a 'no difference' or 'no correlation' $\boldsymbol{H_0}$ that is unlikely to be true in the first place. Basically, in FOST, a Type I error is concluding that a difference or correlation of interest is not in the region of relative or practical equivalence while it actually is part of it, and a Type II error is the opposite (Leppink, 2019).

Considerations around different types of errors have also contributed to quite a bit of debate about whether and how we should correct for multiple testing. The problem with many approaches to multiple testing is that they assume $\boldsymbol{H_0}$ to hold in all comparisons—or assign a fairly high prior probability to that (e.g., Westfall, Johnson, & Utts, 1997)—even though that is very unlikely to begin with and, where applicable, appropriate omnibus tests already resulted in the $\boldsymbol{H_0}$ to be rejected (e.g., Perneger, 1998). In a correlation matrix, it is highly unlikely that all correlations are zero in the population of interest, and besides we may well have specific hypotheses to be tested thereby reducing the number of tests needed (e.g., Benjamini, Krieger, & Yekutieli, 2006). In randomised controlled experiments, the presence of specific hypotheses can substantially reduce both the number and nature of tests, and from a FOST perspective we may want to provide 90% CIs (and, in some multiple testing situations, optionally 95% CIs) for each pair of conditions regardless of the outcome of an omnibus test; after all, in FOST, relative equivalence is a valid and interesting outcome (Leppink, 2019).

3.5.4 Sequential One-Sided Testing

Finally, research is not only about large samples but about making the best possible use of resources and not including more participants than necessary as well. This is not only an ethical question but an increasingly important practical question as well. With ever-increasing industries of research, there is an increasing risk of 'over-fishing' of human participants. While it has become easier to contact people in recent years, that same easiness also has resulted in people getting more requests to participate in surveys and other types of research; at some point or another, people get tired and may simply ignore new invitations. Larger samples in single studies can to some extent come at the cost of fewer studies (e.g., Lakens, 2014; Lakens et al., 2018) and that will likely mean fewer replication studies and a reduced generalisability and breadth. A powerful tool that has been around for a while but, at least in the domain of Education, did not yet receive the attention it deserved, is *sequential testing* (Armitage, McPherson, & Rowe, 1969; Dodge & Romig, 1929; Lakens, 2014; Pocock, 1977). Contrary to common research practice, where one fixed sample size is planned before the study, in sequential testing, two or more *blocks* of samples are planned, which may or may not be all of the same size. For example, in a randomised controlled experiment, researchers decide to have two blocks of $N = 60$ each; if they find evidence in favour of the effect of interest after the first block (i.e., statistical significance, information criteria, BF), they will stop data collection and *not* use the second block (e.g., Leppink, 2019). If they fail to find sufficient evidence in favour of the effect of interest after the first block, they proceed with the second block and statistical testing is done on the full sample of two blocks together.

Although the latter means two tests instead of one, these tests are not statistically independent; the first block is used in the first test (i.e., first block only) and second test (i.e., first and second block). To correct for this increased number of though partially dependent tests, we could use $\alpha = 0.0294$ for each block (e.g., Pocock, 1977) or we could use $\alpha = 0.05$ for the first block and an alpha somewhat smaller than $\alpha = 0.0294$ for the second block, depending on which approach we follow (e.g., Fleming, Harrington, & O'Brien, 1984; Lai, Shih, & Zhu, 2006). For larger numbers of blocks, more stringent corrections will be needed (for more details, see: Fleming et al., 1984; Lai et al., 2006; Leppink, 2019; Pocock, 1977).

Moreover, in quite a few studies, researchers already have rather clear expectations with regard to the direction of a particular relation or effect of interest; while they commonly use two-sided testing, one-sided testing would be perfectly defendable, provided that hypotheses calling for one-sided testing were formulated before the start of the study (e.g., preregistration or registered reports). One-sided testing is well known to result in more statistical power with the same sample size or the same statistical power with a smaller sample size for a given effect of interest. For instance, in a two-group experiment, to obtain a statistical power of 0.80 for $d = 0.5$, we would need $n = 64$ per condition when testing two-sided; when testing one-sided, we would need only $n = 51$ per condition. It is also known that sequential testing has a similar effect (e.g., Lakens, 2014). Therefore, when we combine the two into *sequential one-sided testing* (SOST), we may need only 60–

70% of the original sample size for the same statistical power (e.g., Lakens, 2014; Leppink, 2019). It is therefore my prediction that with time more businesses and enterprises will start using SOST, and I hope that Academia will do as well.

References

Abraham, W. T., & Russell, D. W. (2004). Missing data: A review of current methods and applications in epidemiological research. *Current Options in Psychiatry, 17,* 315–321. https://doi.org/10.1097/01.yco.0000133836.34543.7e.

Acock, A. C. (2005). Working with missing values. *Journal of Marriage and the Family, 67,* 1012–1028. https://doi.org/10.1111/j.1741-3737.2005.00191.x.

Agresti, A. (2002). *Categorical data analysis* (2nd ed.). New York, NY: Wiley.

Akaike, H. (1973). Information theory and an extension of the maximum likelihood principle. In B. N. Petrov & F. Csáki (Eds.), *Second International Symposium on Information Theory,* Tsahkadsor, Armenia, USSR, September 2–8, 1971, Budapest: Akadémiai Kiadó (pp. 267–281).

Akaike, H. (1992). Information theory and an extension of the maximum likelihood principle. In S. Kotz & N. Johnson (Eds.), *Breakthroughs in statistics* (pp. 610–624). New York, NY: Springer.

Alani, M. M., Tawfik, H., Saeed, M., & Anya, O. (2018). *Applications of big data analytics: Trends, issues, and challenges.* Cham: Springer. https://doi.org/10.1007/978-3-319-76472-6.

Aldowah, H., Al-Samarraie, H., & Fauzy, W. M. (2019). Educational data mining and learning analytics for 21st century higher education: A review and synthesis. *Telematics and Informatics, 37,* 13–49. https://doi.org/10.1016/j.tele.2019.01.007.

Allison, P. D. (2002). *Missing data* (Vol. 136). Thousand Oaks, CA: Sage.

Armitage, P., McPherson, C. K., & Rowe, B. C. (1969). Repeated significance tests on accumulating data. *Journal of the Royal Statistical Society. Series A (General), 132,* 235–244. https://doi.org/10.2307/2343787.

Azur, M. J., Stuart, E. A., Frangakis, C., & Leaf, P. J. (2011). Multiple imputation by chained equations: What is it and how does it work? *International Journal of Methods in Psychiatric Research, 20*(1), 40–49. https://doi.org/10.1002/mpr.329.

Baker, R. S. (2019). Challenges for the future of educational data mining: The Baker Learning Analytics prizes. *Journal of Educational Data Mining, 11*(1), 1–17.

Bakhshinategh, B., Zaiane, O. R., ElAtia, S., & Ipperciel, D. (2018). Educational data mining applications and tasks: A survey of the last 10 years. *Education and Information Technologies, 23*(1), 537–553. https://doi.org/10.1007/s10639-017-9616-z.

Baraldi, A. N., & Enders, C. K. (2010). An introduction to modern missing data analyses. *Journal of School Psychology, 48*(1), 5–37. https://doi.org/10.1016/j.jsp.2009.10.001.

Barnard, J., & Meng, X. L. (1999). Applications of multiple imputation in medical studies: From AIDS to NHANES. *Statistical Methods in Medical Research, 8,* 17–36. https://doi.org/10.1177/096228029900800103.

Benjamini, Y., Krieger, A. M., & Yekutieli, D. (2006). Adaptive linear step-up procedures that control the false discovery rate. *Biometrika, 93*(3), 491–507. https://doi.org/10.1093/biomet/93.3.491.

Berkey, C. S., Hoaglin, D. C., Mosteller, F., & Colditz, G. A. (1995). A random-effects regression model for meta-analysis. *Statistics in Medicine, 14*(4), 395–411. https://doi.org/10.1002/sim.4780140406.

Bogarín, A., Cerezo, R., & Romero, C. (2018). A survey on educational process mining. *WIREs Data Mining and Knowledge Discovery, 8*(1), e1230. https://doi.org/10.1002/widm.1230.

Burnham, K. P., & Anderson, D. R. (2002). *Model selection and multimodel inference: A practical information-theoretic approach.* New York, NY: Springer.

Burnham, K. P., & Anderson, D. R. (2004). Multimodel inference: Understanding AIC and BIC in model selection. *Sociological Methods & Research, 33,* 261–304. https://doi.org/10.1177/0049124104268644.

Cavanaugh, J. E. (1997). Unifying the deviations of the Akaike and corrected Akaike information criteria. *Statistics & Probability Letters, 31,* 201–208. https://doi.org/10.1016/s0167-7152(96)00128-9.

Claeskens, G., & Hjort, N. L. (2008). *Model selection and model averaging*. Cambridge, MA: Cambridge University Press.

Cole, J. C. (2010). How to deal with missing data: Conceptual overview and details for implementing two modern methods. In J. W. Osborne (Ed.), *Best practices in quantitative methods (Chap. 15)* (pp. 214–238). London: Sage.

Collins, L. M. J. L., Schafer, J. L., & Kam, C. M. (2001). A comparison of inclusive and restrictive strategies in modern missing data procedures. *Psychological Methods, 6*(4), 330–351.

De Rooij, M. (2018). Transitional modeling of experimental longitudinal data with missing data. *Advances in Data Analysis and Classification, 12*(1), 107–130. https://doi.org/10.1007/s11634-015-0226-6.

DerSimonian, R., & Laird, N. (1986). Meta-analysis in clinical trials. *Controlled Clinical Trials, 7* (3), 177–188. https://doi.org/10.1016/0197-2456(86)90046-2.

Dodge, H. F., & Romig, H. G. (1929). A method of sampling inspection. *Bell System Technical Journal, 8*(4), 613–631. https://doi.org/10.1002/j.1538-7305.1929.tb01240.x.

Eekhout, I., De Vet, H. C. W., Twisk, J. W. R., Brand, J. P. L., De Boer, M. R., & Heymans, M. W. (2014). Missing data in a multi-item instrument were best handled by multiple imputation at the item score level. *Journal of Clinical Epidemiology, 67*(3), 335–342. https://doi.org/10.1016/j.jclinepi.2013.09.009.

Enders, C. K. (2010). *Applied missing data analysis*. New York, NY: Guilford Press.

Enders, C. K., & Tofighi, D. (2008). The impact of misspecifying class-specific residual variances in growth mixture models. *Structural Equation Modeling: A Multidisciplinary Journal, 15*(1), 75–95. https://doi.org/10.1080/10705510701758281.

Field, A. (2018). *Discovering statistics using IBM SPSS statistics* (5th ed.). London: Sage.

Fleming, T. R., Harrington, D. P., & O'Brien, P. C. (1984). Designs for group sequential tests. *Contemporary Clinical Trials*. https://doi.org/10.1016/S0197-2456(84)80014-8.

Forster, M. R. (2000). Key concepts in model selection: Performance and generalizability. *Journal of Mathematical Psychology, 44,* 205–231.

Fox-Wasylyshyn, S. M., & El-Masri, M. M. (2005). Handling missing data in self-report measures. *Research in Nursing & Health, 28*(6), 488–495. https://doi.org/10.1002/nur.20100.

Geisser, S. (1975). The predictive sample reuse method with applications. *Journal of the American Statistical Association, 70*(350), 320–328. https://doi.org/10.1080/01621459.1975.10479865.

Gelman, A., & Tuerlinckx, F. (2000). Type S error rates for classical and Bayesian single and multiple comparison procedures. *Computational Statistics, 15*(3), 373–390. https://doi.org/10.1007/s001800000040.

George, B. J., & Aban, I. B. (2016). An application of meta-analysis based on DerSimonian and Laird method. *Journal of Nuclear Cardiology, 23*(4), 690–692. https://doi.org/10.1007/s12350-015-0249-6.

Giraud, C. (2015). *Introduction to high-dimensional statistics*. Boca Raton, FL: CRC.

Graham, J. W., & Schafer, J. L. (1999). On the performance of multiple imputation for multivariate data with small sample size. In R. H. Hoyle (Ed.), *Statistical strategies for small sample size* (pp. 1–29). Thousand Oaks, CA: Sage.

Hacking, I. (1965). *Logic of statistical inference*. Cambridge, MA: Cambridge University Press.

Haitovsky, Y. (1968). Missing data in regression analysis. *Journal of the Royal Statistical Society, 30B*, 67–82. https://www.jstor.org/stable/2984459.

Hayes, R., & McArdle, J. J. (2017). Should we impute or should we weight? Examining the performance of two CART-based techniques for addressing missing data in small sample research with nonnormal variables. *Computational Statistics & Data Analysis, 115,* 35–52. https://doi.org/10.1016/j.csda.2017.05.006.

Hedges, L. V., & Olkin, I. (1985). *Statistical methods for meta-analysis*. San Diego, CA: Academic Press.

Hedges, L. V., & Vevea, J. L. (1998). Fixed- and random-effects models in meta-analysis. *Psychological Methods, 3*(4), 486–504.

Hofmann-Wellenhof, B., Lichtenegger, H., & Collins, J. (2012). *Global positioning system: Theory and practice* (4th rev. ed.). New York: Springer.

Horowitz, J. L., & Manski, C. F. (2000). Nonparametric analysis of randomized experiments with missing covariate and outcome data. *Journal of the American Statistical Association, 95*(449), 77–84. https://doi.org/10.1080/01621489.2000.10473902.

Horton, N. J., & Lipsitz, S. R. (2001). Multiple imputation in practice. *The American Statistician, 55*(3), 244–254. https://doi.org/10.1198/000313001317098266.

Howell, D. C. (2017). *Statistical methods for psychology* (8th ed.). Boston: Cengage.

Hoyle, R. H. (2000). Confirmatory factor analysis. In H. E. A. Tinsley & S. D. Brown (Eds.), *Handbook of applied multivariate statistics and mathematical modeling* (Chap. 16, pp. 465–497). Cambridge, MA: Academic Press. https://doi.org/10.1016/B978-012691360/50017-3.

Hunter, J. E., & Schmidt, F. L. (2004). *Methods of meta-analysis: Correcting error and bias in research findings* (2nd ed.). Newbury Park, CA: Sage.

Hurvich, C. M., & Tsai, C. L. (1989). Regression and time series model selection in small samples. *Biometrika, 76,* 297–307. https://doi.org/10.1093/biomet/76.2.297.

Hussain, S., Dahan, N. A., Ba-Alwib, F. M., & Ribata, N. (2018). Educational data mining and analysis of students' academic performance using WEKA. *Indonesian Journal of Electrical Engineering and Computer Science, 9*(2), 447–459. https://doi.org/10.11591/ijeecs.v9.i2.pp447-459.

Janssen, K. J. M., Donders, A. R. T., Harrell, F. E., Vergouwe, Y., Chen, Q., Grobbee, D. E., & Moons, K. G. M. (2010). Missing covariate data in medical research: To impute is better than to ignore. *Journal of Clinical Epidemiology, 63*(7), 721–727. https://doi.org/10.1016/j.jclinepi.2009.12.008.

Kitchin, R., & McArdle, G. (2016). What makes Big Data, Big Data? Exploring the ontological characteristics of 26 datasets. *Big Data & Society, 3*(1), 1–10. https://doi.org/10.1177/2053951716631130.

Kruschke, J. (2013). Bayesian estimation supersedes the *t* test. *Journal of Experimental Psychology: General, 142*(2), 573–603. https://doi.org/10.1037/a0029146.

Kruschke, J. (2014). *Doing Bayesian data analysis: A tutorial with R, JAGS, and Stan* (2nd ed.). Boston: Academic Press.

Kruschke, J. (2018). BEST: Bayesian estimation supersedes the *t*-test (R package). Retrieved from: https://cran.r-project.org/web/packages/BEST/BEST.pdf. Accessed February 1, 2020.

Kruschke, J., & Liddell, T. M. (2017). The Bayesian new statistics: Hypothesis testing, estimation, meta-analysis, and power analysis from a Bayesian perspective. *Psychonomic Bulletin & Review, 25*(1), 178–206. https://doi.org/10.3758/s13423-016-1221-4.

Kurtz, A. K. (1948). A research test of Rorschach test. *Personnel Psychology, 1,* 41–53. https://doi.org/10.1111/j.1744-6570.1948.tb01292.x.

Lai, T. L., Shih, M. C., & Zhu, G. (2006). Modified Haybittle-Peto group sequential designs for testing superiority and non-inferiority hypotheses in clinical trials. *Statistics in Medicine, 25,* 1149–1167. https://doi.org/10.1002/sim.2357.

Lakens, D. (2014). Performing high-powered studies efficiently with sequential analyses. *European Journal of Social Psychology, 44,* 701–710. https://doi.org/10.1002/ejsp.2023.

Lakens, D. (2017). Equivalence tests: A practical primer for *t* tests, correlations, and meta-analyses. *Social Psychological and Personality Science, 8*(4), 355–362. https://doi.org/10.1177/1948550617697177.

Lakens, D. (2018). TOSTER: Two one-sided tests (TOST) equivalence testing. Retrieved from: https://CRAN.R-project.org/package=TOSTER. Accessed February 1, 2020.

Lakens, D., Adolfi, F. G., Albers, C. J., Anvari, F., Apps, M. A. J., Argamon, S. E., et al. (2018). Justify your alpha. *Nature: Human Behaviour, 2*, 168–171. https://www.nature.com/articles/s41562-018-0311-x.

LeCun, Y., Bengio, Y., & Hinton, G. (2015). Deep learning. *Nature, 521*, 436–444. https://doi.org/10.1038/nature14539.

Leppink, J. (2019). *Statistical methods for experimental research in education and psychology*. Cham: Springer. https://doi.org/10.1007/978-3-030-21241-4.

Leppink, J., & Pérez-Fuster P. (2019). Mental effort, workload, time on task, and certainty: Beyond linear models. *Educational Psychology Review*. https://doi.org/10.1007/s10648-018-09460-2.

Little, R. J. A. (1988). A test of missing completely at random for multivariate data with missing values. *Journal of the American Statistical Association, 83*, 1198–1202. https://doi.org/10.1080/01621459.1988.10478722.

Little, R. J. A., & Rubin, D. B. (2002). *Statistical analysis with missing data*. Hoboken, NJ: Wiley.

Luo, Y., Szolovits, P., Dighe, A. S., & Baron, J. M. (2017). 3D-MICE: Integration of cross-sectional and longitudinal imputation for multi-analyte longitudinal clinical data. *Journal of the American Medical Informatics Association, 25*(6), 645–653. https://doi.org/10.1093/jamia/ocx133.

Marsh, H. W., Morin, A. J. S., Parker, P. D., & Kaur, G. (2014). Exploratory structural equation modelling: An integration of the best features of exploratory and confirmatory factor analysis. *Annual Review of Clinical Psychology, 10*, 85–110.https://doi.org/10.1146/annurev-clinpsy-032813-153700.

McQuarrie, A. D. R., & Tsai, C. L. (1998). *Regression and time series model selection*. Singapore: World Scientific.

Meehl, P. E. (1990). Appraising and amending theories: The strategy of Lakatosian defense and two principles that warrant it. *Psychological Inquiry, 1*(2), 108–141. https://doi.org/10.1207/s15327965pli0102_1.

Molenberghs, G., & Verbeke, G. (2005). *Models for discrete longitudinal data*. Berlin: Springer.

Morris, C. N. (1983). Parametric empirical Bayes inference: Theory and applications. *Journal of the American Statistical Association, 78*(381), 47–55. https://doi.org/10.1080/01621459.1983.10477920.

Mosier, C. I. (1951). Problems and designs of cross-validation. *Educational and Psychological Measurement, 11*, 5–11.

Mulaik, S. (1987). A brief history of the philosophical foundations of exploratory factor analysis. *Multivariate Behavioral Research, 22*(3), 267–305. https://doi.org/10.1207/s15327906mbr2203_3.

Osborne, J. W. (2010). Creating valid prediction equations in multiple regression: Shrinkage, double cross-validation, and confidence intervals around predictions. In J. W. Osborne (Ed.), *Best practices in quantitative methods (Chap. 20)* (pp. 299–305). London: Sage.

Osborne, J. W., Costello, A. B., & Kellow, J. T. (2010). Best practices in exploratory factor analysis. In J. W. Osborne (Ed.), *Best practices in quantitative methods (Chap. 6)* (pp. 86–99). London: Sage.

Paule, R. C., & Mandel, J. (1982). Consensus values and weighting factors. *Journal of Research of the National Bureau of Standards, 87*(5), 377–386.

Perneger, T. V. (1998). What's wrong with Bonferroni adjustments. *BMJ, 316*(7139), 1236–1238. https://doi.org/10.1136/bmj.316.7139.1236.

Peto, R., Pike, M. C., Armitage, P., Breslow, N. E., Cox, D. R., Howard, S. V., et al. (1977). Design and analysis of randomized clinical trials requiring prolonged observation of each patient: II. Analysis and examples. *British Journal of Cancer, 35*, 1–39. https://doi.org/10.1038/bjc.1977.1.

Pocock, S. J. (1977). Group sequential methods in the design and analysis of clinical trials. *Biometrika, 64*(2), 191–199. https://doi.org/10.1093/biomet/64.2.191.

Rajpurkar, P., Irvin, J., Ball, R. L., Zhu, K., Yang, B., Mehta, H., et al. (2018). Deep learning for chest radiograph diagnosis: A retrospective comparison of the CheXNeXt algorithm to practicing radiologists. *PLoS Medicine, 15*(11), e1002686. https://doi.org/10.1371/journal.pmed.1002686.

Raudenbush, S. W. (2009). Analyzing effect sizes: Random effects models. In H. Cooper, L. V. Hedges, & J. C. Valentine (Eds.), *The handbook of research synthesis and meta-analysis* (2nd ed., pp. 295–315). New York, NY: Russell Sage Foundation.

Ray, S., & Saeed, M. (2018). Applications of educational data mining and learning analytics tools in handling big data in higher education. In M. M. Alani, H. Tawfik, M. Saeed, & O. Anya (Eds.), *Applications of big data analytics: Trends, issues, and challenges (Chap. 7)* (pp. 135–160). Cham: Springer. https://doi.org/10.1007/978-3-319-76472-6_7.

Rodrigues, M. W., Isotani, S., & Zárate, L. E. (2018). Educational data mining: A review of evaluation process in the e-learning. *Telematics and Informatics, 35,* 1701–1717. https://doi.org/10.1016/j.tele.2018.04.015.

Roth, P. L. (1994). Missing data: A conceptual review for applied psychologists. *Personnel Psychology, 47*(3), 537–560. https://doi.org/10.1111/j.1744-6570.1994.tb01736.x.

Rouder, J. N., Speckman, P. L., Sun, D., Morey, R. D., & Iverson, G. (2012). Bayesian *t* tests for accepting and rejecting the null hypothesis. *Psychonomic Bulletin & Review, 16*(2), 225–237. https://doi.org/10.3758/PBR.16.2.225.

Royall, R. M. (1997). *Statistical evidence: A Likelihood paradigm*. London: Chapman & Hall.

Royall, R. M. (2004). The likelihood paradigm for statistical evidence. In M. L. Taper & S. R. Lele (Eds.), *The nature of scientific evidence*. Chicago: University of Chicago Press.

Rubin, D. B. (1976). Inference and missing data. *Biometrika, 63*(3), 581–592. https://doi.org/10.1093/biomet/63.3.581.

Rubin, D. B. (1987). *Multiple imputation for nonresponse in surveys*. New York, NY: Wiley.

Samuel, A. (1959). Some studies in machine learning using the game of checkers. *IBM Journal of Research and Development, 3*(3), 210–229. https://doi.org/10.1147/rd.33.0210.

Santos, K. J. O., Menezes, A. G., De Carvalho, A. B., & Montesco, C. A. E. (2019). Supervised learning in the context of educational data mining to avoid university students dropout. In *2019 IEEE 19th International Conference on Advanced Learning Technologies (ICALT)* (pp. 207–208). https://doi.org/10.1109/ICALT.2019.00068.

Schafer, J. L. (1997). *Analysis of incomplete multivariate data*. London: Chapman & Hall.

Schafer, J. L., & Graham, J. W. (2002). Missing data: Our view of the state of the art. *Psychological Methods, 7,* 147–177.

Schumacher, C., & Ifenthaler, D. (2018). Features students really expect from learning analytics. *Computers in Human Behavior, 78,* 397–407. https://doi.org/10.1016/j.chb.2017.06.030.

Schwarz, G. (1978). Estimating the dimensions of a model. *Annals of Statistics, 6,* 461–465.

Sidik, K., & Jonkman, J. N. (2005a). A note on variance estimation in random effects meta-regression. *Journal of Biopharmaceutical Statistics, 15*(5), 823–838. https://doi.org/10.1081/BIP-200067915.

Sidik, K., & Jonkman, J. N. (2005b). Simple heterogeneity variance estimation for meta-analysis. *Journal of the Royal Statistical Society C, 54*(2), 367–384. https://doi.org/10.1111/j.1467-9876.2005.00489.x.

Silberzahn, R., Uhlman, E. L., Martin, D. P., Anselmi, P., Aust, F., Awtrey, E., et al. (2018). Many analysts, one data set: Making transparent how variations in analytic choices affect results. *Advances in Methods and Practices in Psychological Science, 1*(3), 337–356. https://doi.org/10.1177/2515245917747646.

Stone, M. (1974). Crossvalidatory choice and assessment of statistical predictions. *Journal of the Royal Statistical Society, Series B (Methodological), 26,* 111–147. https://www.jstor.org/stable/pdf/2984809.

Tiffin, P. A., & Paton, L. W. (2018). Rise of the machines? Machine learning approaches and mental health: Opportunities and challenges. *The British Journal of Psychiatry, 213,* 509–510. https://doi.org/10.1192/bjp.2018.105.

Tofighi, D., & Enders, C. K. (2007). Identifying the correct number of classes in mixture models. In G. R. Hancock & K. M. Samuelsen (Eds.), *Advances in latent variable mixture models*. Greenwich, CT: Information Age Publishing.

Tshitoyan, V., Dagdelen, J., Weston, L., Dunn, A., Rong, Z., Kononova, O., et al. (2019). Unsupervised word embeddings capture latent knowledge from materials science literature. *Nature, 571,* 95. https://doi.org/10.1038/s41586-019-1335-8.

Twisk, J. W. R., Bosman, L., Hoekstra, T., Rijnhart, J., Welten, M., & Heymans, M. (2018). Different ways to estimate treatment effects in randomised controlled trials. *Contemporary Clinical Trials Communications, 10,* 80–85. https://doi.org/10.1016/j.conctc.2018.03.008.

Twisk, J. W. R., Hoogendijk, E. O., Zwijsen, S. A., & De Boer, M. R. (2016). Different methods to analyze stepped wedge trials designs revealed different aspects of intervention studies. *Journal of Clinical Epidemiology, 72,* 75–83. https://doi.org/10.1016/j.clinepi.2015.11.004.

Van Buuren, S. (2012). *Flexible imputation of missing data*. New York, NY: Chapman & Hall.

Van Buuren, S., & Groothuis-Oudshoorn, K. (2011). Mice: Multivariate imputation by chained equations in R. *Journal of Statistical Software, 45,* 1–67.

Van der Eijk, C., & Rose, J. (2015). Risky business: Factor analysis of survey data—Assessing the probability of incorrect dimensionalisation. *PLoS ONE, 10*(3), 1–31. https://doi.org/10.1371/journal.pone.0118900.

Van der Zee, T., & Reich, J. (2018). Open education science. *AERA Open, 4*(3), 1–15. https://doi.org/10.1177/2332858418787466.

Van Ginkel, J. R., Sijtsma, K., Van der Ark, L. A., & Vermunt, J. K. (2010). Incidence of missing item scores in personality measurement, and simple item-score imputation. *Methodology, 6,* 17–30. https://doi.org/10.1027/1614-2241/a000003.

Viberg, O., Hatakka, M., Bälter, O., & Mavroudi, A. (2018). The current landscape of learning analytics in higher education. *Computers in Human Behavior, 89,* 98–110. https://doi.org/10.1016/j.chb.2018.07.027.

Viechtbauer, W. (2005). Bias and efficiency of meta-analytic variance estimators in the random-effects model. *Journal of Educational and Behavioral Statistics, 30*(3), 261–293. https://doi.org/10.3102/10769986030003261.

Vieira, C., Parsons, P., & Byrd, V. (2018). Visual learning analytics of educational data: A systematic literature review and research agenda. *Computers & Education, 122,* 119–135. https://doi.org/10.1016/j.compedu.2018.03.018.

Westfall, P. H., Johnson, W. O., & Utts, J. M. (1997). A Bayesian perspective on the Bonferroni adjustment. *Biometrika, 84*(2), 419–427. https://doi.org/10.1093/biomet/84.2.419.

White, I. R., & Carlin, J. B. (2010). Bias and efficiency of multiple imputation compared with complete-case analysis for missing covariate values. *Statistics in Medicine, 29,* 2920–2931. https://doi.org/10.1002/sim.3944.

Wilks, S. S. (1938). The large-sample distribution of the likelihood ratio for testing composite hypotheses. *The Annals of Mathematical Statistics, 9*(1), 60–62. https://doi.org/10.1214/aoms/1177732360.

Wood, A. M., White, I. R., & Thompson, S. G. (2004). Are missing outcome data adequately handled? A review of published randomized controlled trials in major medical journals. *Clinical Trials, 1*(4), 368–376. https://doi.org/10.1191/1740774504cn032oa.

Yu, C. H. (2010). Resampling: A conceptual and procedural introduction. In J. W. Osborne (Ed.), *Best practices in quantitative methods (Chap. 19)* (pp. 283–298). London: Sage.

Yuan, K. H., Yang-Wallentin, F., & Bentler, P. M. (2012). ML versus MI for missing data with violation of distribution conditions. *Sociological Methods & Research, 41*(4), 598–629. https://doi.org/10.1177/0049124112460373.

4 Anchoring Narratives

Abstract
Discourse on rather forced and unconstructive quantitative-qualitative divides has made researchers in some fields of Education believe that quality criteria in 'quantitative' research are radically different from those in 'qualitative' research, and that 'quantitative' research uses random sampling while all 'qualitative' research uses non-random sampling, that 'quantitative' research is about linear relations in large samples whereas 'qualitative' research is about nonlinear relations in small samples, and ideas alike. Some have taken these ideas further by stating that all randomised controlled experiments are a waste of money, and that concepts like reliability and validity have a place only in 'quantitative' research. This chapter demonstrates that such quantitative-qualitative divides are not only useless but undermine progress in Education as well. Uniting contemporary validity frameworks, this chapter provides a framework for thinking about evidence in educational settings that is applied in several chapters later on in this book.

4.1 Introduction

Once upon a time, on a Friday night around almost midnight, a 25-year old man was attacked by two other men of similar age. Without asking or saying anything, one of the attackers punched the victim in the face. The victim fell down, the two attackers seized the victim's mobile phone and wallet from his jacket and ran off. There were eight eyewitnesses: a single man in his 70s, a married couple in their 30s, three students in their early 20s who were flatmates, and two other people—a man and a woman, both in their 40s—who did not know each other and, like the single man in his 70s, had never met the other eyewitnesses either. None of the witnesses had seen any of the attackers before that night. That same night, within

J. Leppink, *The Art of Modelling the Learning Process*, Springer Texts in Education,
https://doi.org/10.1007/978-3-030-43082-5_4

the first three hours after the event, the police interviewed five of the eight eyewitnesses in the following order: the single man in his 70s, the married couple in their 30s, the woman in her 40s, and finally the man in his 40s. The two eyewitnesses in their 30s were interviewed as a couple, and—living in the same street as the three students who witnessed the event—they provided the police with the names and address of the three students. The next day, in the early afternoon, two policemen visited the three students for an interview at their place. Based on all these interviews, the single man in his 70s was interviewed again five days after the event, and another time about two weeks after the event.

The three interviews with the single man in his 70s resulted in highly inconsistent statements. Although the story of the married couple and the story of the three students differed in important aspects, there were no disagreements among the couple about their story and there were no disagreements among the students about their story either. The man and the woman in their 40s gave very similar accounts of what happened, even though they did not talk to each other at any point before they were interviewed, and they were interviewed separately. When the man in his 70s and the married couple were asked if they could identify the attackers, they responded that they could not because they had never seen the attackers in town before. The two policemen interviewing the students asked whether they thought the attackers were foreigners, to which the students responded: 'possibly yes'.

4.2 Evidence of Guilt or Innocence

An important principle in international law is *unus testis, nullus testis*, which literally means *one witness is no witness* and more broadly means that decisions ought not to be based on a single piece of evidence (Wagenaar, Van Koppen, & Crombag, 1993). In a criminal case, whether we deal with eyewitnesses, a DNA match, fingerprints, video or other evidence, in isolation they may not provide any evidence; *absolute evidence* does not exist. Even though a DNA match, a video or GPS information from a mobile device constitute potentially very powerful pieces of evidence, their meaning needs to be understood in a broader context. For example, a match in DNA between Suspect A and a piece of cigarette found in the backyard of Victim B whose dead body was found in that backyard cannot in itself be understood as decisive evidence that A killed B; someone may have collected that piece of cigarette from an ashtray, may have killed B and put the old piece of cigarette in the backyard as well (Leppink, 2017). Video can be edited, and mobile devices can be stolen or at least taken away from the owner temporarily.

A witness recognising a robber or attacker in an identification procedure at the local police station can serve as evidence in combination with other pieces of evidence, and equally a failure of recognition may not matter much if other pieces of evidence are available. For instance, suppose a burglar attempts to break into a house on a sunny and dry day in July at 5:00 in the morning, uses a shovel to try to break a window in the back part of the house but the noise wakes up the people living in the house, one of whom sees the burglar through the window just before he runs off. He leaves behind the shovel he used. The people in the house call the police, who turn up quite quickly, and send the Crime Scene Investigation (CSI) team within the next two hours to examine traces on the shovel, window, and perhaps other areas of the house (among others: doors and other windows). At 6:00 the same morning, the police receive a call from another house almost around the corner of where the attempted burglary took place, that someone managed to get into the house, take some money from a room downstairs, and run off before the people living in the house could catch him. Again, left behind is a shovel, which this time was used to open the backdoor. Also left behind is his backpack, because he had to run away very fast to avoid being caught by one of the people living in the house he entered. That backpack helps the police to catch its owner, whose DNA and fingerprints happen to be in a database system because of prior crimes. The DNA and fingerprints on both shovels match with the DNA and fingerprints of the owner of the backpack. Even if none of the people living in either of the two houses recognise the burglar in an identification procedure at the local police station, the combination of backpack (personal material including DNA), two shovels (same method used in two places where the burglar was never seen before), DNA and fingerprint matches, and an inability to provide material evidence of being present in completely different place around the times of the attempted and successful burglary (that would have made it impossible to arrive at either of the crime scenes when the events happened) provide very strong evidence of the suspect's guilt in the two cases.

4.2.1 Independence

Given the absence of absolute evidence, no piece of evidence should be interpreted as providing a 100% probability of a suspect being *guilty* ($\boldsymbol{H_1}$) or a 100% probability of a suspect being *innocent* ($\boldsymbol{H_0}$). However, given two competing hypotheses —$\boldsymbol{H_0}$ versus $\boldsymbol{H_1}$—we can express each piece of evidence (E_x) as a LR:

$$LR_x = P(E_x|\boldsymbol{H_1})/P(E_x|\boldsymbol{H_0}).$$

For example, for a confession by a suspect of a gasoline station robbery (let us call it: E_1), the LR would be:

$$LR_1 = P(E_1|\boldsymbol{H_1})/P(E_1|\boldsymbol{H_0}).$$

If apart from this confession, we also have a video of that robbery from which the suspect can be recognised (let us call it: E_2), the LR of that piece of evidence is:

$$LR_2 = P(E_2|\boldsymbol{H_1})/P(E_2|\boldsymbol{H_0}).$$

If we can treat E_1 and E_2 as independent pieces of evidence, we can multiply LR_1 and LR_2 to obtain the LR of E (i.e., LR_E):

$$LR_E = LR_1 * LR_2.$$

Another way to write this is:

$$LR_E = P(E_1 \,\&\, E_2|\boldsymbol{H_1}) * P(E_1 \,\&\, E_2|\boldsymbol{H_0}).$$

For any E_x, $LR_x > 1$ indicates that the evidence is more likely to have occurred under $\boldsymbol{H_1}$ than under $\boldsymbol{H_0}$ while $LR_x < 1$ indicates that the evidence is more likely to have occurred under $\boldsymbol{H_0}$ than under $\boldsymbol{H_1}$. Pieces that have $LR_x > 1$ contribute to a larger LR_E, while pieces that have $LR_x < 1$ contribute to a larger LR_E. In other words, when all $LR_x > 1$, LR_E is larger than the largest LR_x in the equation; when all $LR_x < 1$, LR_E is smaller than the smallest LR_x in the equation. Finally, in situations where one or more pieces of evidence have $LR_x > 1$ (e.g., DNA match, GPS data) and one or more other pieces of evidence have $LR_x < 1$ (e.g., witness fails to identify suspect, suspect denies involvement, a third party had a motive to kill the victim, evidence that the DNA match resulted from an old piece of cigarette being taken from an ashtray), LR_E lies somewhere in between the largest and the smallest LR_x.

4.2.2 Dependence

The aforementioned formulae and reasoning are valid whenever we can conceive the different pieces of evidence as independent. In practice, there often is some kind of dependence between pieces of evidence, and a correction of some kind has to be applied to the aforementioned formulae which results LR_x to end up at least somewhat closer to 1 than it would be in the case of independence. A suspect of a gasoline station robbery may be more likely to confess in the knowledge that there is a video of the robbery showing his involvement.

Likewise, in the example case we started this chapter with, the eight eyewitnesses cannot be conceived as eight independent pieces of evidence. The single man in his 70s and the man and woman in their 40s may provide three independent pieces of evidence, unless the statements of the ones interviewed later in the sequence are to some extent influenced by questions based on earlier interviews, with other eyewitnesses of the same event, or leading (i.e., suggestive) questions used by the police. As far as the other five eyewitnesses are concerned, the number of independent observations probably lies closer to two than to five.

The independence formulae and correction for dependence wherever applicable should not be thought of as providing concrete numbers in concrete criminal cases; there are hardly any broadly agreed numbers of LR_x for any piece of evidence. However, this LR framework provides a way of *thinking* about the strength of evidence in a particular case.

4.2.3 Reliability and Validity

The strength of a piece of evidence is partly a function of its reliability and validity, and these can be influenced substantially by dependence between pieces of evidence. In the context of eyewitness testimonies, the *reliability* of the piece of evidence (i.e., the eyewitness) can be defined as the degree of consistency of statements from that eyewitness at different occasions, while the *validity* of that piece of evidence is about the degree to which it provides an accurate account of the event of interest (Wagenaar et al., 1993). Reliability is a necessary though not sufficient condition for validity; someone who delivers the same story every time again is reliable but is not necessarily providing an accurate account of the event of interest, while someone who tells a very different story at each subsequent occasion cannot really be thought of as a valid piece of evidence, even though one of the stories told may well be true or each of the different stories have some element(s) of truth. In the example case, for instance, the single man in his 70s is not to be thought of as a reliable eyewitness; the three interviews result in highly inconsistent statements. If we were to express the evidence coming from this eyewitness in a LR, we would need a value much closer to 1 compared to the LR of a more reliable eyewitness.

As a rule of thumb, two eyewitnesses who independently provide consistent stories at two or three occasions that match with each other (i.e., a high degree of overlap between the stories from the two eyewitnesses) provide much more reliable and probably more valid evidence than two eyewitnesses who provide inconsistent stories and/or eyewitnesses who tell the same story probably because they have talked to each other, have common interests, or have been interviewed in a suggestive way and/or have been interviewed together.

4.2.4 Prior Odds

Given that the interest lies in the question which of the competing hypotheses is more likely given the evidence available, some readers may wonder if we should not multiple LR_E with the *prior odds* as per Bayes' theorem (Bayes, 1763; Laplace, 1812) to obtain the *posterior odds*:

$$P(\boldsymbol{H_1}|\mathrm{E})/P(\boldsymbol{H_0}|\mathrm{E}) = [P(\mathrm{E}|\boldsymbol{H_1})/P(\mathrm{E}|\boldsymbol{H_0})] * [P(\boldsymbol{H_1})/P(\boldsymbol{H_0})].$$

In this formula, E represents the combination of pieces of evidence at hand. There is legitimate disagreement on this matter for at least two reasons. First, there is the legal principle of *ei incumbit probation qui dicit, non qui negat*: the burden of proof is on the one who says, not on the one who denies; this principle is also called the *presumption of innocence*. If we take the presumption of innocence literally, $P(\boldsymbol{H_1}$: 'guilt') is 0 and hence $P(\boldsymbol{H_0})$ is 1; assigning any other probabilities to these two possible and mutually exclusive hypotheses can be interpreted as a violation of the presumption of innocence (e.g., Wagenaar et al., 1993). Second, even if we ignore that argument, if we ask five experts to provide estimates of the prior odds in a given case, we will probably see very different outcomes.

Neither of the two arguments provides a sufficient justification against the use of Bayes' theorem. With regard to the presumption of innocence, zero probability of a suspect being guilty is a very extreme perspective. Even if the pool of people who could possibly be guilty is as large as 10,000 people, the prior probability of suspect A being guilty is not exactly 0, and assigning equal probability to all suspects (i.e., 0.0001) may well be reasonable. Different expert opinions resulting in different prior odds estimates is not a problem either; rather, they can help us to estimate the posterior odds under different assumptions. That said, neither LR_E nor posterior odds should be thought of as providing hard numbers to be used to quantify decision making in a given criminal case; rather, they provide us with a framework to qualitatively think about evidence and the role of different pieces in that evidence: LR is the *shift* in likelihood of one hypothesis versus another from *before* seeing the evidence (i.e., *prior*) to *after* seeing the evidence (i.e., *posterior*). Given LR, changes in the prior will result in a different posterior, and given prior, changes in LR will also result in a different posterior. When no reasonable agreement can be found on what reasonable input numbers, a pragmatic solution is to compute the posterior under different priors and under different LRs; doing so can shed light on the degree of uncertainty around inputs, and the extent to which that degree of uncertainty actually influences the outcome.

4.3 Evidence of a Student's Competence

The thinking framework just discussed in a context of forensics can also be applied to thinking about evidence in questions like individual students' competence. Differences between students in competence rated by multiple independent assessors contribute to a within-student between-assessors correlational structure, cf. the concept of *ICC* discussed in Chap. 2. If there were no differences between students, *ICC* should be (approximately) zero. Present differences between students, once we account for these differences, the residual correlations between independent assessors are (approximately) zero. Hence, independent assessors can be thought of as independent pieces of evidence of a student's competence.

4.3.1 Independent Assessors

Suppose, three assessors are to decide, based on a driving test, whether a student is competent enough to be given a driver licence ($\boldsymbol{H_1}$) or does not yet have that competence ($\boldsymbol{H_0}$). Table 4.1 presents tendencies of these three assessors—A, B, and C—for a group of 1000 students. For the sake of simplicity of the example, the group is divided into 500 competent ($\boldsymbol{H_1}$) and 500 not yet competent students ($\boldsymbol{H_0}$), resulting in prior odds of 0.5/0.5 = 1.

Table 4.1 Competence decision tendencies of Assessors A, B, and C for 500 competent and 500 not yet competent students

Assessor	Student competent?	Student is	
		Competent (H_1)	Not competent (H_0)
A	Yes	480	80
	No	20	420
B	Yes	450	50
	No	50	450
C	Yes	400	10
	No	100	490

For Assessor A, we find $P(\text{Yes}|\boldsymbol{H_1}) = 480/500 = 0.96$ and $P(\text{Yes}|\boldsymbol{H_0}) = 80/500 = 0.16$. For Assessor B, we find $P(\text{Yes}|\boldsymbol{H_1}) = 450/500 = 0.90$ and $P(\text{Yes}|\boldsymbol{H_0}) = 50/500 = 0.10$. For Assessor C, we find $P(\text{Yes}|\boldsymbol{H_1}) = 400/500 = 0.80$ and $P(\text{Yes}|\boldsymbol{H_0}) = 10/500 = 0.02$. From these numbers, it becomes clear that A is the most lenient assessor and C is the most stringent assessor. Compared to B and C, A gives competent students the highest chance of a 'competent' judgement, and even not yet competent students have a fair chance of receiving that judgement. With C, not yet competent students are very unlikely to be judged 'competent' and even competent students face a considerable chance of being judged 'not yet competent'. Given the numbers in Table 4.1, the LRs for a 'competent' (i.e., Yes) judgement are: $LR_A = 0.96/0.16 = 6$; $LR_B = 0.90/0.10 = 9$; and $LR_C = 0.80/0.02 = 40$. Thus, although the chance of competent students being judged 'competent' is lowest with Assessor C, LR also takes into account the proportion of incompetent students receiving a 'competent' judgement and that is much lower with C than with A or B. Therefore, a 'competent' judgement given by Assessor C constitutes a shift from prior to posterior odds of 40, which is considerably more than the shift we see with Assessor A or B. However, Assessors A and B combined yields a LR_E higher than LR_C:

$$LR_E = LR_A * LR_B = 6 * 9 = 54.$$

In other words, receiving a 'competent' judgement from both Assessor A and Assessor B means a shift from prior to posterior of 54. Ultimately, if we have three assessors and all say 'confident':

$$LR_E = LR_A * LR_B * LR_C = 6 * 9 * 40 = 2160.$$

We can compute the probability of these series of 'competent' judgements under $\boldsymbol{H_1}$ (competent) and $\boldsymbol{H_0}$ (not yet competent) from LR_E as follows:

$$P(\text{'competent'}|\boldsymbol{H_1}) = \mathrm{LR_E}/(\mathrm{LR_E}+1),$$
$$P(\text{'competent'}|\boldsymbol{H_0}) = 1/(\mathrm{LR_E}+1).$$

As we see, the more independent assessors provide a 'competent' judgement, the more likely these judgements are given under $\boldsymbol{H_1}$ and the less likely they are given under $\boldsymbol{H_0}$. With prior odds of 1, the posterior odds equal $\mathrm{LR_E}$ and hence P('competent'|$\boldsymbol{H_1}$) = $P(\boldsymbol{H_1}|$'competent') and P('competent'|$\boldsymbol{H_0}$) = $P(\boldsymbol{H_0}|$'competent'). With prior odds larger than 1 (i.e., more than 50% competent students), the posterior odds are larger than $\mathrm{LR_E}$, and hence P('competent'|$\boldsymbol{H_1}$) < $P(\boldsymbol{H_1}|$'competent') and P('competent'|$\boldsymbol{H_0}$) > $P(\boldsymbol{H_0}|$'competent'). With prior odds smaller than 1 (i.e., less than 50% competent students), it is exactly the other way around.

We can do the same for 'not yet competent' judgements: $\mathrm{LR_A}$ = 21, $\mathrm{LR_B}$ = 9, and $\mathrm{LR_C}$ = 4.9. The resulting $\mathrm{LR_E}$ is:

$$\mathrm{LR_E} = \mathrm{LR_A} * \mathrm{LR_B} * \mathrm{LR_C} = 21 * 9 * 4.9 = 926.1.$$

Given that this time $\mathrm{LR_E}$ is about 'not yet competent', we can compute the probability of three 'not yet competent' judgments under $\boldsymbol{H_0}$ (not yet competent) and $\boldsymbol{H_1}$ (competent) from $\mathrm{LR_E}$ as follows:

$$P(\text{'not competent'}|\boldsymbol{H_0}) = \mathrm{LR_E}/(\mathrm{LR_E}+1),$$
$$P(\text{'competent'}|\boldsymbol{H_1} = 1/(\mathrm{LR_E}+1).$$

We find: P('competent'|$\boldsymbol{H_1}$) ≈ 0.001, meaning there is only a very small chance a student is competent if all three assessors judge the student as 'not yet competent'. The relation between prior odds and posterior odds remains the same; with prior odds larger than 1 $P(\boldsymbol{H_1}|$'competent') > P('competent'|$\boldsymbol{H_1}$) and $P(\boldsymbol{H_0}|$'competent') < P('competent'|$\boldsymbol{H_0}$), while with prior odds smaller than 1 $P(\boldsymbol{H_0}|$'competent') > P('competent'|$\boldsymbol{H_0}$) and $P(\boldsymbol{H_1}|$'competent') < P('competent'|$\boldsymbol{H_1}$).

The same logic can be applied to situations where there is disagreement between assessors. Suppose, we have a situation where Assessors A and B judge a student as 'competent' while Assessor C judges that student as 'not yet competent': $\mathrm{LR_A}$ = 6, $\mathrm{LR_B}$ = 9, and $\mathrm{LR_C}$ = (1/4.9). For $\mathrm{LR_E}$, we then find:

$$\mathrm{LR_E} = \mathrm{LR_A} * \mathrm{LR_B} * \mathrm{LR_C} = 6 * 9 * (1/4.9) \approx 11.020.$$

With this outcome, we find: P('competent'|$\boldsymbol{H_1}$) ≈ 0.917. With prior odds 1, P('competent'|$\boldsymbol{H_1}$) = $P(\boldsymbol{H_1}|$'competent'). If prior odds were 2 instead of 1 (i.e., two thirds instead of half of the students being competent), the same $\mathrm{LR_E}$ of 11.020 would result in posterior odds of 22.040, and that would mean $P(\boldsymbol{H_1}|$'competent') ≈ 0.957. However, if prior odds were 0.5 (i.e., only one third of the students being competent), the same $\mathrm{LR_E}$ of 11.020 would result in posterior odds of 5.510 and $P(\boldsymbol{H_1}|$'competent') ≈ 0.846. Still a good chance of $\boldsymbol{H_1}$ being true given the data (i.e., the combination of the three assessments), but less so than with prior odds 1 or higher.

If in the aforementioned case Assessor B judged 'not yet competent' (cf. Assessor C) instead of 'competent' (cf. Assessor A), the resulting LR_E would be:

$$LR_E = LR_A * LR_B * LR_C = 6 * (1/9) * (1/4.9) \approx 0.136.$$

Or, we could turn it around: LR_A = (1/6), LR_B = 9, and LR_C = 4.9, and LR_E:

$$LR_E = LR_A * LR_B * LR_C = (1/6) * 9 * 4.9 = 7.35.$$

One LR_E is the inverse of the other, because in the first case we compute LR_E for 'competent' while in the second case we compute LR_E for 'not yet competent', and the product of these two equals 1. With prior odds 1, LR_E = 7.35 for not competent corresponds with $P(\boldsymbol{H_0}|\text{'competent'}) \approx 0.880$. Prior odds of 'competent' of 0.5 corresponds with prior odds of 'not yet competent' of 2 and hence LR_E = 7.35 would result in posterior odds of 14.70 and $P(\boldsymbol{H_0}|\text{'not yet competent'}) \approx 0.936$. Likewise, prior odds of 'competent' of 2 corresponds with prior odds of 'not yet competent' of 0.5 and hence LR_E = 7.35 would result in posterior odds of 3.675 and $P(\boldsymbol{H_0}|\text{'not yet competent'}) \approx 0.786$. The latter is still a good chance of $\boldsymbol{H_0}$ being true, but less so than with prior odds on the other side of 1.

Finally, although for the sake of simplicity the examples discussed thus far involve dichotomous decisions and two competing hypotheses, a similar reasoning—albeit with more complex formulae—applies to multicategory and scale variables (e.g., higher scores being more likely if one is competent) and both the LR_E and Bayesian approach allow for direct testing of more than two hypotheses (e.g., innocent, main perpetrator, complicit; not competent, sufficiently competent, excellent). Even where hard numbers cannot be provided, the LR_E and Bayesian approach provide a thinking framework for how different pieces of evidence can be combined and how different assumptions about these pieces of evidence (and about the prior odds) influence the outcomes.

4.3.2 Time Series and Triangulation

Thus far we have seen that, whether we deal with decisions in a criminal case or with decisions regarding competence of students, different pieces of evidence have to be integrated with each other and anchored into facts and common sense; if this process is successful, it results in a coherent story that provides a reasonable *chain of evidence* in favour of one hypothesis relative to its one or several competing hypotheses (i.e., beyond reasonable doubt; Kane, 2006; Leppink, 2017; Wagenaar et al., 1993). In educational settings, longitudinal assessment provides a great context for accumulating evidence from a variety of sources. For instance, in a longitudinal clerkship, where medical students are placed in a clinical environment for 9–12 months, students see a variety of professionals, patients, and other stakeholders; the experiences of each of these stakeholders can help to shed light on different types of skills on the part of the individual student. When organised and

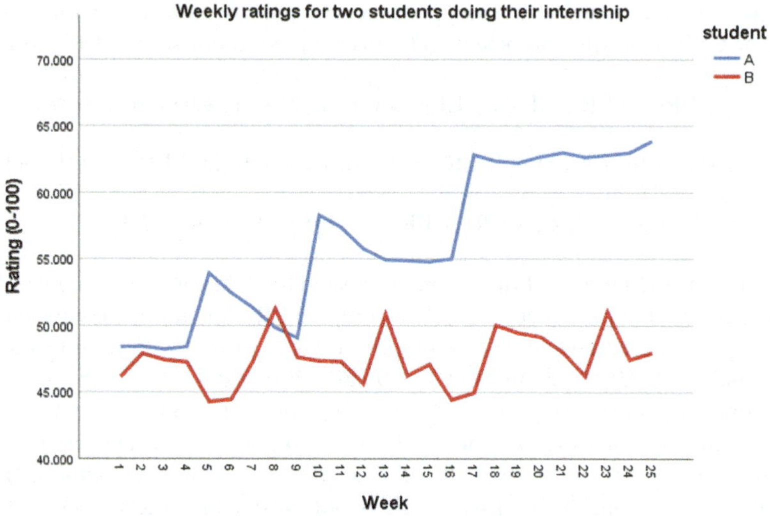

Fig. 4.1 Time series graphs of students' ratings on Skill X (0–100) in the first 25 weeks of their longitudinal clerkship at Hospital X (SPSS)

documented properly, these experiences can result in very powerful narratives about the growth and development of individual students as well as regarding the functioning of teams. Well-developed rating scales may help to structure some of these narratives, and vice versa, some of the narratives may facilitate our understanding of growth or stagnation of individual students in different phases of the clerkship.

Figure 4.1 presents time series graphs of two students who have been doing a longitudinal clerkship in Hospital X for nearly half a year. The students have weekly team meetings, on the Fridays in the early afternoon, where cases, incidents, and developments are discussed, and feedback is provided. Both students receive narrative feedback from two doctors and two nurses in the team and receive ratings on a VAS from 0 (minimum) to 100 (maximum) from the two doctors (i.e., a single rating based on consensus between the two doctors) every Friday morning. Each student receives ratings on a series of skills defined prior to the longitudinal clerkship, in line with the learning outcomes of that clerkship. Figure 4.1 provides the ratings on one of these skills, Skill X.

While Student A demonstrates a clear growth over the 25 weeks, Student B does not. In the case of Student A, we see a clear increase from one week to the next at three points in time: week 5, week 10, and week 17. These happen to be weeks that included an intensive four-hour training session on the Monday afternoon. Student A has always been present, has attended the three trainings, and that is visible in the growth trajectory. However, Student B missed the training in week 5 and was offered a similar training in week 7, missed the training in week 10, and attended the training in week 17 but did not improve by much after that.

Note that we are already using information *not* included in the graph to help to understand each of the two trajectories (i.e., A and B). Other evidence to facilitate the understanding of these trajectories could come from a variety of sources, including: patient feedback during the clerkship, weekly ratings of other skills, weekly narrative feedback provided by the doctors and nurses, and the students' module or block performance assessments in the medical programme. While these graphs cannot be understood in the absence of any kind of context, ratings like these can help different stakeholders put things into context and see how things are developing. Besides, if we asked the students to rate their own skills prior to receiving the ratings from the doctors, that could help to facilitate reflection and discourse on the development of metacognitive skills. As explained in Chap. 1, with the development of metacognitive skills, one would expect initial discrepancies between doctors' ratings of a student's performance and that student's own ratings to decrease with time.

4.4 Review and Meta-Analysis

Where longitudinal assessment can provide a multitude of pieces of evidence that each shed light on somewhat different aspects of individual competence, replications and meta-analytic and review studies provide researchers with very powerful tools for developing *chains of evidence* regarding empirical phenomena of interest in our fields (Leppink & Pérez-Fuster, 2016). As discussed in Chaps. 2 and 3 in this book, sample-to-sample fluctuation in estimates of phenomena of interest is normal and should be expected to be large especially when sample sizes are relatively small. In educational research, small samples are common, and documentation of the study procedure and other choices made is often incomplete. The latter makes it difficult to undertake replication research in the first place, and even where it is possible to replicate a study, with small samples findings can fluctuate considerably from study to study.

4.4.1 Measurements

Apart from group differences, treatment effects, and other phenomena commonly of interest, the very ways in which we measure variables of interest are in need of a chain of evidence. Suppose, we are interested in establishing a chain of evidence for the statement that a new instrument, Test Z, provides a one-dimensional measure of understanding of basic probability calculus among high school students. Test Z presents 20 short cases. In each case, the individual test taker has to filter some information in order to do a simple calculation that results in a simple, single probability as a response to the question. For each case, there is only one correct answer, and any response can be coded as either 'correct' or 'incorrect' (i.e., there is no such a thing as 'partially correct'). If the 'one dimension' statement is true, we can combine item scores into a single test score and interpret that as a measure of understanding of basic probability calculus, with higher scores (i.e., more correct performance) indicating a better understanding. Three types of evidence can provide support for the statement.

First, if the 20 short-case items resemble items used in instruments that are already known to measure understanding of basic probability calculus, this provides initial face-value evidence for the statement. However, without data, we are just another opinion that may be proven wrong once we have data.

Second, once we collect data and we see that a one-latent-variable model fits well, we gain initial evidence for the set of items measuring a single trait or state of interest. With this initial evidence, it is time for a next study where we administer in a large sample of students both Test Z and an instrument that is already reasonably known to measure the variable of interest (e.g., Messick, 1989), here: understanding of basic probability calculus. Let us call this well-established instrument 'Y'. Test Z results in a score *Z* and instrument Y results in score *Y*; if both instruments yield scores that are supposed to reflect better understanding when they are higher, we should find a substantial positive correlation between *Y* and *Z*. The sample should be large enough to counterbalance the order in which the instruments are administered, and we should be able to find a substantial positive correlation between *Y* and *Z* in both order conditions.

Third, provided that we do find evidence for unidimensionality and a positive correlation between *Y* and *Z*, we should now search for an evidence-based effective intervention aimed at improving understanding of basic probability calculus and make that part of a randomised controlled experiment. That is, in a new study, we would randomly allocate a large random sample of students to an intervention (i.e., treatment) and a no-intervention (i.e., control) condition. For reasons of ethics, both groups could be provided the treatment, but the control condition would only receive it *after* completing Test Z and Instrument Y, whereas the treatment condition would receive it *before* completing Test Z and Instrument Y. Provided that we use an intervention that has received good empirical support in terms of its effectiveness to improve high students' understanding of basic probability calculus, we should be able to find positive correlations between *Y* and *Z* in both the treatment and the control condition and performance on both *Y* and *Z* should on average be substantially higher in the treatment condition than in the control condition. Again, we could counterbalance the order in which the instruments are considered, now in both the treatment and control condition, and we should be able to find positive correlations between *Y* and *Z* in both treatment and control condition and on average better performance on both *Y* and *Z* for both instrument orders.7

4.4.2 Arguments

Together, the aforementioned factors—face-value evidence based on comparisons with at least one well-established instrument, empirical support for the correlation between the new instrument and the well-established instrument, and expected differences in response to experimental manipulation—provide a coherent validity argument (Kane, 2006) or chain of evidence (cf. Leppink, 2017; Wagenaar et al., 1993). Although the different studies may not be completely independent and using any hard numbers is likely impossible, in terms of the previously discussed LR_E approach, evidence in favour of all three factors means $LR_x > 1$ for each of these pieces of evidence and that all contributes to a higher LR_E in favour of the statement that Test Z provides a unidimensional measure of the understanding of basic probability calculus.

4.5 Documenting and Storytelling

Quantitative differences are qualitative differences that have been counted or measured, because we came to understand some centuries ago that we can use mathematics and probability to reasonably understand and predict the occurrence and absence of many phenomena, and that this understanding and prediction become easier with more trials (e.g., larger samples of people, larger numbers of measurements from the same people). Many people who do not have a background in Mathematics, Statistics, Econometrics or other fields where probability is important do not understand how probability works and then easily dismiss statistics as 'useless', as 'lies' or labels alike. When Donald J. Trump won the 2016 presidential election in the United States after pollsters had predicted Hillary Clinton would probably win, newspapers wrote about the 'failure' of statistics and people on social media judged accordingly with statements like 'this shows that Big Data is not ready for primetime and in my view it never will be'. If the outcome of a poll is that Hillary Clinton has a 75% chance of winning the elections and Donald J. Trump has a 25% chance of winning, that does not mean that statistics is great if Hillary Clinton wins and it is bad if Donald J. Trump wins. Most of us would probably not board a train that had a 25% of ending in a severe crash, because most of us would consider 25% a serious chance. Likewise, 25% chance of winning an election is a real chance. It is like a game of tossing two fair coins; there are four possible combinations, each with a probability of 25%, and one of these combinations yields two heads (cf. Donald J. Trump winning the election). Although not very likely before the game, in 25% of the cases where people play the game this is the outcome.

Qualitative differences can be conceived as quantitative differences that have been categorised either because the way we have set up our study does not allow us to be more precise or because we have not really found a way to quantify the differences. Where we can quantify pieces of evidence, doing so can help us to enhance our understanding of evidence in a given situation. However, even where we cannot (yet) really quantify pieces of evidence, the laws of mathematics and probability can still provide a thinking framework and help to make sense of the evidence to some degree.

Statistics is not limited to linear relations with large samples; the criminal case, the competence assessment case, and the longitudinal clerkship provide three easy counterexamples. Numbers can help to facilitate and structure discourse, and narrative information can help to understand some of the numbers, in large samples as well as in case studies. National health interview surveys employ different types of random sampling and can ask for all kinds of information, much of which can be quantified and some of which perhaps not yet or at least not easily. Many case studies do not result from random sampling, yet statistics can be very useful in understanding phenomena of interest. In Education, numbers mean nothing in isolation, but is that any different for words? Any kind of information needs to be interpreted in a broader context; whether we talk about a criminal case, the assessment of competence of students, following learners longitudinally, smaller or larger empirical studies, or meta-analytic and review studies, it is all about integrating different pieces of evidence and anchoring them into facts and common sense to provide a coherent chain of evidence or validity argument in favour of one hypothesis relative to one or several competing hypotheses, beyond reasonable doubt. And to be able to make that argument in such a way that it convinces other researchers, professionals in educational practice and/or policymakers, we should carefully document all steps and choices made, so that the reader can decide what to do with the argument or, where applicable and possible, to reasonably *reproduce* the findings and conclusions using the same methods on the same data or to *replicate* the project in their own setting.

References

Bayes, T. (1763). LII. An essay towards solving a problem in the doctrine of chances. By the late Rev. Mr. Bayes, F. R. S. communicated by Mr. Price, in a letter to John Canton, A. M. F. R. S. *Philosophical Transactions*, *53*, 370–418. https://doi.org/10.1098/rstl.1763.0053.

Kane, M. T. (2006). Validation. In R. L. Brennan (Ed.), *Educational measurement* (4th ed., pp. 17–64). Westport: Praeager.

Laplace, P. (1812). *Analytique des probabilités*. Paris: Courcier.

Leppink, J. (2017). Evaluating the strength of evidence in research and education: The theory of anchored narratives. *Journal of Taibah University Medical Sciences, 12*(4), 284–290. https://doi.org/10.1016/j.jtumed.2017.01.002.

Leppink, J., & Pérez-Fuster, P. (2016). What is science without replication? *Perspectives on Medical Education, 5*(6), 320–322. https://doi.org/10.1007/s40037-016-0307-z.

Messick, S. (1989). Validity. In R. L. Linn (Ed.), *Educational measurement* (3rd ed., pp. 13–103). New York: Macmillan.

Wagenaar, W. A., Van Koppen, P. J., & Crombag, H. F. M. (1993). *Anchored narratives: The psychology of criminal evidence*. Hertfordshire, UK: Harvester Wheatsheaf.

Part II
Variable Types

Pass/Fail and Other Dichotomies

5

Abstract

Dichotomous variables are omnipresent in educational research and practice. MCQ performance, for example, is often coded as 'correct' or 'incorrect'. In a broader perspective, many decisions in educational practice are of a 'pass/fail' nature. Dropout—from research or from an educational programme or activity—can be conceived as a dichotomous variable as well. These and other examples of dichotomous outcome variables, some of which are observed once in time and some of which are observed at several occasions during a longer time interval, are discussed in this chapter, with appropriate analytic methods.

5.1 Introduction

Dichotomous variables are very common in educational research and practice, both as outcomes and as predictors. Treatment factors and other grouping variables are common predictor variables. Common outcome variables include pass/fail decisions, correct/incorrect item performance as well as dropout (yes/no) or the occurrence versus absence of missing data (for a brief overview of missing data methods, see also Chap. 3). Examples of these outcome variables are discussed in this chapter.

5.2 Study 1: Predicting Exam Outcomes

Of a group of 235 candidates who signed up for a General Practice licencing exam in a country where English is the official language, 159 are foreign (i.e., come from other countries) and 152 are non-native speakers (i.e., English is their second, third

J. Leppink, *The Art of Modelling the Learning Process*, Springer Texts in Education,
https://doi.org/10.1007/978-3-030-43082-5_5

Table 5.1 Joint distribution of the two grouping variables (foreigner: 0 = no, 1 = yes; language: 0 = native, 1 = non-native) and the outcome variable of interest (exam outcome: 0 = fail, 1 = pass)

		Exam outcome	
Language	Foreigner	Fail (0)	Pass (1)
Native (0)	No (0)	12	25
	Yes (1)	12	34
Non-native (1)	No (0)	12	27
	Yes (1)	65	48

or fourth language). Of this group of 235 candidates, 134 candidates pass the exam, which corresponds with a 57.0% pass rate. However, the organisers of the exam want to know to what extent being a foreigner and/or being a non-native speaker can predict exam performance and in what direction(s). Table 5.1 presents the joint distribution of these two grouping variables and exam outcome (pass vs. fail), which constitutes the outcome variable of interest.

Thus, there are 37 native non-foreigners, 46 native foreigners, 39 non-native foreigners (i.e., candidates who were born in the country but due to the language spoken at home in their early childhood years do not consider themselves native English speakers), and 113 non-native foreigners. Ideally, predictor variables should not correlate. However, unless we deal with carefully designed and well controlled experiments, we rarely find ourselves in that ideal situation, and we may still proceed with the different predictor variables under consideration if the correlation is not too strong.

5.2.1 Measures of Explained Variance for Categorical Outcome Variables

When dealing with outcome variables of interval or ratio level of measurement (Stevens, 1946), squaring Pearson's r (R^2) yields an estimate of the proportion of variance explained in the outcome variable by the predictor or combination of predictor variables in the model, and when several predictor variables are considered some will prefer *adjusted* R^2, which is a bit lower than R^2, to provide a penalty for model complexity. In the case of categorical outcome variables, quite a variety of different R^2-statistics have been proposed in the literature (e.g., Menard, 2000; Mittlbock & Schemper, 1996).

An R^2-statistic that is similar to R^2 for non-categorical outcome variables is McFadden's R^2_{McF} McFadden (1974). Suppose, we want to understand to what extent we can explain being or not being a native English speaker by being or not being a foreigner, using the data provided in Table 5.1. In a model *without* predictor variables, the so-called *null model* (henceforth: Model 0), has a deviance (−2LL) of 305.218, and we find AIC = 307.218 and BIC = 310.678 (*JASP*). In a model *with* the predictor variable of interest (henceforth: Model 1), we find: −2LL = 296.593,

AIC = 300.593, and BIC = 307.512. Model 0 represents $\boldsymbol{H_0}$: 'no relation', whereas Model 1 represents $\boldsymbol{H_1}$: 'being or not being a foreigner and being or not being a native English speaker are related'. Both AIC and BIC prefer Model 1 ($\boldsymbol{H_1}$). With a LR test at $df = 1$ (because the difference between models is a dichotomous predictor variable), we conclude the same: χ^2_1 = [−2LL Model 0] − [−2LL Model 1] = 8.625, $p = 0.003$.

R^2_{McF} can be computed directly from the −2LLs of the two competing models:

$$R^2_{\mathrm{McF}} = 1 - ([-2\mathrm{LL}\,\underline{\mathrm{Model}\,1}]/[-2\mathrm{LL}\,\underline{\mathrm{Model}\,0}]).$$

In this case, we find:

$$R^2_{\mathrm{McF}} = 1 - (296.593/305.218) \approx 0.028.$$

From the computation of χ^2, it follows that another way to compute R^2_{McF} is:

$$R^2_{\mathrm{McF}} = \chi^2/[-2\mathrm{LL}\,\underline{\mathrm{Model}\,0}] = 8.625/305.218 \approx 0.028.$$

Three other R^2-statistics that have enjoyed some popularity are Tjur's R^2_{T} (2009), Cox and Snell's R^2_{CS} (Cox & Snell, 1989; Cragg & Uhler, 1970; Maddala, 1983) and Nagelkerke's R^2_{N} (1991). However, these three alternatives have some undesirable features (e.g., Leppink, 2019a): contrary to what an R^2-statistic is supposed to do, R^2_{T} and R^2_{CS} have upper bounds (i.e., maximum values) below 1, which depend on the marginal probability; R^2_{N} is effectively a correction of R^2_{CS} in that R^2_{CS} is divided by its upper bound, but that can result in rather unrealistically high estimates in many situations. For weaker relations, all three alternatives can provide (unrealistically) high R^2-estimates. For the case at hand, we find (*JASP*): $R^2_{\mathrm{CS}} = 0.036$, $R^2_{\mathrm{N}} = 0.050$, and $R^2_{\mathrm{T}} = 0.134$. While 0.036 is not an unreasonable estimate for the data at hand, 0.050 is already more questionable, and 0.134 is outright unrealistic. Given the easy interpretation of R^2_{McF} and the problems of alternatives, R^2_{McF} probably remains the best R^2-statistic for categorical outcome variables (Kvålseth, 1985; Leppink, 2019a; Menard, 2000).

R^2_{McF} is very attractive in that it can be directly interpreted as a *deviance reduction factor* (DRF): R^2_{McF}-values of 0.10, 0.25 and 0.50, for example, can be interpreted as the model in question reducing −2LL (the deviance) of Model 0 by 10%, 25%, and 50%, respectively. This interpretation has many uses (e.g., Leppink, 2019a), as is also demonstrated in later chapters of this book.

Other useful statistics with regard to the magnitude of a relation of interest are Cramér's V (Cramér, 1946) and the *odds ratio* (OR) and ln(OR) (the latter is also called log OR or logit and is found by taking the natural logarithm, ln, of the OR; Agresti, 2002). When all variables involved are dichotomous, Cramér's V yields the same point estimate as Pearson's r, Spearman's ρ, Kendall's τ coefficients, and coefficient φ (Agresti, 2002; Guilford, 1936), and values of 0.1, 0.3, and 0.5 are commonly interpreted as 'small', 'medium', and 'large' effects, but these labels are associated with larger values when both variables involved have three or more categories (Cohen, 1988; Lipsey & Wilson, 2001).

5.2.2 Multiple Competing Models

The association between being or not being a foreigner and being or not being a native speaker is rather weak and should not stop us from considering models where both predictor variables are present. In the prediction of exam performance, five competing models can be identified:

Model 0: *the null model*, without any predictor variable;
Model 1: being or not being a *foreigner* as predictor;
Model 2: being or not being a *native* speaker as predictor;
Model 3: both *foreigner* and *native* speaker as predictors; and
Model 4: *full model*, Model 3 + a combined (i.e., *interaction*) effect of foreigner and native.

Table 5.2 presents R^2_{McF}, −2LL, AIC, and BIC of each of these five models.

The difference in R^2_{McF} between Model 3 and Model 4, which as we have seen can be computed directly from the difference in −2LL between these two models (i.e., 1 − [301.660/306.857] ≈ 0.017), is indicative of the magnitude of the interaction term, since that is the only term by which Model 3 (no interaction) and Model 4 (interaction) can be distinguished. Given that both foreigner and native are dichotomous variables (i.e., $df = 1$), the interaction term has $df = 1$ as well. The resulting LR test of the interaction effect yields: $\chi^2_1 = 5.197$, $p = 0.023$. AIC also prefers Model 4, but BIC prefers Model 2; the latter is not convinced by the modest increases in R^2_{McF} from Model 2 to Model 3 and Model 4.

What does the interaction pattern look like? As can be computed from Table 5.1, pass rates are 67.6% for non-foreign natives, 73.9% for foreign natives, 69.2% for non-foreign non-natives, and 42.5% for foreign non-natives. In a substantially larger sample, these same percentages would eventually result in BIC preferring the interaction model (Model 4), but for binary logistic regression (Agresti, 2002; Field, 2018) the sample size is fairly 'small' and hence BIC will be convinced by more complexity only if that increase in complexity comes with a more sizeable reduction of −2LL (and hence, a stronger increase in R^2_{McF}). In this case, researchers

Table 5.2 Five competing models in terms of R^2_{McF}, −2LL, AIC, and BIC (JASP)

Model	R^2_{McF}	−2LL	AIC	BIC
0: *null*	0.000	321.130	323.130	326.589
1: *foreign*	0.019	315.059	319.059	325.978
2: *native*	0.033	310.522	314.522	321.441
3: *foreign* + *native*	0.044	306.857	312.857	323.236
4: *full*	0.061	301.660	309.660	323.498

who prefer the LR test or AIC may interpret the interaction effect, whereas researchers who are inclined to prefer BIC will likely refrain from interpreting the interaction effect.

5.3 Study 2: Predicting Dropout

In a MOOC, large groups of individuals can sign up to learn about a topic of interest. Although the extent of dropout varies considerably across settings, dropout is a problem and understanding it may help to reduce dropout. A group of researchers interested in this phenomenon of dropout in MOOCs have access to a random sample of $N = 682$ individuals who have signed up for a MOOC on problem-based learning. Although the vast majority of individuals who usually sign up for this MOOC have a background in Education, there is substantial interest in this MOOC among people who do not (yet) have that background as well. In the sample of $N = 682$, $n = 481$ participants (70.5%) have at least a Bachelor's degree in Education while the remaining $n = 201$ participants (29.5%) do not meet that criterion. The researchers are interested in the extent to which background (Education vs. other) can help to explain and predict dropout.

5.3.1 Dropout Versus Completion

In both groups, 46 participants drop out of the MOOC. However, *proportionally*, this number looks different for the two groups: about 9.56% of 481 participants in the Education group versus around 22.89% of 201 participants in the non-Education group. For Model 0 (i.e., *null model*), we find: −2LL = 539.587, AIC = 541.587, and BIC = 546.112. For Model 1 (i.e., groups model), we find: −2LL = 519.630, AIC = 523.630, and BIC = 532.680. The LR test yields: $\chi^2_1 = 19.957, p < 0.001$. In short, all criteria prefer Model 1. For R^2_{McF} of Model 1, we find 0.037. The *OR* is 2.806 with a 90% CI of [1.927; 4.087] (ln(OR) = 1.032 with 90% CI of [0.656; 1.408]), and Cramér's $V = 0.178$.

5.3.2 Dropout and Time

The duration of the full MOOC is 24 weeks, and each week a different subtopic of problem-based learning is covered. Figure 5.1 presents the histograms of the distribution of the number of weeks completed among the dropouts in both groups.

The number of weeks completed among dropouts varies from 10 to 23 ($M = 15.804$, $SD = 2.802$) in the Education group and from 11 to 21 ($M = 16.043$, $SD = 2.413$) in the non-Education group. This results in $d = 0.091$ with a 90% CI of [−0.252; 0.434].

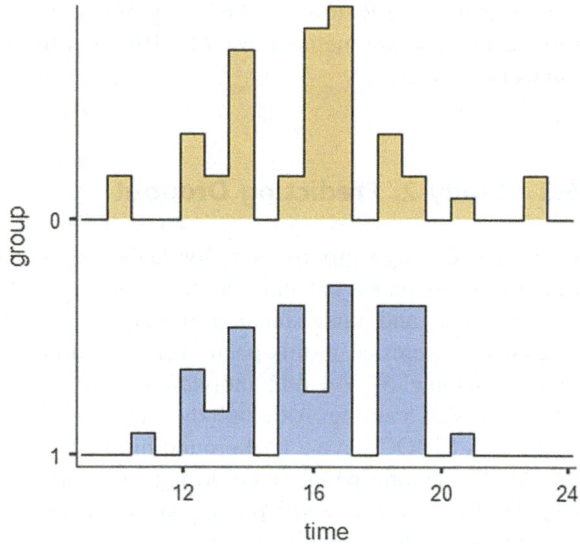

Fig. 5.1 Distribution of number of weeks completed among dropouts in the Education (group = 0) and non-Education group (group = 1) (*Jamovi*)

Figure 5.2 displays the *survival curve* (Kaplan & Meier, 1958) of the completion (i.e., survival) rates in the two groups (*Jamovi*). The survival rate in group *X* is found by dividing the number of participants surviving longer than time point *t* by the total number of participants in group *X*.

Another way to plot the difference between groups is in terms of *cumulative hazard* (Peterson, 1977). As long as the survival is 1 (100%), the cumulative hazard

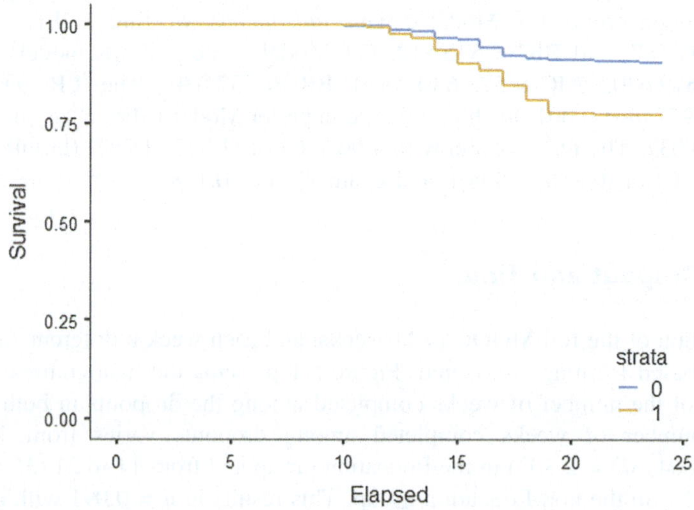

Fig. 5.2 Survival plot of Study 2 (0 = Education, 1 = non-Education) (*Jamovi*)

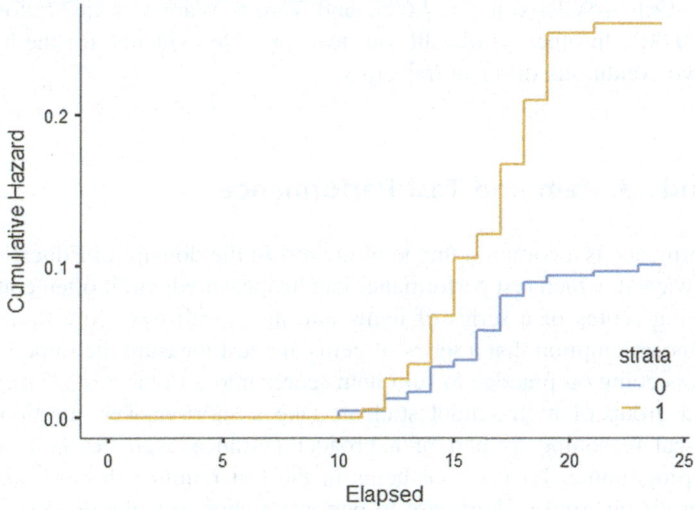

Fig. 5.3 Cumulative hazard function of Study 2 (0 = Education, 1 = non-Education) (Jamovi)

equals 0. Once we start to see dropouts, the survival rate goes down to 1, while the cumulative hazard starts to go up from 0. The cumulative hazard, which is also referred to as the *conditional failure rate*, is the event at time point *t* conditional on surviving up to or beyond time *t*. Figure 5.3 presents the cumulative hazard function for Study 2.

Figures 5.2 and 5.3 illustrate that, apart from the very beginning of dropout, the proportion of dropout is higher in the non-Education group than in the Education group throughout the trajectory. Different tests can be used to study the difference between groups in this trajectory of dropout in terms of statistical significance: the nonparametric *log-rank* test (Mantel, 1966; Mantel & Haenszel, 1959), the Gehan-Wilcoxon test (Gehan, 1965), the Peto-Peto test (Peto & Peto, 1972), and the Tarone-Ware test (Tarone & Ware, 1977). Key assumption in the use of the log-rank test is the *proportional hazard assumption*: the hazard ratio of the groups compared is proportional across time. When that assumption is not realistic, the other three options, which are based on the Wilcoxon *signed-rank test* (Wilcoxon, 1945) and for that reason are also called *generalised Wilcoxon tests*, are usually better; they differ from the log-rank test as well as from each other in how they deal with multiple dropouts at a given time point *t* and the extent to which they give more weight to earlier than to later dropouts (i.e., in the log-rank test, all accidents have the same weight). The classical test is more efficient than its alternatives whenever the proportional hazard assumption is realistic, whereas the alternatives are more efficient in the case of (substantial) departures from that assumption (Harrington & Fleming, 1982). When in doubt, reporting all four tests is always an option. Doing so, in Study 2, we find (Jamovi): log-rank $z = 4.657$, Peto-Peto

$z = 3.968$, Gehan-Wilcoxon $z = 4.605$, and Tarone-Ware $z = 4.632$; for all four tests, $p < 0.001$. In other words, all four tests provide evidence for the hypothesis that the two conditions differ in trajectory.

5.4 Study 3: Item and Test Performance

Test performance is a common theme of interest in the domain of Education. There are many ways in which test performance can be measured, but it often comes down to combining scores of a series of items into an overall test score. For example, based on the assumption that a series of items in a test measure the same variable of interest, it is common practice to sum item scores into a (total) test score. Suppose, we have a group of high school students take a short-answer questions test on mathematical reasoning as part of a broader entrance exam to an International Business programme. Each of ten items in the test requires the test taker to use some information from a short case to perform a short calculation. Based on previous research that has been carefully documented in the literature, it is reasonable to treat the ten items in the test as one set of items measuring mathematical reasoning, even though these items do differ somewhat in difficulty.

Whether a student is allowed to take the entrance exam, of which the mathematical reasoning test is part, is to some extent a matter of lottery: although the top 10% performing students in the national high school central state exam in mathematics are admitted to the International Business programme without any entrance exam, all other students interested in the programme enter a lottery which results in a random sample of students having to take the entrance exam. This year, that is a group of 283 students. Due to logistic constraints, the students have to be randomly allocated to either a computer version of the mathematical reasoning test ($n = 139$) or a paper version of that test ($n = 144$).

5.4.1 Models for Group Differences in Test and Item Performance

One of the questions of concern in this situation is whether the two delivery formats of the test can reasonably be considered *parallel* or of 'the same' difficulty. An easy way to do this, which is common across fields in Education, is to compute the sum score of test performance from the ten items for the two groups and compare the two groups. Given ten items, each of which can result in an incorrect answer (coded: 0) or a correct answer (coded: 1), the sum score (i.e., test score) of a candidate can range from 0 to 10. Figure 5.4 presents the histograms of the distribution of test scores in the two groups.

In the computer group, test performance ranges from 2 to 9 with $M = 5.367$ and $SD = 1.716$. In the paper group, test performance ranges from 0 to 10 with $M = 5.368$ and $SD = 1.913$. For the difference between groups, we find $d \approx 0$ with

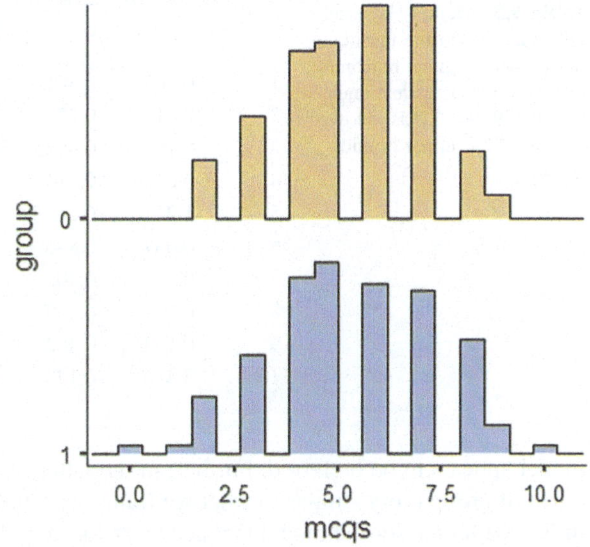

Fig. 5.4 Distribution of test scores in the two groups in Study 3 (0 = computer, 1 = paper) (*Jamovi*)

a 90% CI of [−0.196; 0.195] and $p = 0.996$. In short, it seems fairly safe to treat the two delivery formats as relatively or practically equivalent. Using a default JZS prior in *JASP* (Rouder, Speckman, Sun, Morey, & Iverson, 2012), BF in favour of $\boldsymbol{H_0}$: 'formats are equivalent' versus $\boldsymbol{H_1}$: 'formats are *not* equivalent' (i.e., BF_{01}) is 7.652, which provides positive evidence in favour of $\boldsymbol{H_0}$ (Jeffreys, 1961; Kass & Raftery, 1995), and the 95% CRI of d is [−0.227; 0.224]. In sum, whether we use TOST, ROPE or FOST, the outcomes are in support of our interpretation of the group difference in test performance as relatively or practically equivalent.

Alternative approaches to the question of group differences lie in *item* rather than overall *test* performance. Even if groups do not differ significantly in overall test performance, if important information in one or some of the questions was presented in a considerably poorer quality on paper than on screen, this may well have contributed to performance differences between groups on one or several items. If the two delivery formats can be considered equal, we should find evidence in favour of no group-by-item interaction, that is: the difference between groups in performance (here: proportion correct response) should not differ (significantly) across items. The resulting model is a *two-level* (i.e., upper level: student; lower level: item) *mixed-effects* (i.e., combining fixed and random effects) binary logistic regression model. In its easiest form, we assume that differences between students in mathematical reasoning ability result in a residual correlation across item pairs that is proportional to these differences. This residual covariance structure is also known as *compound symmetry* (CS) structure (e.g., Leppink, 2019a; Tan, 2010).

SPSS returns $p = 0.526$ for the interaction effect and AICc = 12508.484 and BIC = 12573.740 for the model that includes the interaction term (i.e., full factorial model) and AICc = 12491.498 and BIC = 12556.790 for the model *without* interaction term (i.e., main-effects-only model). In other words, the *no interaction*

Table 5.3 Mantel-Haenszel DIF analysis on the ten items in the mathematical reasoning test in Study 3: χ^2-test and OR with 95% CI (LB = lower bound, UB = upper bound) (Stata)

Item	χ^2_1	p	*OR*	95% CI LB	95% CI UB
1	0.767	0.381	1.380	0.749	2.542
2	0.410	0.522	0.762	0.394	1.473
3	0.191	0.662	0.852	0.494	1.469
4	0.012	0.914	1.008	0.587	1.732
5	1.221	0.269	1.396	0.822	2.371
6	0.037	0.848	0.921	0.557	1.525
7	0.695	0.405	0.772	0.457	1.304
8	0.031	0.859	0.923	0.554	1.539
9	0.704	0.402	0.757	0.435	1.318
10	2.416	0.120	1.637	0.930	2.883

model appears to be preferred. Further, in the latter, we find $p = 0.988$ for the main effect of group (very similar to what we found with the sum score comparison), and in line with that, for the model that accounts for item differences only (i.e., assumes the groups to be equal across items) we find AICc = 12487.257 and BIC = 12552.553. In other words, the latter model yields lower AICc and BIC values than the other two models and is therefore preferred in this comparison. We turn to differences between items in a bit.

A slightly different approach to detecting potential item bias is found in the Mantel-Haenszel approach to *differential item functioning* (DIF; Holland & Thayer, 1985, 1988; Mantel & Haenszel, 1959). Briefly put, this approach comes down to the following. If item A measures a variable of interest consistently, students from different groups who have the same mathematical reasoning *ability* (i.e., same position on the latent continuum from very low to very high ability) should have the same probability of a correct response to item A. In other words, students with ability X from the delivery formats should have the same probability P of responding to item A correctly. If this is not the case, there might be some form of bias and the item should undergo review. This logic can be applied to each item and in statistical practice results in an *OR* and χ^2-test for each item which tests $\boldsymbol{H_0}$: 'no DIF' against $\boldsymbol{H_1}$: 'DIF'. Table 5.3 presents the outcomes of that analysis, using Stata.

None of the items indicate any DIF. This in line with other group comparisons supports our decision to treat the group of $N = 283$ students as one group in the remainder of the analysis.

5.4.2 Item and Test Information

It is common practice to compute Cronbach's alpha (1951), which is the same as Guttman's lambda-3 (1945) and in the case of dichotomous items yields the same outcome as Kuder-Richardson's KR-20 coefficient for dichotomous items (Kuder &

Richardson, 1937), over a set of test items, and interpret this as an indicator the 'internal consistency' or 'reliability' of a test. Doing so for the data set at hand, we find 0.379. This practice may be useful when the different items are of more or less the same difficulty and the correlation is more or less the same across item pairs (cf. CS). In the case of dichotomous variables, the variance σ^2 is a direct function of the proportion π:

$$\sigma^2 = \pi * (1-\pi).$$

SD is the square root of the variance. From this formula, it becomes clear that considerable heterogeneity in item difficulty results in different *SD*s for different items. Moreover, in the case of dichotomous variables, that heterogeneity also contributes to differences in correlation across item pairs. These are two key violations of CS that tend to result in alpha underestimating test reliability (e.g., Leppink, 2019a, 2019b). For items that can be conceived as of at least interval level of measurement, several alternatives have been provided (for a review, see: Revelle & Zinbarg, 2009), including the Greatest Lower Bound (GLB; e.g., Peters, 2014; Sijtsma, 2009), variance-adjusted alpha (Leppink, 2019a, 2019b) and McDonald's omega (ω: e.g., Crutzen & Peters, 2017; Deng & Chan, 2017; Dunn, Baguley, & Brunsden, 2014; Green & Yang, 2009; Leppink, 2019a, 2019b; Peters, 2014; Revelle & Zinbarg, 2009; Trizano-Hermosilla & Alvarado, 2016; Watkins, 2017; Zhang & Yuan, 2016). However, these alternatives are not really suitable for dichotomous items, because some of the assumptions associated with them (e.g., approximately Normal distributions of residuals) do not hold. Besides, reliability is a function of test information (which is a function of item information), and test information is rarely if ever constant across the range of *ability*. Item response theory (IRT; e.g., Embretson & Reise, 2000; Hambleton, Swaminathan, & Rogers, 1991) can help us to estimate item and test information across the range of *ability* (θ).

Several types of IRT models exist, three of which are the *one-parameter logistic* (1PL), the *two-parameter logistic* (2PL), and the *three-parameter logistic* (3PL) model (e.g., Hambleton et al., 1991; Lord & Novick, 1968). In the 1PL model, *item difficulty* is allowed to vary across items; any item can be conceived as a battle between the item respondent with ability θ and the (difficulty of the) item, and more difficult items are less likely to be beaten (i.e., a lower probability of a correct response). In the 2PL model, both item difficulty and *item discrimination* are allowed to vary across items; the latter is the extent to which an item discriminates between students with a lower θ and students with a higher θ. For some items, the probability of a correct response may increase only very gradually with increasing θ (i.e., low discrimination parameter), while for other items that increase may be stronger (i.e., higher discrimination parameter). In the 3PL model, a *guessing* parameter is added to account for the probability of guessing a correct response.

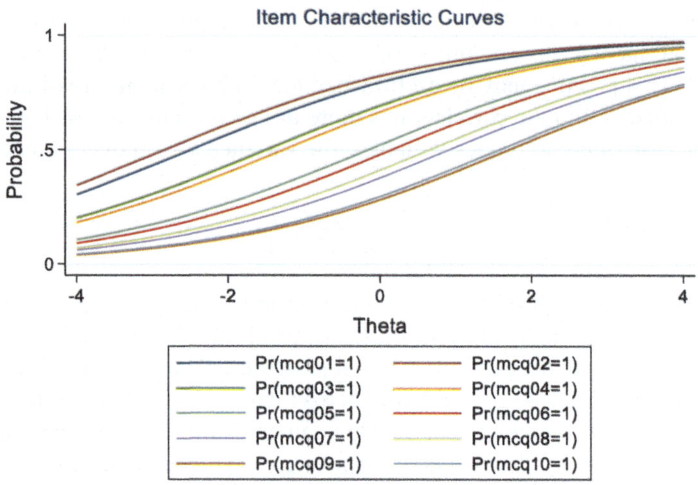

Fig. 5.5 Item characteristic curves according to the 1PL model in Study 3 (<u>*Stata*</u>)

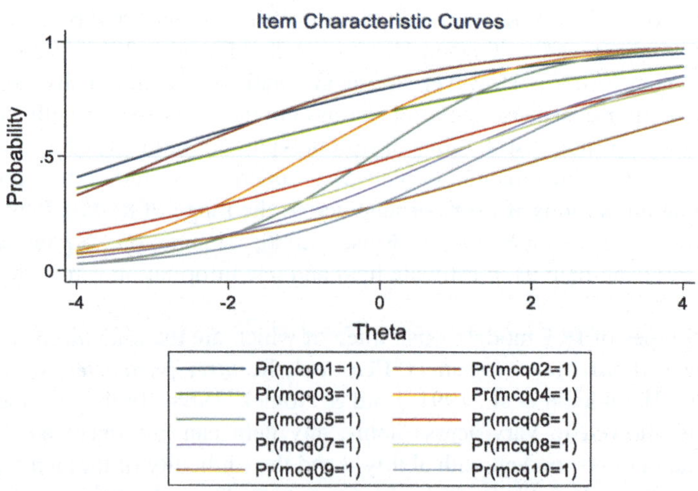

Fig. 5.6 Item characteristic curves according to the 2PL model in Study 3 (<u>*Stata*</u>)

The latter does not really make sense in our mathematical reasoning test, but the 1PL and 2PL model are worth exploring. Figures 5.5 and 5.6 present the item characteristic curves obtained with the 1PL and 2PL model, respectively, using <u>*Stata*</u>.

In Fig. 5.5, the slopes of the curve are equal at probability 0.5 (i.e., probability of a correct response being 1/2), while in Fig. 5.6 these slopes vary because the discrimination parameter varies across items. In both figures, item difficulty is the θ-value at probability 0.5: the ability at which one is expected to have 50% chance to

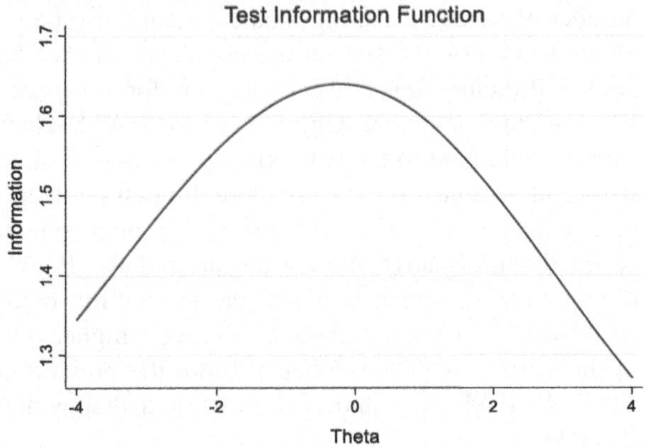

Fig. 5.7 TIF according to the 1PL model in Study 3 (<u>*Stata*</u>)

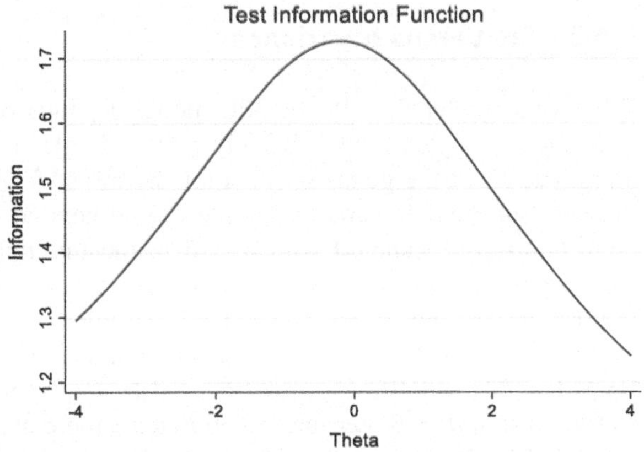

Fig. 5.8 TIF according to the 2PL model in Study 3 (<u>*Stata*</u>)

win the battle against the item. There are many other types of graphs we can obtain, but one of the important graphs is the so-called *test information function* (TIF) plot, which tells us how much information a test provides us with at different levels of θ. Figures 5.7 and 5.8 present the TIF for the 1PL and 2PL model, respectively, using <u>*Stata*</u>.

TIF can be used to compute the *SE* of measurement (SEM) and reliability (ρ):

$$\text{SEM} = 1/\sqrt{\text{TIF}}; \text{ and}$$
$$\rho = 1 - \text{SEM}^2 = 1 - (1/\text{TIF}).$$

In our case, the maximum TIF is slightly left of $\theta = 0$, because the items are on average slightly easier than a probability of 0.5: 1.640 in the 1PL model (SEM = 0.781, $\rho = 0.390$) and 1.727 in the 2PL model (SEM = 0.761, $\rho = 0.421$). However, the further we go towards the left or right of the θ-distribution, the lower the TIF and ρ. For higher TIF and ρ we could do two things. First, increasing the number of items measuring mathematical reasoning ability would help. Second, if all students took the test on the computer and we had a large bank of items with known difficulty level, we could opt for *computerised adaptive testing* (CAT; Wainer, 2000; Weiss & Kingsbury, 1984). With adaptive testing, items are sampled from an item bank such that correct performance on item A, or a sequence of items, will result in a next item being more difficult while incorrect performance on item A or a sequence of items will result in a next item being less difficult. Items are optimally informative if they are around the θ-level of the individual test taker (here: student), which is where the probability of a correct response is 50%. As such, with CAT we are likely to achieve a higher ρ with the same number of items or the same ρ with fewer items. From the previous formulas, it follows that with TIF = 4, SEM = 0.5 and $\rho = 0.750$, and that with TIF = 10, SEM $\approx$ 0.316 and $\rho = 0.900$.

5.4.3 Fit Versus Invariance

Whether to prefer the 1PL or 2PL model depends on a number of questions. To start, more complex models usually require larger samples. With the data at hand, Stata reaches convergence in just a few iterations for both the 1PL and 2PL model, but with substantially smaller samples going beyond 1PL may not work. Although there is no gold standard with regard to the minimum required sample size, one should probably not use the 1PL (model) with $N < 100$ and one should probably not use the 2PL model (let alone, more complex) with $N < 200$, and the larger the sample size the better. Next, for the situation at hand, we can do a LR test as usual: for 1PL, −2LL = 3492.143; for 2PL, −2LL = 3488.819; $\chi^2_9 = 3.324$, $p = 0.950$. It is a χ^2_9-test at $df = 9$, because given k items there are $k - 1$ more parameters to be estimated in the 2PL model than in the 1PL model. Reason for that is that in the 1PL one discrimination parameter is estimated that is supposed to hold for all items while in the 2PL model each item has its own discrimination parameter. The LR test indicates that we have insufficient evidence to prefer the 2PL model over the 1PL model.

However, there is another important reason to consider the 1PL model, or better: the older cousin of the 1PL model known as the *Rasch model* (Andrich, 2004; Bond & Fox, 2007; Rasch, 1960; Wright & Stone, 1979). To start, 1PL and 2PL (and its extensions into 3PL and beyond) are *probit* models (i.e., they use an inverse Normal link function), whereas the Rasch model is a logit model (i.e., it uses the logit link function, which is also used in *logistic regression*). Proponents of the 1PL model and its extensions generally argue that we should compare different models in terms of fit and opt for 2PL or 3PL (or even beyond) if the 1PL model does not fit well or extensions fit substantially better. However, proponents of the Rasch model argue that it is *not* about fitting models to data; rather, the Rasch model provides a mathematically robust measurement model that can help us to make sense of a particular theoretical framework and provide *invariant measures* (e.g., Engelhard, 1994) of the degree of θ of both participants and items. The rationale behind these measures is that a test taker with a higher θ should be more likely to correctly respond to an item than a test taker with a lower θ (regardless of which items are encountered), and that the probability of correct item response is lower for items of higher θ than for items of lower θ. For multicategory or polytomous (i.e., non-dichotomous) items, there is a variety of extensions of the Rasch model to choose from, including the *rating scale model* (Andrich, 1978; Embretson & Reise, 2000; Wright & Masters, 1982) and the *partial credit model* (Embretson & Reise, 2000; Masters, 1982; Masters & Wright, 1996). Other extensions of the Rasch model include the *binomial trials model* (Wright & Masters, 1982), the *Poisson model* (Rasch, 1960), the *Saltus model* (Wilson, 1989), the *many-faceted Rasch measurement model* (Linacre, 1989), the *linear logistic test model* (Fischer, 1973), and the *mixed Rasch model* (Rost, 1990, 1991). The latter combines principles of the Rasch model and *latent class analysis* (Ding, 2018; Hagenaars & McCutcheon, 2002; McCutcheon, 1987; see next paragraph), meaning that the Rasch model is applied within each class and the parameters obtained from the Rasch model are allowed to vary across classes.

Software packages like GR provide a range of options for Rasch modelling; they can provide θ-estimates for items as well as for different sum scores (i.e., different test takers) as well as person-specific and overall residual-based item fit statistics and a variety of plots including item characteristic curves and TIF curves. For example, Fig. 5.9 presents the TIF function (upper graph) and individual item information functions (lower graphs) obtained with GR.

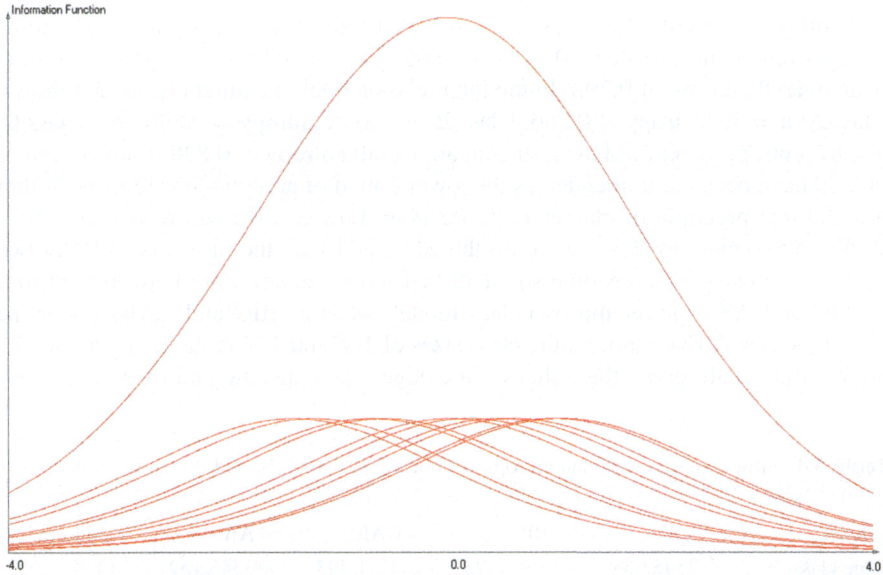

Fig. 5.9 TIF and item information functions in Study 3 (GR): information function (vertical) versus θ (horizontal)

This kind of graphs helps to understand that individual items have limited information, but a series of items give more information, and where the TIF is most informative depends on where (most of) the items are most informative.

5.4.4 Latent Classes

Another thing that software packages like GR enable us to do is *latent class analysis*. In the Rasch model, as well as in the 1PL model and its extensions, we treat the group of test takers as (a sample from) one class (i.e., coming from one population). However, there are situations where the test takers are best viewed as coming from two or more classes, and Rasch analysis may then be applied to each of these classes (cf. mixed Rasch as in Rost, 1990, 1991). Table 5.4 presents information criteria and entropy, a fit criterion in latent class analysis, for the one-class, two-class, and three-class solution returned by GR.

CAIC is an extension of AIC developed by Bozdogan (1987) that, somewhat like BIC, provides a stricter penalty for adding more parameters and as such reduces the likelihood of too complex models being selected when many parameters can be estimated. Entropy values provide an indication of the accuracy of classification. With only one class, accuracy is 100% (hence: entropy = 1), because there is no misclassification. When more than one class is involved, there will virtually always be some misclassification. In the two-class model, 135 of the 283 test takers are classified into Class A and the other 148 test takers are classified into Class B. That is, each individual receives latent class probabilities, and the class where that probability is highest is the class to which that individual is assigned. GR returns class-specific entropy values: 0.788 for Class A and 0.807 for Class B. This results in an overall entropy of 0.798. In the three-class model, the numbers are as follows: Class A: $n = 49$, entropy = 0.766; Class B: $n = 167$, entropy = 0.846; and Class C: $n = 67$, entropy = 0.827. This results in an overall entropy of 0.828. Entropy values of 0.80 have been recommended as the lower bound of acceptable values for further use and interpretation of classes (e.g., Pearson, Lawless, Brown, & Bravo, 2015). With the two-class model, we are on the edge, and with the three-class model two of the three class sizes become so small that most outcomes are hard to interpret.

AIC and AICc prefer the two-class model, whereas BIC and CAIC prefer the one-class model. Even though the class sizes of 148 and 135 in the two-class model are not that small, given the rather on-the-edge (class-specific and overall) entropy

Table 5.4 Information criteria and entropy for one-class, two-class, and three-class solutions in Study 3 (GR)

Model	AIC	BIC	CAIC	AICc	Entropy
One class	3545.038	3581.493	3591.493	3545.152	1
Two classes	3528.562	3605.117	3626.117	3528.808	0.798
Three classes	3536.906	3653.560	3685.560	3537.294	0.828

Table 5.5 Estimated probabilities of correct response per item for the one-class and the two-class model (*GR*)

	One-class model	Two-class model	
Item	*P*(correct)	Class A, *P*(correct)	Class B, *P*(correct)
1	0.784	0.862	0.713
2	0.813	0.916	0.719
3	0.686	0.763	0.615
4	0.661	0.829	0.508
5	0.523	0.706	0.356
6	0.484	0.590	0.388
7	0.389	0.511	0.277
8	0.420	0.537	0.314
9	0.297	0.383	0.218
10	0.311	0.459	0.176

estimates and the lack of a theoretical justification for the presence of two classes, I would be inclined to prefer the one-class solution in this case. However, for the sake of the example, Table 5.5 presents the estimated probabilities of correct response per item for the one-class and the two-class model (*GR*).

The estimates of the one-class model are simply the observed probabilities correct response in the entire sample of 283 students. In the two-class model, the probability correct is consistently higher in Class A than in Class B. Again, although there are situations where this two-class approach is useful, in the absence of theory as well as the absence of other variables that can help to explain class membership to a reasonable extent, it is difficult to interpret in this situation. Moreover, while in the situation at hand the two-class model results in classes of almost equal proportions (47.7% of the students are classified as A, and the remaining 52.3% of the students are classified as B), the more class membership percentages go down the larger the sample size required to obtain meaningful estimates.

References

Agresti, A. (2002). *Categorical data analysis* (2nd ed.). New York: Wiley.

Andrich, D. (1978). Application of a psychometric model to ordered categories which are scored with successive integers. *Applied Psychological Measurement*, *2*, 581–594. https://doi.org/10.1177/014662167800200413.

Andrich, D. (2004). Controversy and the Rasch model: A characteristic of incompatible paradigms? In E. V. Smith Jr., & R. M. Smith (Eds.), *Introduction to Rasch measurement* (pp. 143–166). Maple Grove, MN: JAM Press.

Bond, T., & Fox, C. M. (2007). *Applying the Rasch model: Fundamental measurement in the human sciences*. Mahwah, NJ: *Erlbaum*. https://doi.org/10.1186/1471-2377-13-78..

Bozdogan, H. (1987). Model selection and Akaike's Information Criterion (AIC): The general theory and its analytical extensions. *Psychometrika, 52*(3), 345–370. https://doi.org/10.1007/BF02294361.

Cohen, J. (1988). *Statistical power analysis for the behavioural sciences*. New York: Routledge.

Cox, D. R., & Snell, E. J. (1989). *Analysis of binary data* (2nd ed.). New York: Chapman & Hall.

Cragg, J. G., & Uhler, R. S. (1970). The demand for automobiles. *The Canadian Journal of Economics, 3*(3), 386–406. https://doi.org/10.2307/133656.

Cramér, H. (1946). *Mathematical methods of statistics*. Princeton, NJ: Princeton University Press.

Cronbach, L. J. (1951). Coefficient alpha and the internal structure of tests. *Psychometrika, 16*(3), 297–334. https://doi.org/10.1007/BF02310555.

Crutzen, R., & Peters, G. J. Y. (2017). Scale quality: Alpha is an inadequate estimate and factor-analytic evidence is needed first of all. *Health Psychology Review, 11*(3), 242–247. https://doi.org/10.1080/17437199.2015.1124240.

Deng, L., & Chan, W. (2017). Testing the difference between reliability coefficients alpha and omega. *Educational and Psychological Measurement, 77*(2), 185–203. https://doi.org/10.1177/0013164416658325.

Ding, C. S. (2018). *Fundamentals of applied multidimensional scaling for educational and psychological research*. New York: Springer. https://doi.org/10.1007/978-3-319-78172-3.

Dunn, T. J., Baguley, T., & Brunsden, V. (2014). From alpha to omega: A practical solution to the pervasive problem of internal consistency estimation. *British Journal of Psychology, 105*(3), 399–412. https://doi.org/10.1111/bjop.12046.

Embretson, S. E., & Reise, S. P. (2000). *Item response theory for psychologists*. Mahwah, NJ: Erlbaum.

Engelhard, G. (1994). Historical views of the concept of invariance in measurement theory. In M. Wilson (Ed.), *Objective measurement: Theory into practice* (Vol. 2, pp. 73–99). Norwood, NJ: Ablex.

Field, A. (2018). *Discovering statistics using IBM SPSS statistics* (5th ed.). London: Sage.

Fischer, G. H. (1973). The linear logistic test model as an instrument in educational research. *Acta Psychologica, 37*, 359–374. https://doi.org/10.1016/0001-6918(73)90003-6.

Gehan, E. (1965). A generalized Wilcoxon test for comparing arbitrarily singly-censored samples. *Biometrika, 52*(1/2), 203–223. https://doi.org/10.2307/2333825.

Green, S. G., & Yang, Y. (2009). Commentary on coefficient alpha: A cautionary tale. *Psychometrika, 74*, 169–173. https://doi.org/10.1007/s11336-008-9098-4.

Guilford, J. (1936). *Psychometric methods*. New York: McGraw-Hill.

Guttman, L. (1945). A basis for analyzing test-retest reliability. *Psychometrika, 10*(4), 255–282. https://doi.org/10.1007/BF02288892.

Hagenaars, J. A., & McCutcheon, A. L. (2002). *Applied latent class analysis*. Cambridge: Cambridge University Press.

Hambleton, R. K., Swaminathan, H., & Rogers, H. J. (1991). *Fundamentals of item response theory*. London: Sage.

Harrington, D. P., & Fleming, T. R. (1982). A class of rank test procedures for censored survival data. *Biometrika, 69*(3), 553–566. https://doi.org/10.1093/biomet/69.3.553.

Holland, P. W., & Thayer, D. T. (1985). *An alternative definition of the ETS delta scale of item difficulty* (ETS Program Statistics Research Technical Report No. 85–64). Princeton, NJ: ETS.

Holland, P. W., & Thayer, D. T. (1988). Differential item functioning and the Mantel-Haenszel procedure. In H. Wainer & H. I. Braun (Eds.), *Test validity* (pp. 129–145). Hillsdale, NJ: Erlbaum.

Jeffreys, H. (1961). *Theory of probability*. Oxford: Oxford University Press.

Kaplan, E. L., & Meier, P. (1958). Nonparametric estimation from incomplete data. *Journal of the American Statistical Association, 53*(282), 457–481. https://doi.org/10.2307/2281868.

Kass, R. E., & Raftery, A. E. (1995). Bayes factors. *Journal of the American Statistical Association, 90*(430), 773–795. https://doi.org/10.1080/01621459.1995.10476572.

Kuder, G. F., & Richardson, M. W. (1937). The theory of the estimation of test reliability. *Psychometrika, 2*(3), 151–160. https://doi.org/10.1007/BF02288391.

Kvålseth, T. O. (1985). Cautionary note about R^2. *The American Statistician, 39*, 279–285. https://doi.org/10.1080/00031305.1985.10479448.

Leppink, J. (2019a). *Statistical methods for experimental research in education and psychology*. Cham: Springer. https://doi.org/10.1007/978-3-030-21241-4.

Leppink, J. (2019b). How we underestimate reliability and overestimate resources needed: Revisiting our psychometric practice. *Health Professions Education, 5*(2), 91–92. https://doi.org/10.1016/j.hpe.2019.05.003.

Linacre, J. M. (1989). *Many-faceted Rasch measurement*. Chicago: MESA Press.

Lipsey, M., & Wilson, D. (2001). *Practical meta-analysis*. Thousand Oaks: Sage.

Lord, F. M., & Novick, M. R. (1968). *Statistical theories of mental test scores*. Reading, MA: Addison Wesley.

Maddala, G. S. (1983). *Limited dependent and qualitative variables in econometrics*. Cambridge: Cambridge University Press.

Mantel, N. (1966). Evaluation of survival data and two new rank order statistics arising in its consideration. *Cancer Chemotherapy Reports, 50*(3), 163–170. https://doi.org/10.1093/jnci/22.4.719.

Mantel, N., & Haenszel, W. (1959). Statistical aspects of the analysis of data from retrospective studies of disease. *Journal of the National Cancer Institute, 22*(4), 719–748.

Masters, G. N. (1982). A Rasch model for partial credit scoring. *Psychometrika, 47*(2), 149–174. https://doi.org/10.1007/BF02296272.

Masters, G. N., & Wright, B. D. (1996). The partial credit model. In W. J. Van der Linden & R. K. Hambleton (Eds.), *Handbook of modern item response theory* (pp. 101–122). New York: Springer.

McCutcheon, A. L. (1987). *Latent class analysis*. London: Sage.

McFadden, D. (1974). Conditional logit analysis of qualitative choice behaviour. In P. Zarembka (Ed.), *Frontiers in econometrics*. Berkeley, CA: Academic Press.

Menard, S. (2000). Coefficients of determination for multiple logistic regression analysis. *The American Statistician, 54*(1), 17–24. https://doi.org/10.1080/00031305.2000.10474502.

Mittlbock, M., & Schemper, M. (1996). Explained variation in logistic regression. *Statistics in Medicine, 15*, 1987–1997. https://doi.org/10.1002/(SICI)1097-0258(19961015)15:19<1987::AID-SIM318>3.0.CO;2-9.

Nagelkerke, N. J. D. (1991). A note on a general definition of the coefficient of determination. *Biometrika, 78*(3), 691–692.

Pearson, M. R., Lawless, A. K., Brown, D. B., & Bravo, A. J. (2015). Mindfulness and emotional outcomes: Identifying subgroups of college students using latent profile analysis. *Personality and Individual Differences, 76*, 33–38. https://doi.org/10.1016/j.paid.2014.11.009.

Peters, G. J. Y. (2014). The alpha and the omega of scale reliability and validity: Why and how to abandon Cronbach's alpha and the route towards more comprehensive assessment of scale quality. *European Health Psychologist, 16*(2), 56–69.

Peterson, A. V. (1977). Expressing the Kaplan-Meier estimator as a function of empirical subsurvival functions. *Journal of the American Statistical Association, 72*(360), 854–858. https://doi.org/10.2307/2286474.

Peto, R., & Peto, J. (1972). Asymptotically efficient rank invariant test procedures. *Journal of the Royal Statistical Society. Series A (General), 135*(2), 185–207. https://doi.org/10.2307/2344317.

Rasch, G. (1960). *Probabilistic models for some intelligence and achievement tests*. Copenhagen: Danish Institute for Educational Research.

Revelle, W., & Zinbarg, R. E. (2009). Coefficients alpha, beta, omega, and the glb: Comments on Sijtsma. *Psychometrika, 74*, 145–154. https://doi.org/10.1007/s11336-008-9102-z.

Rost, J. (1990). Rasch models in latent classes: An integration of two approaches to item analysis. *Applied Psychological Measurement, 14*, 271–282. https://doi.org/10.1177/014662169001400305.

Rost, J. (1991). A logistic mixture distribution model for polytomous item responses. *British Journal of Mathematical and Statistical Psychology, 44*, 75–92. https://doi.org/10.1111/j.2044-8317.1991.tb00951.x.

Rouder, J. N., Speckman, P. L., Sun, D., Morey, R. D., & Iverson, G. (2012). Bayesian *t* tests for accepting and rejecting the null hypothesis. *Psychonomic Bulletin & Review, 16*(2), 225–237. https://doi.org/10.3758/PBR.16.2.225.

Sijtsma, K. (2009). On the use, the misuse, and the very limited usefulness of Cronbach's alpha. *Psychometrika, 74*, 107–120. https://doi.org/10.1007/s11336-008-9101-0.

Stevens, S. S. (1946). On the theory of scales of measurement. *Science, 103*, 677–680. https://www.jstor.org/stable/1671815.

Tan, F. E. S. (2010). Best practices in analysis of longitudinal data: A multilevel approach. In J. W. Osborne (Ed.), *Best practices in quantitative methods* (Chap. 30, pp. 451–470). London: Sage.

Tarone, R. E., & Ware, J. (1977). On distribution-free tests for equality of survival distributions. *Biometrika, 64*, 156–160. https://doi.org/10.93/biomet/64.1.156.

Tjur, T. (2009). Coefficients of determination in logistic regression models—A new proposal: The coefficient of discrimination. *The American Statistician, 63*(4), 366–372. https://doi.org/10.1198/tast.2009.08210.

Trizano-Hermosilla, I., & Alvarado, J. M. (2016). Best alternatives to Cronbach's alpha reliability in realistic conditions: Congeneric and asymmetrical measurements. *Frontiers in Psychology, 7*, 769. https://doi.org/10.3389/fpsyg.2016.00769.

Wainer, H. (2000). *Computerized adaptive testing: A primer* (2nd ed.). Mahwah, NJ: Erlbaum.

Watkins, M. W. (2017). The reliability of multidimensional neuropsychological measures: From alpha to omega. *The Clinical Neuropsychologist, 31*(6–7), 1113–1126. https://doi.org/10.1080/13854046.2017.1317364.

Weiss, D. J., & Kingsbury, G. G. (1984). Applications of computerized adaptive testing to educational problems. *Journal of Educational Measurement, 21*(4), 361–375. https://doi.org/10.1111/j.1745-3984.1984.tb01040.x.

Wilcoxon, F. (1945). Individual comparisons by ranking methods. *Biometrics Bulletin, 1*(6), 80–83. https://doi.org/10.2307/3001968.

Wilson, M. (1989). Saltus: A psychometric model for discontinuity in cognitive development. *Psychological Bulletin, 105*, 276–289.

Wright, B. D., & Masters, G. N. (1982). *Rating scale analysis*. Chicago: MESA Press.

Wright, B. D., & Stone, M. H. (1979). *Best test design*. Chicago: MESA Press.

Zhang, Z. Y., & Yuan, K. H. (2016). Robust coefficients alpha and omega and confidence intervals with outlying observations and missing data: Methods and software. *Educational and Psychological Measurement, 76*(3), 387–411. https://doi.org/10.1177/0013164415594658.

Multicategory Nominal Choices

6

Abstract

Although they appear somewhat less common than the other types of outcome variables discussed in this book, multicategory nominal choice variables relevant in educational settings include the choice of elective modules and internships, the experience of different types of emotions that may not be easily captured on a unidimensional (e.g., negative-positive, good-bad) continuum, as well as choices relating to what peers or groups to interact with. This type of outcome variables is discussed in this sixth chapter, with appropriate analytic methods. Through common statistical concepts, comparisons with examples from Chap. 5 are provided.

6.1 Introduction

Suppose, an online learning environment presents a wide range of learning tasks in four different modules that represent four different content domains: A, B, C, and D. In each of the modules, the variety and depth in content and learning tasks is such that it could easily keep learners busy for an entire year. Anyone with access to internet based anywhere in the world can sign up, but for logistic reasons the organisers of this environment have decided to, at least for the first year that it is used, randomly sample from a much larger waiting list of people interested. The learning environment is fully in English, and once granted access, learners can freely choose which of four domains to focus on.

J. Leppink, *The Art of Modelling the Learning Process*, Springer Texts in Education,
https://doi.org/10.1007/978-3-030-43082-5_6

6.2 Single-Time and Multiple-Time Choices

A total of $N = 2690$ learners, divided into native English speakers ($n = 1078$) and non-native English speaker ($n = 1612$), choose either module A, module B, module C or module D. Among the native speakers, 305 choose A (28.3%), 70 choose B (6.5%), 124 choose C (11.5%), and 579 choose D (53.7%). Among non-native speakers, 453 choose A (28.1%), 103 choose B (6.4%), 183 choose C (11.4%), and 873 choose D (54.2%). If we are interested in the question of differences between native and non-native speakers in choices, we can perform *multinomial logistic regression* (Anderson & Rutkowski, 2010), for instance in Stata or Jamovi. Doing so on the data in this example, Model 0 has −2LL = 5992.871 and Model 1 has −2LL = 5992.815. The resulting LR test is: $\chi^2_3 = 0.056$, $p = 0.997$. This is a χ^2-test at $df = 3$, because given a choices and b groups, the difference between the two models in df is:

$$df = (a - 1) * (b - 1) = 3.$$

6.2.1 Different Estimates in Different Software Packages

We can also compute R^2_{McF}: we find a value of almost 0.00001, very small. If the differences between groups were a bit more substantial, we could also compute AIC, BIC or criteria alike, but for this situation there is no need. With regard to the computation of R^2_{McF}, and alternatives discussed in Chap. 5, it is worth noting that there are differences between software packages. Leppink (2019) provides examples of how SPSS provides substantially higher estimates of R^2_{McF}, R^2_{CS}, and R^2_N than Stata and Jamovi (e.g., SPSS returning $R^2_{McF} = 1$ where Stata and Jamovi return $R^2_{McF} = 0.5$ or $R^2_{McF} = 0.58$; SPSS returning $R^2_{CS} = 0.048$ and $R^2_N = 0.052$ where Jamovi returns $R^2_{CS} = 0.012$ and $R^2_N = 0.026$) and why for multinomial logistic regression Stata and Jamovi are to be preferred over SPSS.

6.2.2 Change with Time

Now that we have insufficient ground to assume any kind of group differences, there is no reason to follow up with module-specific group differences (for examples of such follow-up analyses, see Anderson & Rutkowski, 2010; Leppink, 2019). However, suppose that learners in the online environment can choose A, B, C, or D several times instead of once, and that—given the variety and depth in content and learning tasks—it is possible to choose the same module two, three or even four times. Learners who have broad interests or have more of a generalist attitude may choose three or four different modules in the four periods, whereas learners who come with a very specific interest or want to specialise into one particular domain may choose the same module three or four times. Given four choice moments and

Table 6.1 Choices of modules A, B, C, and D in four consecutive rounds (Rnd. 1–4)

Rnd. 1	Rnd. 2		Rnd. 2	Rnd. 3		Rnd. 3	Rnd. 4	
A (758)	**A**	563	**A**	**A**	561	**A**	**A**	565
	B	94		**B**	36		**B**	39
	C	32		**C**	23		**C**	23
	D	69		**D**	131		**D**	135
B (173)	**A**	31	**B**	**A**	96	**B**	**A**	30
	B	28		**B**	30		**B**	30
	C	29		**C**	22		**C**	36
	D	85		**D**	184		**D**	169
C (307)	**A**	75	**C**	**A**	24	**C**	**A**	21
	B	43		**B**	27		**B**	24
	C	17		**C**	11		**C**	18
	D	172		**D**	70		**D**	49
D (1452)	**A**	82	**D**	**A**	81	**D**	**A**	151
	B	167		**B**	172		**B**	73
	C	54		**C**	56		**C**	160
	D	1149		**D**	1166		**D**	1167

four modules, there are $4^4 = 256$ possible combinations, some of which will likely occur more frequently than others. We already know the choices of the first term, which for the two groups (i.e., native and non-native speakers) are: 758 for A (28.2%), 173 for B (6.4%), 307 for C (11.4%), and 1452 for D (54.0%). Table 6.1 lists the numbers of choices in each subsequent round given the module in the current round.

We could present the same table in percentages as well, but the numbers provide insight in possible small-number cells and percentages can be computed directly from them. Two observations stand out. First, although all four modules are chosen by over 4% of the learners in any of the rounds, module D is the most frequently chosen module, followed by module A. Second, from one round to the next, for both modules A and D, 74% of the learners or a bit more than that choose the same module in the next round. There are 1250 learners who choose the same module in all four rounds: 819 learners choose D throughout (30.4% of 2690), 430 learners choose A throughout (16.0% of 2690), 1 learner chooses B throughout, and no learners choose C throughout. In other words, almost half of the sample choose either A or D throughout.

There are several options for more detailed analysis, partly depending the questions different researchers may have, such as the *nominal response model* (i.e., an IRT model for variables of nominal level of measurement; Bock, 1972, 1997) and *mixed-effects multinomial logistic regression* models (i.e., an extension of mixed-effects binary logistic regression discussed in Chap. 5; e.g., Dey, Raheem, & Lu, 2016; Hedeker, 2003). Mixed-effects multinomial logistic regression also provides a straightforward way to test for group-by-round interaction. As we have seen, with a single round, the group factor (i.e., language) requires 3 *df*, because the difference between groups can be estimated for each comparison of module *X* with the reference category. The main effect of round has 9 *df*:

$$df = (\text{rounds} - 1) * (\text{module choice} - 1) = (4 - 1) * (4 - 1) = 9.$$

The same goes for the group-by-round interaction, because for group $df = 1$. For the data at hand, using effectively the same fixed and random effects as in Chap. 5 but with a multicategory outcome variable instead of a binary one, we find for the full factorial model, which includes group main effect, round main effect, and group-by-round interaction effect: AICc = 130369.031 and BIC = 130390.873, and for the interaction effect, we find $p = 0.431$. For the two-main-effects model (i.e., no interaction), we find: AICc = 130311.004 and BIC = 130332.848, and for the group effect, we find: $p = 0.636$. Finally, for the module that accounts only for differences over time, we find: AICc = 130291.240 and BIC = 130313.085, and for the time effect, we find: $p < 0.001$. Altogether, these findings justify a preference for a no-group-differences model.

Another straightforward way to understand which choices from which rounds tend to go together, and—if there was still any doubt—to what extent being a native or non-native English speaker helps to explain differences in choice behaviour, can be found in *multiple correspondence analysis* (Greenacre, 2007; Greenacre & Blasius, 2006; Le Roux & Rouanet, 2004). Multiple correspondence analysis can be conceived as a cousin of principal component analysis; where the latter can help to make decisions with regard to which variables of interval or ratio level of measurement can be grouped together, multiple correspondence analysis can help to model structures in data of nominal level of measurement. One of several useful things multiple correspondence analysis can provide is a low-dimensional (often two or three dimensions) plot of coordinates that helps to understand which choices are similar. Figure 6.1 presents that plot for the data at hand, acquired through multiple correspondence analysis in *SPSS*.

This plot nicely depicts the patterns discussed previously: there is a fairly strong tendency among learners who chose module A or module D to stick with that choice in later rounds, while there is no such a pronounced tendency for module B or module C.

While in the example at hand we deal with learners' choices of modules, the same methods can be applied in studies where for instance information is presented and people are asked to indicate from a series of options which is their dominant emotion in response to that information. While some emotions may be easily ranked on a single dimension, that is not always the case (e.g., Leppink, 2019: indifferent, embarrassed, surprised or disappointed). Things do become trickier when multiple choices can be made within a round, or when people are allowed to select multiple emotions in response to the aforementioned question. In such cases, more complex mixed-effects binary logistic models and latent class models may still work, but multinomial models are based on the idea of only a single choice being made by the individual at a given time.

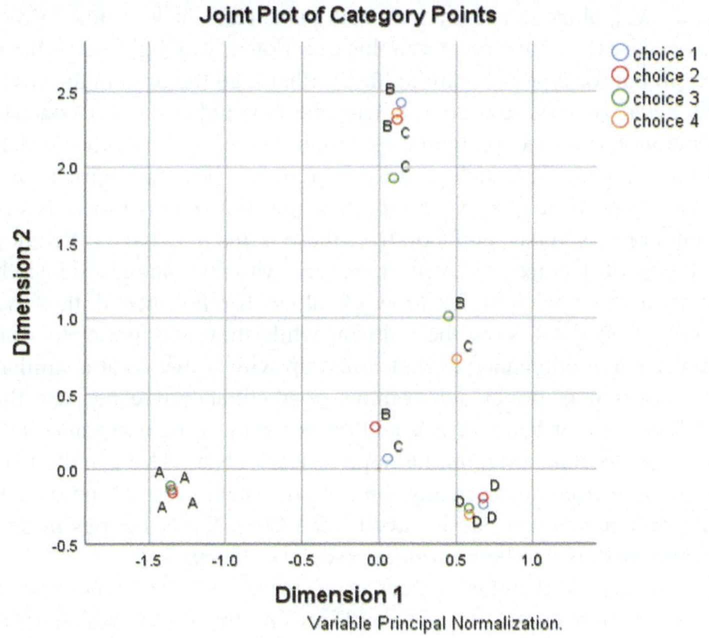

Fig. 6.1 Joint plot of category points in the module choice study (SPSS)

6.3 Autonomous Versus Collaborative Versus No Preference

Suppose, each of the modules A, B, C, and D has four types of learning tasks. Before the next cohort of $N = 3073$ students choose their first module, we ask them to complete a questionnaire that asks among others to indicate for each of the four types of learning tasks if they prefer to do it by themselves (autonomously), in collaboration with a peer or they do not have a preference. Some might treat this as ordinal data, but that assumes a consistent order of the three options, for example: autonomous (self), no preference (neither self nor peer), collaboration (peer). However, it is well possible that these three options have different meanings for different learners and can therefore not be captured in three consistent categories. On the one hand, learners who are inclined to work alone may well indicate a preference for autonomous for most or all four types of learning tasks, while learners who are inclined to study together may indicate a preference for collaboration for most if not all four types of learning tasks. On the other hand, no preference may mean several things. Some learners may work well alone as well as with peers and would be okay either way, having to complete a task alone or with a peer. Other learners may have no preference either because they (know that they) do neither study well alone nor study well with peers (e.g., lack of time or motivation) or simply because they have not given this question any thought yet or have given it some thought but for types of learning tasks other than the ones in the environment. Given this heterogeneity, it is unclear why there would be a clear consistent order such as 'autonomous—no preference—collaborative' or any other order for that matter. In the absence of such a consistent order, it is appropriate to treat the categories as nominal. In fact, one might even question whether there is a consistent order in autonomous versus collaborative; these terms may have different means to different types of learners as well. Learners who are already somewhat more advanced in a topic may prefer to work alone for instance if they worry that working with a peer will slow them down, while they may prefer to work with a peer if they see a good chance to be teamed up with someone at a similar stage in the topic. Others may prefer autonomous over collaborative because they know they have little time or learn slowly and do not want to be a nuisance to peers, or they may prefer to collaborate in the hope to learn faster. These and other possible reasons to choose from question any kind of consistent order of options. That said, if there are researchers who are in favour of treating the categories in a consistent order, ordinal models can be considered (see also Chap. 7).

Given four tasks with three choices each, there are $3^4 = 81$ possible combinations. However, in this case, only six combinations are chosen, which are displayed in Table 6.2.

The vast majority consistently (86.2%) consistently make the same choice, and the remaining 13.8% is composed by four smaller groups, two of which (together 4.8%) have a clear preference in all except for the first type of task (Task 1: no preference). Only 9.0% of the respondents indicate no preference in at least two of the tasks. Finally, note that none of the respondents choose 'self' for some tasks and 'with peer' for other tasks. Figure 6.2 presents the joint plot of category points for the data at hand, acquired through multiple correspondence analysis in SPSS.

In the plot, '?' indicates no preference. The 'self' and 'peer' tendency seen in the vast majority of respondents is clearly visible in this plot, but the 'no preference' choices are more scattered out.

Table 6.2 Choice patterns (combinations): all autonomous (self), all collaborative (peer), and other

Pattern	Frequency (%)
All tasks with peer	1847 (60.1)
All tasks self	803 (26.1)
Tasks 1 and 3 with peer, rest no preference	185 (6.0)
Task 1 no preference, rest with peers	107 (3.5)
Task 2 self, rest no preference	91 (3.0)
Task 1 no preference, rest self	40 (1.3)

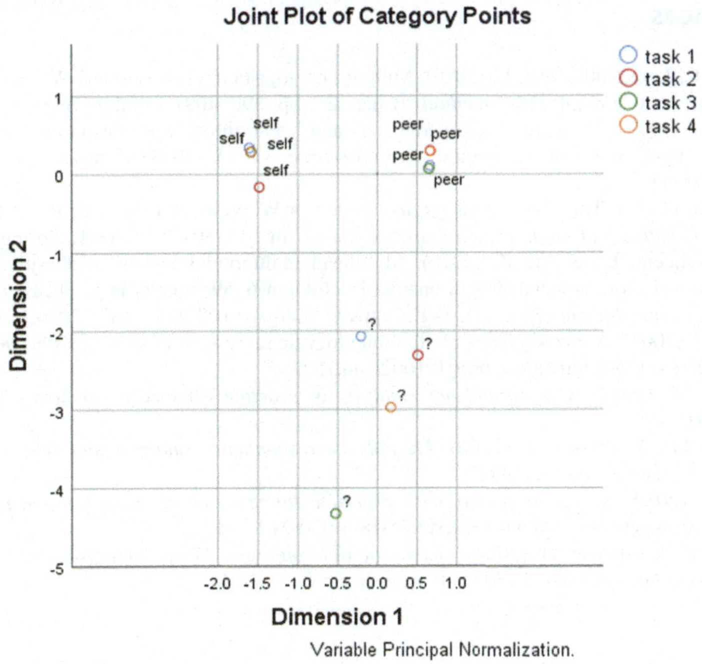

Fig. 6.2 Joint plot of category points in the preference (self vs. peer vs. no preference) choice study (*SPSS*)

6.4 Latent Classes

The latent class analysis approach discussed in Chap. 5 can also be of use when dealing with multinomial variables. The only differences are that with multinomial variables a multinomial logit link function is used (cf. the difference between binary and multinomial logistic regression) and that multicategory variables put higher demands on sample size than binary variables. Besides, when there are only few combinations altogether or only few combinations that have a sufficiently large sample size, latent class analysis will most likely not be feasible. In the case of the different module choices, a two-class model could work but a three-class model would probably not work well due to small class sizes for B- or C-choices in at least some of the rounds. Finally, a two-class model would not really tell us anything that we cannot see already: a clear preference for module A in one class and a clear preference for module D in the other class; what remains difficult to explain are the B- and C-choices. That said, there are certainly situations where studies with sample sizes similar to the ones in our examples result in two- or three-class models that help us to better understand what kind of data we are dealing with.

References

Anderson, C. J., & Rutkowski, L. (2010). Multinomial logistic regression. In J. W. Osborne (Ed.), *Best practices in quantitative methods* (Chap. 26, pp. 390–409). London: Sage.

Bock, R. D. (1972). Estimating item parameters and latent ability when responses are scored in two or more nominal categories. *Psychometrika*, *37*(1), 29–51. https://doi.org/10.1007/BF02291411.

Bock, R. D. (1997). The nominal categories model. In W. Van der Linden & R. K. Hambleton (Eds.), *Handbook of modern item response theory* (pp. 33–50). New York: Springer.

Dey, S., Raheem, E., & Lu, Z. (2016). Multilevel multinomial logistic regression model for identifying factors associated with anemia in children 6–59 months in northeastern states of India. *Cogent Mathematics*, *3*(1), 1–12. https://doi.org/10.1080/23311835.2016.1159798.

Hedeker, D. (2003). A mixed-effects multinomial logistic regression model. *Statistics in Medicine*, *22*(9), 1433–1446. https://doi.org/10.1002/sim.1522.

Greenacre, M. (2007). *Correspondence analysis in practice* (2nd ed.). London: Chapman & Hall/CRC.

Greenacre, M., & Blasius, J. (2006). *Multiple correspondence analysis and related methods*. London: Chapman & Hall/CRC.

Leppink, J. (2019). *Statistical methods for experimental research in education and psychology*. Cham: Springer. https://doi.org/10.1007/978-3-030-21241-4.

Le Roux, B., & Rouanet, H. (2004). *Geometric data analysis: From correspondence analysis to structured data analysis*. Dordrecht: Kluwer.

Ordered Performance Categories

7

Abstract

Many performance ratings in educational research are of an ordinal nature. Examples include global ratings in clinical examination on a scale like 'excellent', 'pass', 'borderline', and 'fail' and overall internship assessments such as 'good', 'sufficient' or 'poor'. Both series of categories have in common that categories can be ordered in terms of performance, but the difference between 'excellent' and 'pass' may not be the same as that between 'borderline' and 'fail', and the difference between 'good' and 'sufficient' is not necessarily the same as that between 'sufficient' and 'poor'. These and other examples of multicategory ordinal outcome variables, some of which are observed once in time some of which are observed at several occasions during a longer time interval, are discussed in this chapter, with appropriate analytic methods. Through common statistical concepts, similarities and differences between methods discussed in this chapter and those discussed in Chaps. 5 and 6 are discussed.

7.1 Introduction

While with nominal variables there is no consistent order in the different categories, such an order does exist in the case of ordinal variables. Different types of ordinal variables can be distinguished (e.g., Kampen & Swyngedouw, 2000), but they all have in common that treating them as if they were of interval level of measurement often means trouble (Kampen, 2019). Although in an attempt to justify the treatment of ordinal data such as Likert data (i.e., Likert, 1932) as interval, a common argument is that Spearman's correlation coefficient ρ (Spearman, 1904) and Pearson's r are often more or less equal if not exactly equal (e.g., Norman, 2010), this argument is problematic because with ρ we are *still* treating data as interval instead

J. Leppink, *The Art of Modelling the Learning Process*, Springer Texts in Education,
https://doi.org/10.1007/978-3-030-43082-5_7

of as truly ordinal (Leppink, 2019; Tacq & Nassiri, 2011). That is, ρ is actually r on ranked data; although we transform our original data into ranks, we then square distances in the rank data as if the rank data is of interval level of measurement (!). For a true ordinal treatment of ordinal data, we have Kendall's τ (rank) coefficients (Kendall, 1938, 1962): these coefficients use the numbers of concordant (i.e., agreeing) and discordant (i.e., disagreeing) pairs and, in some coefficients, the number of ties (i.e., pairs that are neither concordant nor discordant) (e.g., Agresti, 2010; Berry, Johnston, Zahran, & Mielke, 2009; Kruskal, 1958). This is also where some of the 'quantitative-qualitative' discourse comes in again. The work by Pierre Bourdieu (e.g., Bourdieu, 1984) on power relations, financial means, and other factors that help to distinguish the dominant class, the middle class, and the working class is in 'qualitative' arenas sometimes used as an example of how relations between classes and other variables of interest cannot really be quantified but needs to be studied qualitatively. Although the different classes indeed cannot be treated as some kind of interval level of measurement variable, τ coefficients provide us with one of several tools to treat this kind of data as truly ordinal (Leppink, 2019). Let us take a closer look at this with an example.

7.2 Ordinality in Data and Analysis

Suppose, in a survey study, we ask a random sample of $N = 1605$ people living in the United Kingdom to respond to six statements with regard to six particular pro-Brexit candidates to speak in public. For each of six candidates (i.e., each of six statements), respondents can choose from three options: (1) *disagree*, (2) *neutral* or (3) *agree*. Table 7.1 presents frequencies for each response option for each statement as well as Pearson's r, Spearman's ρ, and Kendall's τ_b for each pair of statements.

No differences between r and ρ can be seen in the first three decimals for any of the statement pairs, and this finding was to be expected. All that happens with r is that we treat the three response options as *equidistant*: the distance between *disagree* (1) and *neutral* (2) is the same as the distance between *neutral* (2) and *agree* (3) (i.e., $3 - 2 = 2 - 1$) and therefore the distance between *disagree* and *agree* is twice the *disagree-neutral* or *neutral-agree* distance. It is a bit like treating *mice, hedgehogs*, *cats*, *bears*, and *elephants* as equidistant in weights: it makes no sense (Leppink, 2019). What are the scores '1', '2', and '3' in r are the ranks '1', '2', and '3' in ρ, and given that ρ is effectively r on ranks, we should come up with the same outcomes. Using two coefficients that treat the data as interval cannot be used as a justification of treating the data as interval. When we include in the comparison a coefficient that actually treats the data as ordinal, we see some differences; although the correlations remain high, they are somewhat lower than the ones obtained with r and ρ.

Table 7.1 Frequencies per statement (S1-S6) and correlations for all statement pairs in the Brexit study (*Jamovi*)

		S1	S2	S3	S4	S5	S6
Freq.	Disagree	651	667	665	658	677	678
	Neutral	270	265	275	272	247	249
	Agree	684	673	665	675	681	678
S2	r	0.887					
	ρ	0.887					
	τ_b	0.831					
S3	r	0.880	0.875				
	ρ	0.880	0.875				
	τ_b	0.822	0.814				
S4	r	0.884	0.884	0.884			
	ρ	0.884	0.884	0.884			
	τ_b	0.827	0.828	0.828			
S5	r	0.887	0.881	0.876	0.884		
	ρ	0.887	0.881	0.876	0.884		
	τ_b	0.830	0.822	0.815	0.826		
S6	r	0.888	0.882	0.882	0.892	0.883	
	ρ	0.888	0.882	0.882	0.892	0.883	
	τ_b	0.832	0.823	0.823	0.838	0.823	

The distributions of the different statements are clearly bimodal: for each statement, response percentages for both the agree and the disagree option are in the low 40s, and the remaining 15.4–17.1% go to the neutral option. This may indicate that what is thought of as a random sample from a single population can be conceived as a random sample from a mixture of two or more populations. A two-class model in *Mplus* yields the following outcomes: an overall entropy value of 0.989, with 806 respondents in Class A (50.2%) and 799 respondents in Class B (49.8%). In Class A, the probability of 'agree' is zero across items, whereas in Class B, the probability of 'disagree' is zero across items. Table 7.2 presents the estimated probabilities for the other categories per class.

Table 7.2 Response probabilities per option per statement per class in the Brexit study (*Mplus*)

	Class A probabilities		Class B probabilities	
	Disagree	Neutral	Neutral	Agree
S1	0.817	0.183	0.153	0.847
S2	0.837	0.163	0.167	0.833
S3	0.834	0.166	0.177	0.823
S4	0.826	0.174	0.165	0.835
S5	0.849	0.151	0.157	0.843
S6	0.851	0.149	0.161	0.839

In other words, in Class A, there is a general tendency towards *not* letting each of the six candidates speak in public, while in Class B, there is general tendency towards letting each of these candidates speak. Although in practical survey studies, which may be of a considerably larger size, response option probabilities of zero or one or not common, the presence of two or more different classes in a sample is, when dealing with opinion data, such as whether or not to allow different types of people to speak in public, not uncommon (e.g., Hagenaars & McCutcheon, 2002; McCutcheon, 1987).

7.3 Task-to-Task Transition

In the Brexit study, transition in opinion from one statement to the next is rather unlikely, because of the polarised topic that Brexit has been over the past years; Remain voters in the 2016 Brexit referendum see a variety of advantages of remaining in the European Union and are mostly tired of hearing pro-Brexit arguments, whereas a common argument among Leave voters in the 2016 referendum has been that the United Kingdom should have exited the European Union on the 29th of March 2019 and that a failure to exit the European Union, with or without deal, is not respecting democracy (in the end, the United Kingdom exited the European Union on the 31st of January 2020). However, there are certainly situations where transition from item to item is possible, longitudinal studies constituting one example (e.g., people changing their views about Brexit over time in one direction or another).

7.3.1 Ordered Performance Categories

A common type of ordinal variables in educational settings is found in ordered performance categories, such as: *poor*, *satisfactory*, *good*, and *excellent*. Satisfactory is better than poor, good is better than satisfactory, and excellent is better than good, but why would the distance between adjacent performance categories always be the same? This kind of assessment ratings is encountered in many settings, including in simulation training settings. Suppose, a team of Medical Education researchers are interested in the effectiveness of a particular type of instructional support on students' performance in simulation training settings. They decide to randomly allocate a random sample of $N = 220$ to a treatment condition that receives the support ($n = 110$) and a control condition that does not receive the support (i.e., simulation training as usual: $n = 110$). Both conditions then perform the same sequence of three tasks, which are effectively the same task but with different simulated patients. Although some might argue that 'something works better than nothing', literature on the effects of instructional support on performance are mixed and includes both positive and negative effects. In both conditions, students work individually. Each task performance is scored, by two clinicians who are blind to any kind of expectations with regard to the effectiveness of support, as a consensus judgement of either *poor*, *satisfactory*, *good* or *excellent*.

7.3.2 Condition-by-Task Interaction

In Chap. 5, we have an example of how mixed-effects binary logistic regression can help us to study group-by-item interaction, and in Chap. 6, we have an example of mixed-effects multinomial logistic regression for multicategory nominal instead of binary outcome variables. In this chapter, where we deal with ordinal outcome variables, we can use *mixed-effects ordinal logistic regression* (e.g., Bauer & Sterba, 2011; Hedeker & Gibbons, 1994, 1996; Hox, Moerbeek, & Van de Schoot, 2017; Liu, 2016). Table 7.3 presents the frequencies of performance categories per condition per task.

Figure 7.1 presents *estimated marginal means* (*EMM*) plots of the probabilities of category occurrence in the two conditions per task (*Jamovi*), which use the information from Table 7.3.

While we do not see much of a task-to-task transition in the control condition, we do see some transition for the better in the treatment condition. Moreover, on the first task, the control condition appears to perform better than the treatment condition; there are fewer 'poor' and 'satisfactory' but more 'good' and 'excellent' ratings in the control than in the treatment condition. On the third task, the pattern is almost the reverse, and on the second task it appears that the conditions do about equally well. From the patterns in Fig. 7.1, it appears that for each task, the *cumulative ORs*—that is: odds ratios for higher versus lower categories—are *proportional*: the *OR* for 'higher than 0' versus '0', the *OR* for '2 or 3' versus '0 or 1', and the *OR* for '3' versus '2 or lower' do not differ much from each other. This is also known as the *proportional odds assumption* (for more details, see: Agresti, 2002; Leppink, 2019; McCullagh, 1980). Some software programmes enable researchers to test that assumption through a LR test. For task 1 (t0), *SPSS* returns −2LL = 26.594 under proportional odds and −2LL = 24.253 under disproportional odds; the resulting LR test yields (difference in third decimal due to roundoff error): $\chi^2_2 = 2.340 = 0.310$. For task 2 (t1), we find −2LL = 30.895 under proportional odds and −2LL = 27.057 under disproportional odds; the resulting LR test yields

Table 7.3 Frequencies of performance categories per condition per task

		Performance categories			
Task	Condition	Poor	Satisfactory	Good	Excellent
1	Control	10	54	38	8
	Treatment	20	63	26	1
2	Control	18	35	42	15
	Treatment	8	42	41	19
3	Control	15	50	28	17
	Treatment	11	21	34	44

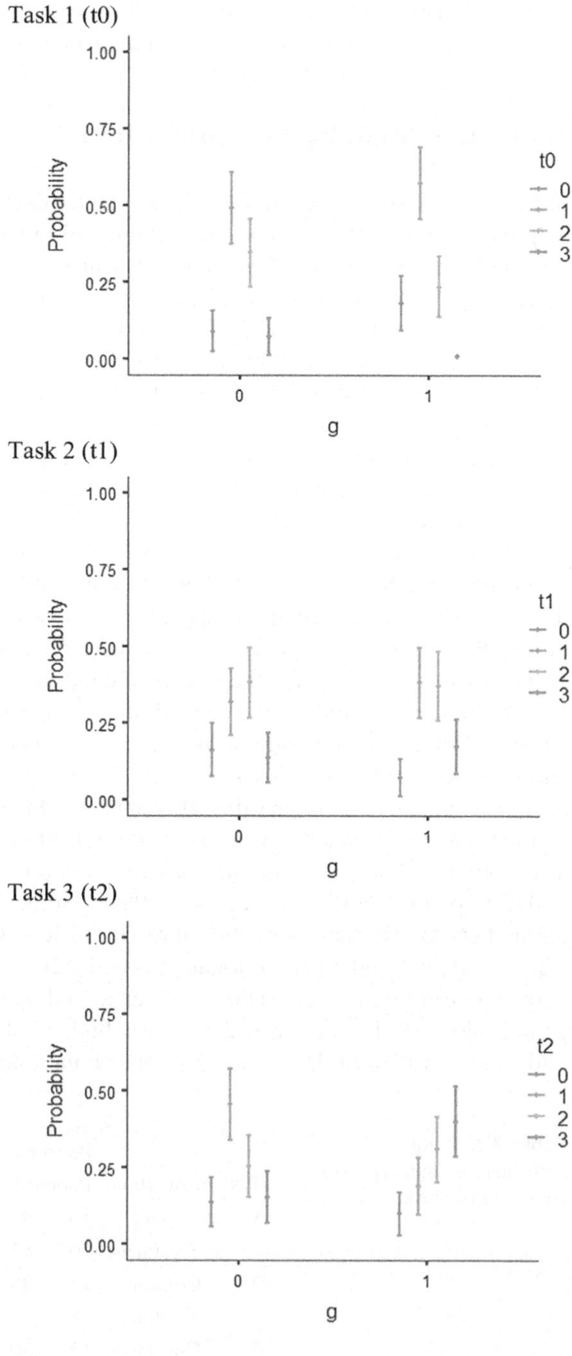

Fig. 7.1 EMM plots of the probabilities of category occurrence in the two conditions per task (*Jamovi*): 0 = poor, 1 = satisfactory, 2 = good, 3 = excellent; $g = 0$ is control and $g = 1$ is treatment condition

(difference in third decimal due to roundoff error): $\chi^2_2 = 3.839 = 0.147$. Finally, for task 3 (t2), we find −2LL = 32.245 under proportional odds and −2LL = 27.224 under disproportional odds, and the resulting LR test yields: $\chi^2_2 = 5.021 = 0.081$. In these tests, *df* = 2, because under the proportional odds assumption we need only *one df* for that common proportional odds, while under disproportional odds we need three *df*, one for each of the three aforementioned cumulative *OR*s. In our case, we find no convincing evidence to reject the proportional odds assumption. Broadly speaking, the proportional odds assumption is often realistic and is useful because it results in fewer parameters to be estimated. It therefore constitutes the default option in ordinal regression models in software packages such as *SPSS*, *Stata*, and *Jamovi*.

Next step is to test the condition-by-task interaction effect through a mixed-effects ordinal logistic regression model. Using effectively the same fixed and random effects as in our mixed-effects examples in earlier chapters with dichotomous (Chap. 5) and multicategory nominal (Chap. 6) outcome variables but now with an ordinal outcome variable (*Stata*), we find −2LL = 1387.004 for the full factorial model and −2LL = 1460.785 for the main-effects-only model. Given that there are two conditions (*df* = 1), three tasks (*df* = 2), and we assume proportional odds (*df* = 1), for the condition-by-task interaction effect: *df* = 1 * 2 * 1 = 2. In the case of disproportional odds, we would be back to a mixed-effects multinomial regression treatment where we would need *df* = 3 for disproportional odds and hence the condition-by-task interaction effect would have *df* = 1 * 2 * 3 = 6 (for an example, see Chap. 6). In this case, we assume proportional odds, and therefore need *df* = 2 for the interaction effect. The resulting LR test yields: $\chi^2_2 = 1460.785 - 1387.004 = 73.781$, $p < 0.001$. Table 7.4 presents the outcomes of the full factorial model computed by *Stata*.

In this model, all estimates are *b*-values are *ln*(*OR*)-values (i.e., natural logarithm of *OR*) that are also called *logits* and are interpreted as regression coefficients on the logit scale, except for the participant variance which is a variance estimate that can be estimated since we have three tasks for each participant. Negative *b*-values correspond with *OR*s smaller than 1, while positive *b*-values correspond with *OR*s larger than 1.

Table 7.4 Full factorial mixed-effects ordinal logistic regression model in simulation training experiment (0 = control, 1 = treatment): point estimates and 95% CIs (*Stata*)

Term	Estimate	95% CI LB	95% CI UB
Condition	−1.361	−2.295	−0.427
Task 2	0.315	−0.251	0.881
Task 3	0.714	−0.496	0.639
Condition * Task 2	1.995	1.165	2.825
Condition * Task 3	3.716	2.813	4.619
Threshold 1	−3.588	−4.375	−2.801
Threshold 2	0.671	0.002	1.340
Threshold 3	3.861	3.080	4.642
Participant variance	7.451	5.337	10.403

The *b*-estimate for 'Condition' of −1.361 is about the difference between the two conditions at task 1 (t0 in Fig. 7.1: intercept). Given the coding of conditions (0 = control, 1 = treatment), a negative *b*-estimate indicates that the treatment condition performed *worse* than the control condition on the first task (cf. t0 in Fig. 7.1). The *b*-values of 'Task 2' and 'Task 3' indicate changes (here: statistically non-significant from zero) from Task 1 to Task 2 and Task 3, respectively. The 'Condition * Task' estimates indicate the *difference in change* between conditions from Task 1 to Task 2 and Task 3, respectively. Again, given the coding of conditions, positive changes indicate a stronger increase in performance in the treatment condition relative to the control condition. In short, the treatment condition starts off worse than the control condition (i.e., initial negative effect of support) but performs much better than the control condition on the third task (i.e., positive effect of support on the third task). For R^2_{McF}, *Jamovi* returns $R^2_{\mathrm{McF}} = 0.021$ for the first task, $R^2_{\mathrm{McF}} = 0.002$ for the second task, and $R^2_{\mathrm{McF}} = 0.035$ for the third task. Finally, the thresholds in Table 7.4 indicate cut-off points on a logit scale for the transition from one performance category to the next.

7.4 Categorical Variables: A Recap

The concepts of R^2_{McF} and its alternatives (including the note of caution with regard to different software packages yielding substantially different outcomes for the same statistics), *OR* and *ln*(*OR*) apply to binary, multinomial, and ordinal logistic regression models, and methods like latent class analysis and IRT can be useful for dichotomous, multicategory nominal, and multicategory ordinal variables. In the Brexit study, latent class analysis provides a useful tool. In the experiment, had the sample size been much larger, we could have considered extensions of the Rasch model discussed in Chap. 5. A potential advantage of dichotomous variables over multicategory nominal and ordinal variables is that generally they are somewhat less sample size demanding. However, when more precise classification through multicategory nominal or ordinal variables is possible, a drawback of dichotomous variables is a loss of information. For example, we probably have assessment scales like *poor-satisfactory-good-excellent* for a reason; reducing them into a dichotomous variable—whether it is poor versus the rest, the lowest two versus the highest two categories, or excellent versus the rest—generally means a substantial loss of information and, in both research and educational practice, an increased likelihood of incorrect decisions being made. At the same time, in cases where there are more categories than can be distinguished, we may create a situation in which respondents who actually differ in categories give the same response and/or respondents who actually belong to the same category respond differently; in such cases, the level of measurement appears not even nominal (e.g., Leppink, 2019).

Treating ordinal variables as if they were of interval level of measurement should also be expected to result in incorrect conclusions. Even if we use the sum or average of a series of items, that does not magically transform series of ordinal measurements into an interval level of measurement score. Suppose, we have ratings of the type: *disagree* (1), *neutral* (2), *agree* (3). The numbers '1', '2', and '3' are just ordinal labels, meaning they should not be interpreted as equidistant as in interval level of measurement variables. Even if different people have *exactly* the same conceptualisation of *disagree*, *neutral*, and *agree*, and we can stick numbers to them, if they are not really equidistant, we run into trouble. For instance, suppose that the actual numbers are: *disagree* (1), *neutral* (2), and *agree* (3.5). We now sum four statements for each of three participants:

Participant A: *neutral, neutral, neutral, neutral*;
Participant B: *disagree, agree, disagree, agree*;
Participant C: *disagree, neutral, neutral, agree.*

In the interval approach, the sum score of all three participants is 8. In the ordinal approach, the sum score of participant A is 8, the sum score of participant B is 9, and the sum score of participant C is 8.5. In other words, in the ordinal world, not only '3'− '2' ≠ '2'− '1', but one sum score '8' is not necessary equal to another sum score '8' either (i.e., one *M* of 2 is not necessarily the same as another *M* of 2).

Finally, researchers sometimes unintendedly treat ordinal variables as multi-category nominal variables, by choosing one reference category (e.g., poor, or excellent) and comparing all other categories with that reference category. Doing so, we lose the ordinality information and miss an opportunity to save *df* through the proportional odds assumption discussed in this chapter.

References

Agresti, A. (2002). *Categorical data analysis* (2nd ed.). New York, NY: Wiley.

Agresti, A. (2010). *Analysis of ordinal categorical data* (2nd ed.). New York: Wiley.

Bauer, D. J., & Sterba, S. K. (2011). Fitting multilevel models with ordinal outcomes: Performance of alternative specifications and methods of estimation. *Psychological Methods, 16*(4), 373–390. https://doi.org/10.1037/a0025813.

Berry, K. J., Johnston, J. E., Zahran, S., & Mielke, P. W. (2009). Stuart's tau measure of effect size for ordinal variables: Some methodological considerations. *Behavior Research Methods, 41*(4), 1144–1148. https://doi.org/10.3758/brm.41.4.1144.

Bourdieu, P. (1984). *Distinction: A social critique of the judgment of taste*. Cambridge, MA: Harvard University Press.

Hagenaars, J. A., & McCutcheon, A. L. (2002). *Applied latent class analysis*. Cambridge, MA: Cambridge University Press.

Hedeker, D., & Gibbons, R. D. (1994). A random-effects ordinal regression model for multilevel analysis. *Biometrics, 50*(4), 933–944. https://doi.org/10.2307/2533433.

Hedeker, D., & Gibbons, R. D. (1996). MIXOR: A computer program for mixed-effects ordinal regression analysis. *Computer Methods and Programs in Biomedicine, 49*(2), 157–176. https://doi.org/10.1016/0169-2607(96)01720-8.

Hox, J. J., Moerbeek, M., & Van de Schoot, R. (2017). *Multilevel analysis: Techniques and Applications* (3rd ed.). New York, NY: Taylor & Francis.

Kampen, J. (2019). Reflections on and test of the metrological properties of summated Likert, and other scales on sums of ordinal variables. *Measurement, 137,* 428–434. https://doi.org/10.1016/j.measurement.2019.01.083.

Kampen, J., & Swyngedouw, M. (2000). The ordinal controversy revisited. *Quality & Quantity, 34* (1), 87–102. https://doi.org/10.1023/A:1004785723554.

Kendall, M. G. (1938). A new measure of rank correlation. *Biometrika, 30*(1–2), 81–89. https://doi.org/10.1093/biomet/30.1-2.81.

Kendall, M. G. (1962). *Rank correlation methods.* New York: Hafner.

Kruskal, W. H. (1958). Ordinal measures of association. *Journal of the American Statistical Association, 53*(284), 814–861. https://doi.org/10.2307/2281954.

Leppink, J. (2019). *Statistical methods for experimental research in education and psychology.* Cham: Springer. https://doi.org/10.1007/978-3-030-21241-4.

Likert, R. (1932). A technique for the measurement of attitudes. *Archives of Psychology, 140,* 1–55.

Liu, X. (2016). *Applied ordinal logistic regression using Stata: From single-level to multilevel modeling*. New York, NY: Sage.

McCullagh, P. (1980). Regression models for ordinal data. *Journal of the Royal Statistical Society. Series B (Methodological), 42*(2), 109–142. https://www.jstor.org/stable/2984952.

McCutcheon, A. L. (1987). *Latent class analysis.* London: Sage.

Norman, G. (2010). Likert scales, levels of measurement and the "laws" of statistics. *Advances in Health Sciences Education, 15,* 625–632. https://doi.org/10.1007/s10459-010-9222-y.

Spearman, C. (1904). The proof and measurement of association between two things. *American Journal of Psychology, 15*(1), 72–101. https://doi.org/10.2307/1412159.

Tacq, J. J. A., & Nassiri, V. (2011). How ordinal is ordinal in ordinal data analysis? In *Proceedings of the 58th World Statistical Congress*, Dublin, Ireland. http://2011.isiproceedings.org/papers/950432.pdf.

Quantifiable Learning Outcomes

8

Abstract

Educational researchers and practitioners use many types of quantitative or qualitative outcome variables that differ not only in how they are measured but differ in the score distributions they tend to generate as well. This has implications for the types of models we should use. For example, exam performance, response time (i.e., time from starting to see a question until a response is verbalised), and number of attempts needed to pass an exam are three different types of outcome variables that each call for different models. These and other quantitative variables, some of which are observed once in time some of which are observed at several occasions during a longer time interval, are discussed in this chapter, with appropriate analytic methods. Examples are provided for appropriate and not so appropriate ways of dealing with 'outliers' and skewness in the distribution of an outcome variable. For instance, response time may well form a unimodal distribution with a clear skew to the right; the use of suboptimal methods of dealing with that right skew may result in a relation between that time variable and another variable of interest appearing more or less linear while it is actually clearly nonlinear.

8.1 Introduction

A commonly heard phrase in educational research as well as in research in some other domains is that when there is no Normally distributed data, we cannot analyse correlations between variables of interest or any kind of differences between groups on one or several variables of interest. This chapter demonstrates why this phrase is incorrect and misleading and is likely to result in not so useful choices in data analysis.

J. Leppink, *The Art of Modelling the Learning Process*, Springer Texts in Education,
https://doi.org/10.1007/978-3-030-43082-5_8

8.2 Lost the Count

One of the types of outcome variables that is commonly mistreated is that of *counts*. For example, suppose that researchers of an online learning environment are interested in estimating the difference between native English and non-native English speakers in terms of the number of redo attempts needed in an exam to complete an online learning module on a complex topic. In a sample of $N = 385$ students, with $n = 243$ native and $n = 142$ non-native speakers, the distribution of the number of redo attempts is as presented in Table 8.1.

Count is not a nominal variable; the different categories can be ordered without any kind of meaningful discussion being needed. Count is not just an ordinal variable either, since it is defendable to treat the distance between adjacent counts as equal (i.e., 1 more redo attempt for each next number in the count). Not only does count meet the requirements to be called a variable of interval level of measurement, it is legitimate to consider this count a variable with a natural 0 and hence to consider 2 redo attempts twice as many as 1 redo attempt, 4 as twice as many as 2, 6 as twice as many as 3, et cetera. In other words, it is defendable to treat this variable as of ratio level of measurement. Researchers who recognise this may not look at contingency tables but order histograms or other graphs, even though the contingency table essentially provides all information we need to proceed, and all other statistics can be computed from there. Nevertheless, in line with convention, Fig. 8.1 presents the histograms of the count distribution for native and for non-native speakers.

Some might order box plots as well or instead of histograms, so in Fig. 8.2 the boxplots of the count distribution per group.

8.2.1 Common Mistreatment of Counts

Based on the information provided in Table 8.1, Fig. 8.1, and/or Fig. 8.2, one group of researchers would argue that although the count distribution is skewed to the right, it is skewed to the right in both groups, the sample is large enough for the probability distributions of the group *M*s and of the difference in *M* between groups (often also referred to as sampling distributions) to approach a Normal distribution, and we can therefore ignore the skewness and compare the groups in *M* and *SD*

Table 8.1 Distribution of number of redo attempts in online environment among native and non-native speakers

	Count (i.e., 0 = pass first sit, no redo needed)						
	0	1	2	3	4	5	6
Native English speakers	69	87	57	23	6	1	0
Non-native English speakers	27	47	41	14	9	2	2

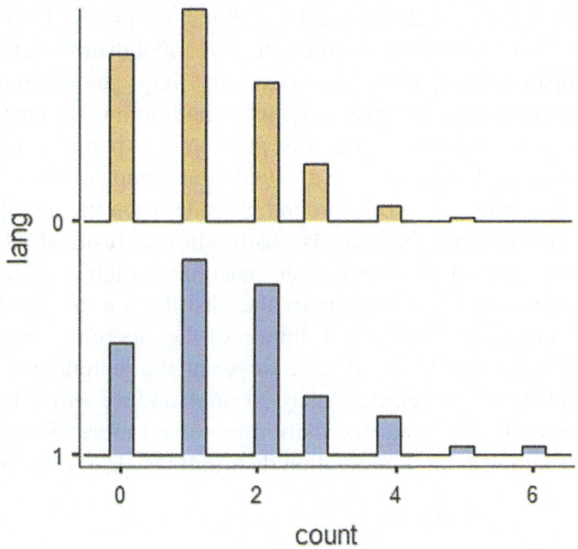

Fig. 8.1 Histogram of count distribution for native (lang = 0) and non-native (lang = 1) speakers (*Jamovi*)

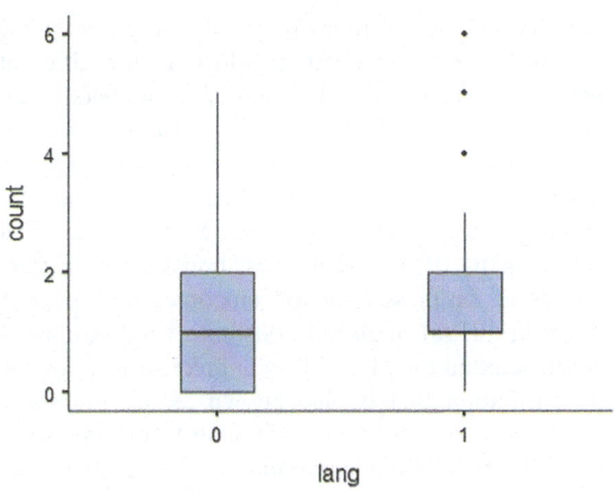

Fig. 8.2 Boxplot of count distribution for native (lang = 0) and non-native (lang = 1) speakers (*Jamovi*)

with a *t*-test. A second group of researchers might interpret cases who need five or six attempts as 'outliers' and delete them from the analysis. A third group of researchers might argue that we cannot use a *t*-test, because even if we delete the 'outliers' we do not have a Normal distribution of data; this group would take a nonparametric alternative to the *t*-test that converts the data into ranks. A fourth group of researchers would apply a square root or logarithmic *transformation* to obtain distributions that are less skewed and perform a *t*-test on the transformed data.

Although it appears to be wisdom of the crowds that data must follow a Normal distribution for *t*-tests and other parametric tests to be used, if that was the case, we could in educational settings almost *never* use a *t*-test because data rarely if ever follows a Normal distribution. A Normal distribution is a mathematical, continuous distribution, while the best we may get in our samples in practice is a non-continuous fairly symmetric and unimodal approximation of a Normal distribution. Besides, Normality assumptions pertain—in some models—to the distribution of *residuals* in a *population* sampled from, and unless we deal with the distribution of scores around a single mean the distribution of sample scores rarely has the same shape as the distribution of residuals. For example, in a study where we attempt to predict an outcome variable with a grouping variable and a non-categorical covariate, the distribution of residuals may be approximately Normal even if the distribution of the outcome variable clearly deviates from that. Finally, for *SE*s and *CI*s, we want the sampling distribution of an estimator of interest to be approximately Normal, and we know that with ever-increasing sample size the sampling distribution more and more closely approximates a Normal distribution even if population distributions clearly deviate from a Normal distribution.

8.2.2 Treating Counts as Counts

The aforementioned four groups of researchers would make inappropriate choices and likely draw incorrect conclusions for different but all wrong reasons and treatments. There is a fifth group of researchers, who treat counts as they should be counted: as counts (e.g., Nussbaum, Elsadat, & Khago, 2010). For other types of quantifiable variables, nonparametric (e.g., Fay & Proschan, 2010; Mann & Whitney, 1947; Mantel, 1966; Mantel & Haenszel, 1959) or robust (e.g., Algina, Keselman, & Penfield, 2005; Mair & Wilcox, 2018; Wilcox, 2017; Wilcox & Tian, 2011; Yuen, 1974) alternatives, transformation (e.g., Field, 2018), analysing the data as is, or presenting the outcomes with a combination of approaches (e.g., Leppink, 2019a) might all constitute valid options. However, each of the approaches discussed thus fair fail to appreciate that counts tend to follow a specific type of distribution that is also known as the *Poisson distribution* (i.e., the Poisson distribution is named after Siméon-Denis Poisson, 1790–1840; e.g., Nussbaum et al., 2010). While it is true that for frequently occurring events, where zero counts are unlikely and there is no stringent restriction in lower or upper limit of counts otherwise, the Poisson distribution may somewhat resemble a Normal distribution, for events like the one discussed in the example at hand, the probability distribution of counts is clearly skewed to the right with a hard limit at 0 and high counts occurring relatively infrequently. Just like we have different members of the *logistic regression* family for *categorical* outcome variables and we have *linear regression* for many different kinds of quantifiable outcome variables, we have *Poisson regression* (e.g., Agresti, 2002; Nussbaum et al., 2010) and variants of it for dealing with count outcome variables. The problem with linear regression on the kind of data encountered in the situation at hand is that the skewness comes with inflated *SD*s and *SE*s and that results in a substantial loss of statistical power for detecting differences of interest and results in unnecessarily wide CIs.

For the data at hand, $M = 1.230$ and $SD = 1.066$ (variance = 1.137) in the native speaker group and $M = 1.613$ and $SD = 1.287$ (variance = 1.657) in the non-native speaker group. As we see, in both groups, the variance is approximately equal to the M of that group. This situation is called *no overdispersion* and is an important condition of obtaining valid Poisson regression estimates (e.g., Agresti, 2002). If there is clear overdispersion, we can opt for a variant of Poisson regression (i.e., a quasi-Poisson model) that applies a correction for this overdispersion (Frome & Checkoway, 1985; Le, 1998) or regression models that are based on the *negative binomial distribution*, which is similar to the Poisson distribution but can deal much better with events that generally have an infrequent occurrence (e.g., 0 or 1) but exponentially smaller probabilities of occurrence for increasingly larger counts (e.g., Leppink, 2019a).

For cases where there is no or minimal overdispersion, like the situation at hand, a Poisson model assuming no overdispersion and a Poisson model correcting for overdispersion will yield about the same results, and there is no need to consider negative binomial regression models. For the data at hand, *Jamovi* returns for the Poisson model assuming no overdispersion: LR test $\chi^2_1 = 9.350$, $p = 0.002$, and for the group difference, $b = 0.271$ with a 95% CI of [0.098; 0.442]. For the Poisson model that corrects for eventual overdispersion, *Jamovi* returns: LR test $\chi^2_1 = 9.718$, $p = 0.002$, and for the group difference, $b = 0.271$ with a 95% CI of [0.101; 0.439]. In short, almost the same outcomes under the two models. The exponent of b, e^b, is about 1.311 and is also known as the *relative risk* ratio (e.g., Nussbaum et al., 2010). It is important to note that this is *not* the same as an *OR* in the categorical outcome variable models discussed in the previous chapters; *OR*s are ratios of *odds*, whereas *relative risk ratios* are ratios of *probabilities*. The ratio of 1.311 indicates that, on average, the number of attempts is about 31.1% higher in the non-native speaker group than in the native speaker group.

8.3 Test Performance at Different Institutions

In our next example, three universities decide to join forces and form a consortium for research methods education in their Bachelor in the health sciences programmes. In their programmes, they already cover the same methods in the same years and during the same periods of the academic year. They also share a concern about students approaching research methods with mixed motivation; some students are very motivated and appear to have a genuine interest in learning more and in applying it in their group projects throughout the Bachelor programme, whereas others see it as a 'necessary evil' that needs to be dealt with in order to get the degree. There is preoccupation among staff of the three universities that many students, especially in the latter category, cram the minimum necessary content in the days prior to the exam and hope that is enough to pass the exam 'hurdle'. To study the development in students' knowledge of research methods throughout the Bachelor programme, the three universities agree to develop an item bank for a joint progress testing programme, which comes down to all students from all years of all three Bachelor programmes sitting down three times a year and take the same 100-item MCQ test as their peers. The test is designed around the end goals of the final, third year of the Bachelor programme; what a graduating Bachelor student is supposed to know about research methods. They now have their first 100-item MCQ test (five alternatives per item) ready and want to administer that to a random sample from Year 3 from the three different Bachelor programmes, each of which hosts in between 400 and 500 students every year. All 100 items have resulted from example items partly adapted from old Year 3 exams partly modified from other sources, using a method that will also be used for rapid expansion of the item bank: *automatic item generation* (AIG; e.g., Blum & Holling, 2018; Bormuth, 1969; Gierl & Haladyna, 2012; Gierl & Lai, 2012; Glas, Van der Linden, & Geerlings, 2010). In AIG, experts create templates called item models, which are then used by computer algorithms to generate test items.

Given that the programmes of the different universities are, for the research methods component, the same, and staff of the three universities have no reasons to assume any kind of differences between the Bachelor populations otherwise that might contribute to differences in test performance between the three universities, they expect $\boldsymbol{H_0}$: '*M* performance is the same across programmes' to be preferred over $\boldsymbol{H_1}$: '*M* performance is *not* the same across programmes (i.e., at least one programme has a different *M* than the others)'. Besides, to examine test-retest reliability, they decide to ask students to come for a test twice: on a Monday morning in one week, and on the Monday morning the week after. Students are told they will complete a new progress test but are not explicitly told they will have the same test at both occasions. Students are not allowed to take the test home after any of the two sits.

The universities decide to randomly sample $n = 100$ Year 3 students from each institution to complete this test. All in total $N = 300$ students agree to participate and complete the test at two occasions. A group of psychometricians from the three universities perform Rasch analysis on the items (cf. Chap. 5) and, based on that analysis, decide to let the test score be the sum of correct responses (i.e., every item has two possible scores: 0 = incorrect; 1 = correct). In other words, a student's test score can range from 0 (minimum) to 100 (maximum). For the sake of simplicity of the example, let us use the sum score of the two tests and use that for comparison between the universities (i.e., leave the items out of the analysis; including them could be done in a three-level mixed-effects binary logistic model). The psychometricians check histograms, boxplots and scatterplots and conclude that all is fine to proceed (i.e., no Hawaii-vs.-US-mainland distance extreme cases or groups of cases that might affect *M*s, inflate *SD*s and affect correlation coefficients). Table 8.2 presents *M*s and *SD*s of performance at the two test occasions and performance difference (i.e., test 2 minus test 1) per university.

As Table 8.2 indicates, differences between the institutions are small.

Table 8.2 *M*s and *SD*s of performance on test 1, test 2, and the difference (test 2 minus test 1) per university

University	Test 1: *M* (*SD*)	Test 2: *M* (*SD*)	Test 2-1: *M* (*SD*)
A	60.190 (9.810)	59.070 (11.919)	−1.120 (7.444)
B	60.730 (9.742)	60.240 (12.097)	−0.490 (6.841)
C	59.300 (10.603)	58.420 (13.438)	−0.880 (7.174)

8.3.1 Random Effects

What we are dealing with here is a two-level design: students constitute the upper level, and the tests—which are stations to be passed by the students—constitute the lower level. This enables us to estimate student-level random effects (i.e., random part) and fixed effects of interest (i.e., fixed part): the main effect of occasion (i.e., test 1 vs. test 2), the main effect of institution (A, B, C), and the institution-by-occasion interaction effect. For the estimation of random effects, we use REML (e.g., Tan, 2010; Verbeke & Molenberghs, 2000). An easy way to model the random part of the model is CS: one estimate of the correlation between residuals (r_{RES}) of the two tests, and one estimate of the residual variance (V_{RES}) that is assumed to hold for the two tests. An alternative structure is to use one estimate of r_{RES} but *two* V_{RES}-estimates, one for each test; this structure, where we allow for varying V_{RES}, is also known as CS heterogenous (henceforth: CSH). The latter requires one more *df* but pays off if the difference in residual variance between the two tests is large enough. To not overestimate any of the random part, it is important we also include our fixed part in our model while we estimate the random part (e.g., Leppink, 2019a).

Under FIML, which we use to estimate the fixed part of a mixed-effects model (e.g., Tan, 2010; Verbeke & Molenberghs, 2000), we can use AIC, BIC, and criteria alike to decide which fixed effects we should include and which ones we may as well leave out. However, under REML this a problem, at least as far as BIC is concerned since this criterion uses the sample size as part of the penalty of adding more parameters to reduce the likelihood of overfitting. However, in mixed-effects models, sample size is open to discussion and the correction applied by BIC is often too severe and that will then result in way too simple random parts (e.g., Delattre, Lavielle, & Poursat, 2014; Fitzmaurice, Laird, & Ware, 2004; Hedeker & Gibbons, 2006). Besides, under REML, different software packages yield different AIC and BIC estimates (e.g., Delattre et al., 2014) and some packages do not even provide BIC under REML (e.g., Jamovi). However, we *can* still use the LR test under REML, as long as we only compare nested models (see Chap. 3 for definition and examples of nested models) only and all under REML. In other words, when we are modelling the fixed part, we use FIML as estimator and we can use LR tests to compare models that differ—in a nested way—in their *fixed* part, and when we are modelling the random part, we use REML as estimator and we can use LR tests to compare models that differ in their *random* part. What we should *not* do is compare one model estimated with FIML and another model estimated with REML, because the −2LL returned by FIML is not the same as the −2RLL (R for 'restricted').

For CS, we find −2RLL = 4294.091, while for CSH, we find −2RLL = 4253.411 (*SPSS*). The difference in *df* between the two models is 1, and the resulting LR test yields: $\chi_1^2 = 40.680, p < 0.001$. In other words, the more complex model is to be preferred. The correlation between the residuals of the two test occasions is 0.820 and can be interpreted as an estimator of test-retest reliability. In the CS model, this estimate would be 0.801, slightly lower than in the CSH model as is to be expected in the face of substantial variation in V_{RES} (e.g., Leppink, 2019a, 2019b).

8.3.2 Fixed Effects

Now that we have decided on the random part, we take care of the fixed part. Table 8.3 presents the −2LL, AIC, and BIC of the null model (Model 0), the occasions main effect model (Model 1), the institutions main effect model (Model 2), the occasions and institutions main effects model (Model 3), and the full factorial model which includes the institution-by-occasion interaction effect as well (Model 4).

AIC prefers Model 1, whereas BIC prefers Model 0. The LR test for the difference between these two models yields: $\chi_1^2 = 4.043, p = 0.044$. DRF_{10} (i.e., DRF of Model 1 vs. Model 0) is nearly 0.001, in short, very small. Besides, what all criteria agree on is that we do not need to account for differences between institutions, neither through the interaction effect nor through the institutions main effect.

8.4 Nonlinearity

We tend to think in terms of linear models, because it is easier to think in linear terms, outcomes from linear models are easier to explain to a broad audience, linear models in many cases do perform reasonably well, and in some cases either the study design or the sample size stand in the way of exploring non-linear models. However, a family of useful non-linear models is found in *polynomial* models, such as the *quadratic* (i.e., to the power 2) and *cubic* (i.e., to the power 3) model; *linear* is the

Table 8.3 Five competing models: −2LL, AIC, and BIC (*SPSS*)

Model	−2LL	AIC	BIC
0 (null)	4267.898	4275.898	4293.485
1 (occasions)	4263.855	4273.855	4295.840
2 (institutions)	4266.875	4278.875	4305.256
3 (main effects)	4262.832	4276.832	4307.611
4 (full factorial)	4262.434	4280.434	4320.006

simplest form of a polynomial model. Although the first-order derivative of a quadratic model and the second-order derivative of a cubic model are linear models as well, the great thing about these only slightly more sophisticated cousins of the linear model allow us to interpret relations between learning-relevant variables of interest in terms other than a straight line without using many more *df*. Given a predictor variable and an outcome variable of interest, the quadratic model uses only 1 *df* more than the linear model (i.e., to estimate the quadratic term) and the cubic model uses 1 *df* more than the quadratic model (i.e., to estimate the cubic term).

When it comes to interrelations between assessments, such as scores from different exams in a Bachelor or Master programme, linear models often perform quite well, and more sophisticated polynomial models hardly add anything to the explanation of differences in scores. However, there certainly are learning-related phenomena where for more sophisticated polynomial models appear to outperform linear models. One recent example of a quadratic model is found in the relation between *mental effort* invested in a question presented and *response time* or time needed from the start of seeing a question to the moment of response (Leppink & Pérez-Fuster, 2019). Figure 8.3 presents an example of the type of quadratic model in that relation.

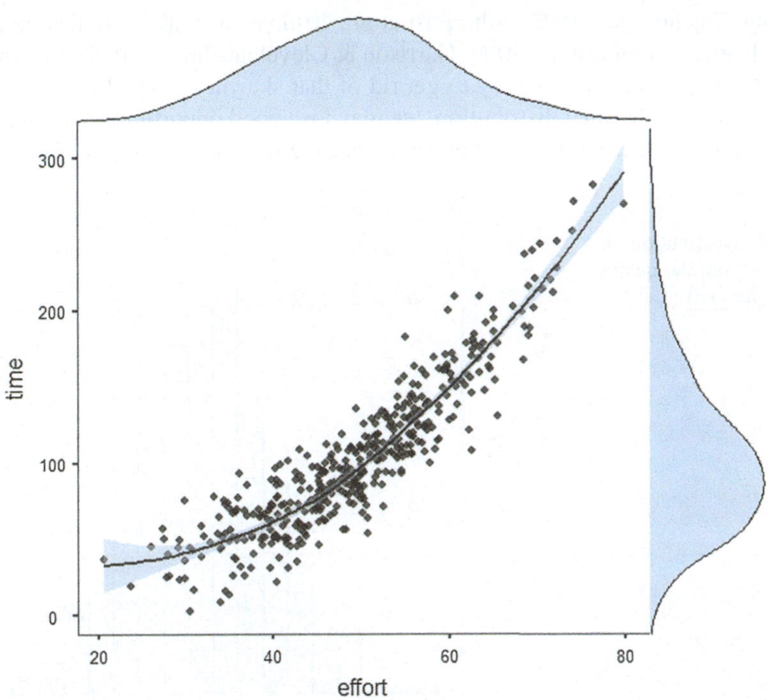

Fig. 8.3 Quadratic relation between mental effort (VAS: 0–100) and response time (seconds) (*Jamovi*)

The blue shade around the best fitting line represents the *SE* around that best fitting line, and the curves around it indicate the density of the distributions of mental effort (horizontally) and response time (vertically). Mental effort is fairly symmetrically distributed, not that much different from Normal, whereas response time is clearly skewed to the right. Researchers who believe that data must follow a Normal distribution and/or who interpret some of the high response time values as 'outliers' may remove some of the high response time values, fit a linear model to the remaining data, and conclude that a linear pattern fits well. In fact, even if we do not remove any 'outliers', packages like Stata and SPSS return $R^2 = 0.818$ for the linear model. However, when we fit a quadratic model in these packages, we find $R^2 = 0.866$. For the *linear* model, we find AIC = 3751.284 and BIC = 3763.404, while for the *quadratic* model, we find AIC = 3625.240 and BIC = 3641.401. In other words, both criteria prefer the quadratic model. Figure 8.4 displays the distribution of *residuals* from the quadratic model.

The residuals are more or less symmetrically and unimodally distributed (skewness: 0.031; kurtosis: 0.234) with $M = 0$ (median = 0.142) and $SD =$ 17.966 s. The residuals from a linear model would be somewhat more skewed to the right (skewness: 0.345; kurtosis: 0.114) with $M = 0$ (median = −0.772) and $SD = 20.925$ s.

In time variables, which are increasingly common in studies involving *eye-tracking* (Duchowski, 2016; Holmqvist et al., 2011) as well as in studies involving online learning (Finkelstein, 2009; Garrison & Cleveland-Innes, 2005), skewness to the right is normal, and if we try to get rid of that skewness to make a distribution more similar to a Normal distribution, we may lose good opportunities to model and understand nonlinear relations between learning-relevant variables. The mental

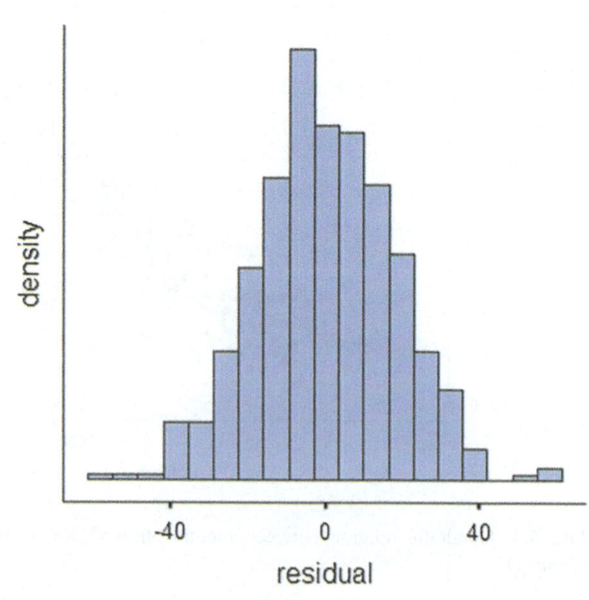

Fig. 8.4 Distribution of residuals from the quadratic model (Jamovi)

effort-response time case provides a clear example of how an outcome variable of interest may be distributed in a way that clearly deviates from Normal, but the residuals are not that bad of an approximation of a Normal distribution.

References

Agresti, A. (2002). *Categorical data analysis* (2nd ed.). New York, NY: Wiley.

Algina, J., Keselman, H. J., & Penfield, R. D. (2005). An alternative to Cohen's standardized mean difference effect size: A robust parameter and confidence interval in the two independent groups case. *Psychological Methods, 10*(3), 317–328.

Blum, D., & Holling, H. (2018). Automatic generation of figural analogies with the IMak Package. *Frontiers in Psychology, 9*(1). https://doi.org/10.3389/fpsyg.2018.01286.

Bormuth, J. (1969). *On a theory of achievement test items*. Chicago, IL: University of Chicago Press.

Delattre, M., Lavielle, M., & Poursat, M. A. (2014). A note on BIC in mixed-effects models. *Electronic Journal of Statistics, 8*, 456–475. https://doi.org/10.1214/14-EJS890.

Duchowski, A. T. (2016). *Eye tracking methodology* (3rd ed.). New York, NY: Springer.

Fay, M. P., & Proschan, M. A. (2010). Wilcoxon-Mann-Whitney or *t*-test? *Statistics Surveys, 4*, 1–39. https://doi.org/10.1214/09-SS051.

Field, A. (2018). *Discovering statistics using IBM SPSS statistics* (5th ed.). London: Sage.

Finkelstein, J. E. (2009). *Learning in real time: Synchronous teaching and learning online*. San Francisco, CA: Jossey-Bass.

Fitzmaurice, G. M., Laird, N. M., & Ware, J. H. (2004). *Applied longitudinal analysis*. New York, NY: Wiley.

Frome, E. L., & Checkoway, H. (1985). Use of Poisson regression models in estimating rates and ratios. *American Journal of Epidemiology, 121*(2), 309–323. https://doi.org/10.1093/oxfordjournals.aje.a114001.

Garrison, D. R., & Cleveland-Innes, M. (2005). Facilitating cognitive presence in online learning: Interaction is not enough. *American Journal of Distance Education, 19*(3), 133–148. https://doi.org/10.1207/s15389286ajde1903_2.

Gierl, M. J., & Haladyna, T. M. (2012). *Automatic item generation, theory and practice*. New York, NY: Routledge Chapman & Hall.

Gierl, M. J., & Lai, H. (2012). The role of item models in automatic item generation. *International Journal of Testing, 12*(3), 273–298. https://doi.org/10.1080/15305058.2011.635830.

Glas, C. A. W., Van der Linden, W. J., & Geerlings, H. (2010). Estimation of the parameters in an item-cloning model for adaptive testing. In W. J. Van der Linden & C. A. W. Glas (Eds.), *Elements of adaptive testing* (pp. 289–314). https://doi.org/10.1007/978-0-387-85461-8_15.

Hedeker, D., & Gibbons, R. D. (2006). *Longitudinal data analysis*. Hoboken, NJ: Wiley.

Holmqvist, K., Nyström, M., Andersson, R., Dewhurst, R., Jarodzka, H., & Van de Weijer, J. (2011). *Eye tracking: A comprehensive guide to methods and measures*. Oxford: Oxford University Press.

Le, C. T. (1998). *Applied categorical data analysis*. New York, NY: Wiley.

Leppink, J. (2019a). *Statistical methods for experimental research in education and psychology*. Cham: Springer. https://doi.org/10.1007/978-3-030-21241-4.

Leppink, J. (2019b). How we underestimate reliability and overestimate resources needed: Revisiting our psychometric practice. *Health Professions Education, 5*(2), 91–92.

Leppink, J., & Pérez-Fuster P. (2019). Mental effort, workload, time on task, and certainty: Beyond linear models. *Educational Psychology Review*. https://doi.org/10.1007/s10648-018-09460-2.

Mair, P., & Wilcox, R. R. (2018). *WRS2: A collection of robust statistical methods*. R package version 0.10–0. Retrieved from: https://cran.r-project.org/web/packages/WRS2/index.html. Accessed February 1, 2020.

Mann, H. B., & Whitney, D. R. (1947). On a test of whether one of two random variables is stochastically larger than the other. *Annals of Mathematical Statistics, 18*(1), 50–60.

Mantel, N. (1966). Evaluation of survival data and two new rank order statistics arising in its consideration. *Cancer Chemotherapy Reports, 50*(3), 163–170. https://doi.org/10.1093/jnci/22.4.719.

Mantel, N., & Haenszel, W. (1959). Statistical aspects of the analysis of data from retrospective studies of disease. *Journal of the National Cancer Institute, 22*(4), 719–748.

Nussbaum, E. M., Elsadat, S., Khago, A. M. (2010). In J. W. Osborne (Ed.), *Best practices in quantitative methods* (Chap. 21, pp. 306–323). London: Sage.

Tan, F. E. S. (2010). Best practices in analysis of longitudinal data: A multilevel approach. In J. W. Osborne (Ed.), *Best practices in quantitative methods (Chap. 30)* (pp. 451–470). London: Sage.

Verbeke, G., & Molenberghs, G. (2000). *Linear mixed models for longitudinal data*. New York, NY: Springer.

Wilcox, R. R. (2017). *Introduction to robust estimation and hypothesis testing* (4th ed.). Burlington, MA: Elsevier.

Wilcox, R. R., & Tian, T. (2011). Measuring effect size: A robust heteroscedastic approach for two or more groups. *Journal of Applied Statistics, 38*(7), 1359–1368. https://doi.org/10.1080/02664763.2010.498507.

Yuen, K. K. (1974). The two sample trimmed *t* for unequal population variances. *Biometrika, 61* (1), 165–170. https://doi.org/10.1093/biomet/61.1.165.

Part III
Variable Networks

Instrument Structures

9

Abstract

Chapter 4 briefly mentions concepts of instrument validity and reliability but in conceptual terms rather than in terms of statistical methods. In this chapter, different statistical methods for the statistical validity and reliability of our psychometric instruments are discussed, including some already introduced in the context of examples in Chaps. 3 (factor analysis), 5 (reliability estimators, IRT and latent class analysis), 7 (latent class analysis), and 8 (mixed-effects models for test-retest reliability). Some of these methods involve latent variables, whereas other methods do not. Relative pros and cons of the different methods included in this chapter are discussed, and a general mixed-effects variable network approach is proposed for the study of statistical validity and reliability. Examples in this chapter include multi-item questionnaires, specific time variables, and exam performance rated by multiple assessors.

9.1 Introduction

Researchers have a wide variety of methods available to study the psychometric structures of the instruments they use, and given a particular situation, some methods may be more appropriate than other methods. There have been important developments in recent years, in both methods and in software that implement these methods, that have implications for what we can do. This chapter presents a range of situations with likely candidate methods and concludes with a general approach that lies at the core of next chapters in this book.

J. Leppink, *The Art of Modelling the Learning Process*, Springer Texts in Education,
https://doi.org/10.1007/978-3-030-43082-5_9

9.2 Residual Covariance Models for Sets of Items

To start with a fairly simple example, suppose we have $N = 250$ students complete a learning task and respond to three interrelated statements relating to the complexity of the task on a VAS from 0 (minimum) to 100 (maximum) about that task. All three items yield fairly symmetric and unidimensional score distributions with $M = 40.323$ ($SD = 5.893$) for item 1, $M = 40.780$ ($SD = 9.889$) for item 2, and $M = 40.649$ ($SD = 9.570$) for item 3. For Pearson's r, we find $r = 0.593$ for items 1 and 2, $r = 0.662$ for items 1 and 3, and $r = 0.405$ for items 2 and 3. In a one-factor model, we obtain standardised loadings of 0.984 for item 1, 0.602 for item 2, and 0.672 for item 3. Many researchers would now use Cronbach's alpha (α) to estimate the internal consistency or reliability of the scale of three items. For the data at hand, we obtain $\alpha = 0.744$. One way to compute α is as follows:

$$\alpha = (k * ICC)/[1 + ((k-1) * ICC)].$$

In this formula, k is the number of items, and in the computation of ICC we assume CS. As discussed previously, CS assumes r to be equal across item pairs and SD to be equal across items. When SD varies considerably across items, α is likely to underestimate scale reliability and V_{RES}-adjusted α—which adjusts for that varying SD—can be an easy alternative, at least if differences in r across item pairs are small (e.g., Leppink, 2019a, 2019b). While α assumes CS, V_{RES}-adjusted α assumes CSH. That is, ICC in α results from a two-level (i.e., student upper level, item lower level) mixed-effects linear regression model with item as fixed effect and student-level random intercept (RI) as random effect (i.e., CS). CSH is a more flexible variant of that model, in that V_{RES} is not assumed constant but can vary across items. For the data at hand, we find $-2\text{RLL} = 5192.290$ for CS and $-2\text{RLL} = 5069.162$ for CSH. The difference in df is 2, because we use $df = 1$ for V_{RES} in CS versus $df = 3$ (i.e., given three items) for V_{RES} in CSH. The resulting LR test yields: $\chi^2_2 = 123.128$, $p < 0.001$. Under CS, ICC is estimated to be 0.492; under CSH, ICC is estimated to be 0.555. When we enter the latter as ICC in the above formula, we obtain V_{RES}-adjusted $\alpha = 0.789$ (Leppink, 2019a, 2019b).

Two other residual covariance models that use the same number of df as CSH but operate slightly differently are Huynh-Feldt (HF: Huynh & Feldt, 1970, 1976) and first-order ante-dependence (AD1: Eyduran & Akbaş, 2010). In HF, all r_{RES}s are a function of the V_{RES}s of the two items that constitute a pair and a constant factor λ that holds for all pairs. In AD1, we allow V_{RES} to vary across items and we estimate a r_{RES} for each pair of adjacent tasks; r_{RES} of any pair of non-adjacent tasks is the product of all adjacent correlations in between. For the data at hand, we find $-2\text{RLL} = 5103.692$ for HF and $-2\text{RLL} = 5133.401$. Although these values also indicate a significant reduction in -2RLL relative to CS, and we cannot perform LR tests on the differences between CSH, HF, and AD1 given that these do not count as nested models, the decrease in -2RLL with CSH is stronger than that achieved with HF or AD1.

Finally, we have a covariance structure that is called *unstructured* (UN: e.g., Lu & Mehrotra, 2009). In UN, we use as many *df* as there are r_{RES}s (i.e., number of item pairs) and V_{RES}s (i.e., number of items) to estimate. For three items, this comes down to three *df* for r_{RES}s and three *df* for V_{RES}s, so $df = 6$ in total. For the data at hand, we find −2RLL = 5034.505 for UN. The difference between UN and any of the three other alternatives to CS discussed is 2 *df*, and each of the four alternatives to UN discussed can be seen as a special (i.e., simple, nested) case of UN. Given the difference in −2RLL between UN and any of the alternatives, all LR tests yield $p < 0.001$, meaning that UN is to be preferred.

Cronbach's α is based on CS, which is in practice often too restrictive. Alternative reliability estimators, which are based on UN or other residual covariance structures discussed in Chaps. 10 and 11, are more flexible. An increasingly popular alternative to α is found in McDonald's ω, which for this data is 0.807. For a broader discussion of α, ω, and other reliability estimates, see for instance (Crutzen & Peters, 2017; Dunn et al., 2014; Leppink, 2019a, 2019b; Peters, 2014; Revelle & Zinbarg, 2009), but I hope this example illustrates why it is useful to look beyond α.

9.3 Latent Variables and Networks

Latent variable models treat items or observed scores otherwise as manifest indicators of not directly observed latent variables. The rationale behind these models is that after we account for the latent variable(s) that are supposed to be measured by the set(s) of manifest variables, the correlations between the residuals of the manifest variables should be (approximately) zero (i.e., *local independence*; e.g., Iramaneerat, Smith, & Smith, 2010). Besides, there should be a *monotonous* relation (which is not necessarily a linear relation) between the manifest variables and the latent variable(s) measured by these manifest variables. For instance, if three items in a questionnaire are supposed to measure intrinsic motivation, students who have more intrinsic motivation should score higher on the items, and not sometimes higher sometimes lower, than students who are less intrinsically motivated.

Another, emerging perspective on measurement is found in *network analysis* (e.g., Borsboom & Cramer, 2013; Cramer, Waldorp, Van der Maas, & Borsboom, 2010; Epskamp, Borsboom, & Fried, 2018; Golino & Epskamp, 2017). The rationale behind network analysis stems from *mutualism* (i.e., reciprocal causation, interaction; Van der Maas et al., 2006): just like groups of animals do not need a latent animal telling them where to go or how not to bump into each other, groups of items formulated in particular ways do not need a latent variable to explain why they tend to result in correlated scores. If a set of items all focus on the complexity of a task, as in the example this chapter starts with, this will likely result in a fully connected *clique* of items in a network. Figure 9.1 presents the network of the three items in the starting example of this chapter (*JASP*).

Fig. 9.1 A network of three positively correlated items (i1, i2, i3) (*JASP*)

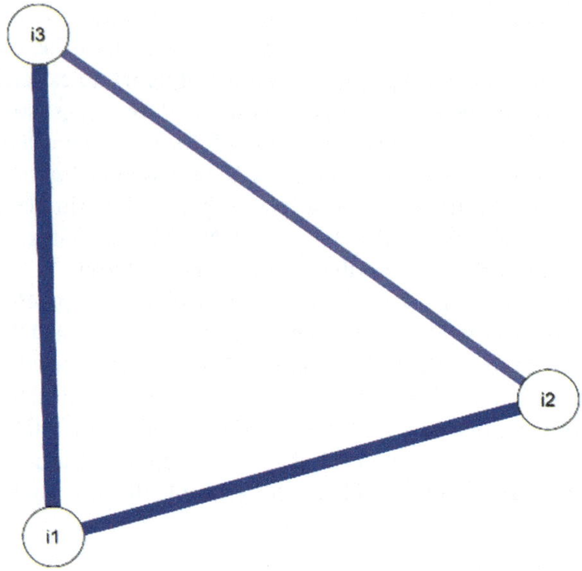

The lines are blue because the correlations are positive; negative correlations would be presented in red. The thicker the lines, the stronger the correlation: the line connecting items 2 and 3 (i.e., i2 and i3) is visibly thinner than the other two lines, because the correlation between items 2 and 3 is only $r = 0.405$, while the other two correlations are $r = 0.593$ and $r = 0.662$.

9.3.1 Manifest Groups and Latent Profiles

Sometimes, we have to account for the presence of different groups when we estimate correlations; failing to do so may result in incorrect conclusions. Suppose, we have the same task as in the previous example but now a total sample of $N = 495$ is composed of students (novices in the topic: $n = 244$) and experts (who have 10+ years of experience in the topic: $n = 251$). Both groups respond to the same set of three items about task complexity right after they complete the task. In both groups, the score distributions are fairly symmetric and unimodal, but the *M*s and *SD*s of the three items are as displayed in Table 9.1.

Figure 9.2 presents the scatterplot of the joint distribution of scores for each pair of items per group.

Table 9.1 *M*s and *SD*s of item response among students and experts

Group	Item 1: *M* (*SD*)	Item 2: *M* (*SD*)	Item 3: *M* (*SD*)
Students	40.285 (5.894)	39.454 (10.521)	40.247 (9.524)
Experts	20.171 (2.911)	20.718 (5.005)	20.089 (5.198)

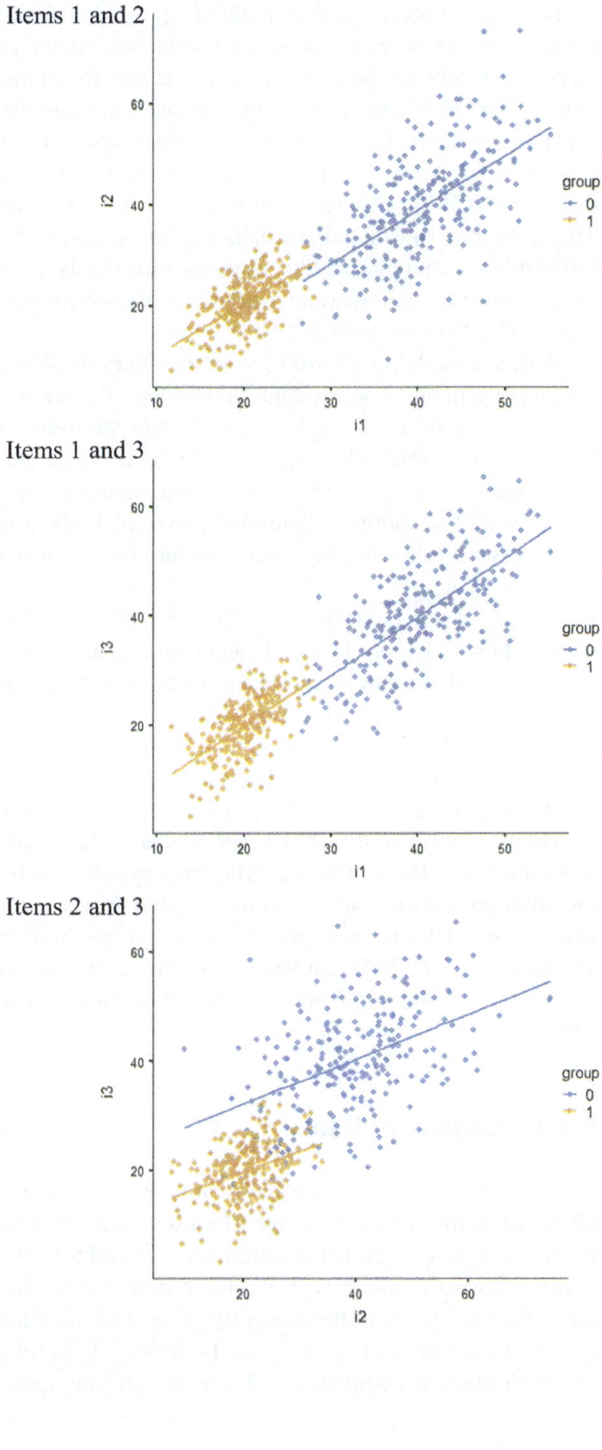

Fig. 9.2 Scatterplot of the joint distribution of scores for each pair of items per group (0 = students, 1 = experts) (*Jamovi*)

There is not much overlap in item response between the two groups. If we ignore the presence of these two groups, we will find inflated correlations for the three item pairs: $r = 0.849$ for items 1 and 2, $r = 0.889$ for items 1 and 3, and $r = 0.773$ for items 2 and 3. When we, as is appropriate, compute the correlations for each group separately, we obtain: $r = 0.600$ for items 1 and 2, $r = 0.668$ for items 1 and 3, and $r = 0.456$ for items 2 and 3, for the students; and we obtain $r = 0.592$ for items 1 and 2, $r = 0.592$ for items 1 and 3, and $r = 0.359$ for items 2 and 3, for the experts. These are still substantial correlations, but of course considerably smaller than the inflated ones that ignore the obvious bimodality in the distributions due to the presence of two very distinct groups. Figure 9.3 presents the resulting network plot for each of the two groups.

With a bimodality as strong as in the example at hand, even if we did not know which participants were students and which ones were experts, we could reasonably cluster the groups through *latent profile analysis* (Ding, 2018; Hagenaars & McCutcheon, 2002; McCutcheon, 1987); while latent class analysis can be used when items are categorical, latent profile analysis can be used when items are not categorical. The rationale behind the two methods is that if there are two or more latent classes, this will likely translate into fairly consistent differences in responses —different categories or different scores—on a set of items supposed to measure the latent variable of interest. IRT and factor analysis treat latent variables as *continuous*, whereas latent class and latent profile analysis treat latent variables as *discontinuous*, albeit that in the case of discontinuity within classes the latent variables of interest are continuous (e.g., the idea behind the mixed Rasch model, which comes down to using latent class analysis to classify respondents into groups to then use Rasch model for each group).

Figure 9.4 presents an *EMM* plot of two latent profiles with the data at hand.

Mplus classifies $n = 234$ respondents (47.3% of 495) as Class 1 and the remaining $n = 261$ as Class 2. The entropy value is 0.965, and when we compare the solution with the actual group membership, we see that Class 2 comprises *all* experts and 10 students, and Class 1 has the remaining 234 students. The 10 students (4.1% of 244) that landed in Class 2 are the ones who provided low scores on the items and could therefore—based on these items—not be separated from the experts.

9.3.2 Cliques of Items

Thus far in this chapter, we have only seen examples of a single factor or single clique of items. In practice, we often deal with instruments where more than one trait or state of interest is measured, and we end up with two or more factors or item cliques. Suppose, along with the three items about the complexity of the task, we have three items about the difficulty of the task instructions; these two aspects may be correlated but need not necessarily be (e.g., Leppink & Hanham, 2019). We have $N = 336$ students complete a task and the six-item questionnaire. In this study, each

Fig. 9.3 Network plot of items 1–3 (i1, i2, i3) for students and experts (JASP)

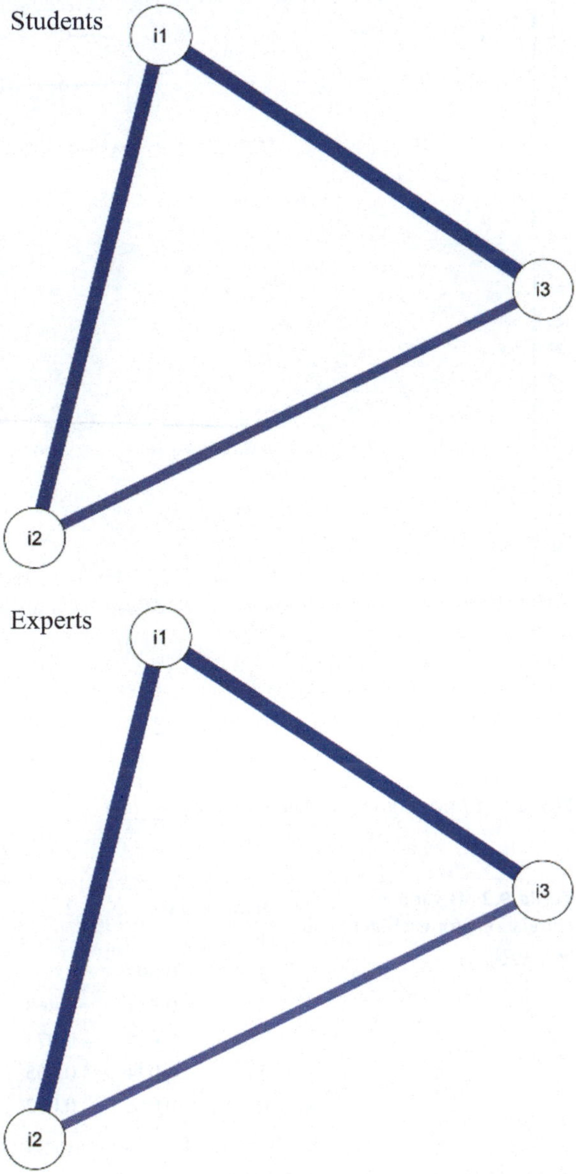

of six items is rated on an integer scale from 0 (minimum) to 10 (maximum). The score distributions are fairly symmetric and unimodal, and the bivariate correlations are as presented in Table 9.2.

With this data, *Jamovi* returns a well-fitting confirmatory two-factor model (i.e., all residual correlations well within the [−0.1; 0.1] range) with loadings of 0.857 for item 1, 0.692 for item 2, and 0.678 for item 3 on factor 1, loadings of 0.871 for item

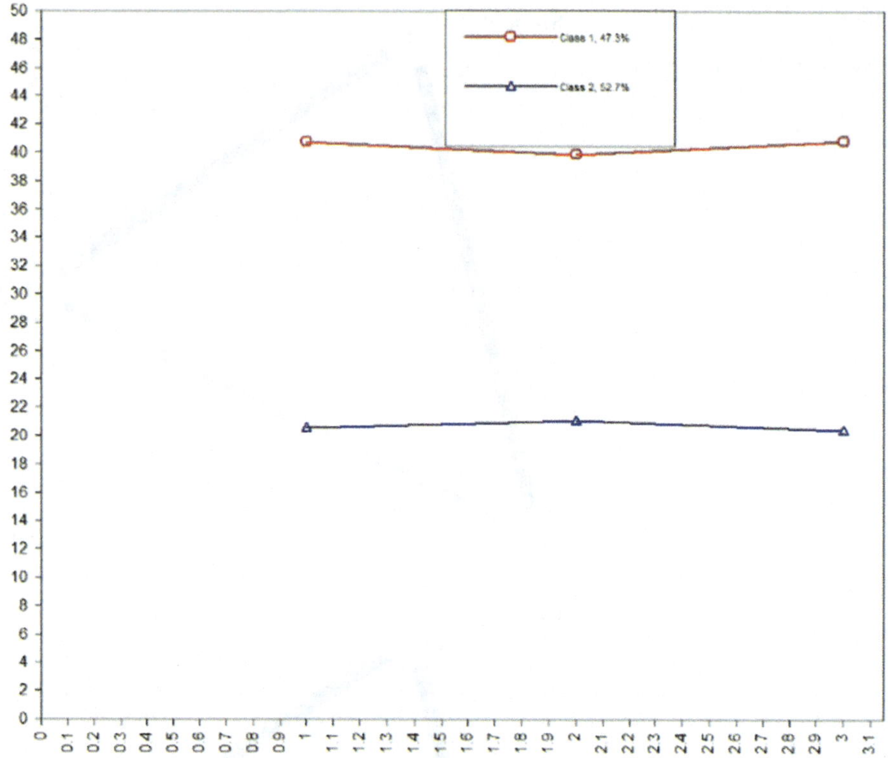

Fig. 9.4 EMM plot of two latent profiles (*Mplus*)

Table 9.2 Bivariate correlations for each item pair (*Jamovi*)

Item	1	2	3	4	5
1					
2	0.593				
3	0.581	0.468			
4	0.035	0.074	0.016		
5	0.034	0.065	0.048	0.563	
6	0.058	0.072	−0.009	0.532	0.392

4, 0.645 for item 5, and 0.610 for item 6 on factor 2, and a correlation between factors of 0.069. Figure 9.5 presents the network plot for this study.

We see two clear cliques of well-connected items in line with the correlation matrix and two-factor model. The network models presented thus far in this chapter are based on *bivariate* correlations, for example as per correlation matrix in Table 9.2. While these network plots provide useful information, there is one drawback: even though some connections are so weak that we can barely see them, all items are connected because none of the correlations is 0 (yes, some are very

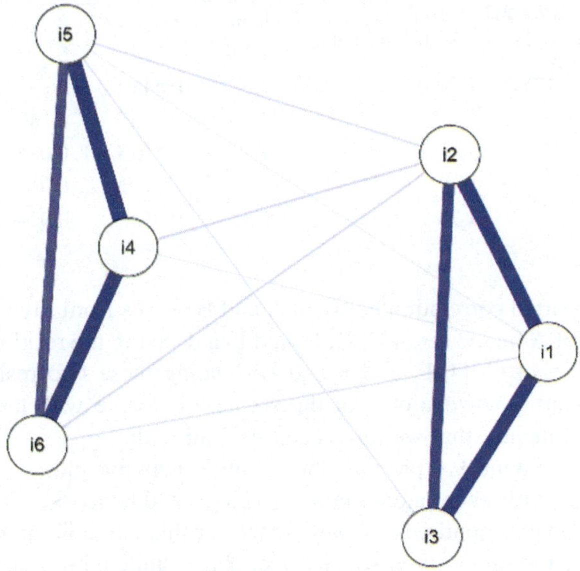

Fig. 9.5 Network plot for six items that can be grouped as two groups of three items (*JASP*)

close to zero, and therefore hard to see in the network plot). Given *k* variables, the number of edges (E) in the plot (i.e., the number of correlations) that can be estimated is:

$$E = k * (k - 1)/2.$$

In the network model in Fig. 9.5, there are no zero correlations, so all 15 edges are estimated (i.e., all edges are non-zero edges). One can barely see it, but even between items 3 and 6 there is a faint red line ($r = -0.009$). Given that all edges are estimated, the *sparsity* (S) of this model is 0; S is the complement of the ratio of actually estimated edges (E_E) and E:

$$S = 1 - (E_E/E).$$

9.3.3 Partial Correlations and Testing

Apart from the bivariate correlations used thus far, we can also compute *partial correlations* (e.g., Howell, 2017). Let us consider an example where we have three items, A, B, and C. To obtain the partial correlation between A and B, we have to take the following steps. We first regress A on C and save the residuals. We then regress B on C and save the residuals. The partial correlation between A and B is then the correlation between the residuals from the regressions of A on C and of B on C. The same logic applies for the partial correlation of any other pair of items. When there are more than three items, for instance six in the case of Fig. 9.5, the

Table 9.3 Partial correlations for the six items (SPSS)

Item	1	2	3	4	5
1					
2	0.443				
3	0.430	0.189			
4	−0.015	0.034	−0.008		
5	−0.025	0.011	0.051	0.453	
6	0.055	0.024	−0.068	0.407	0.135

partial correlation between A and B results from saving the residuals of a regression of A on the set of C, D, E, and F and saving the residuals of a regression of B on the set of C, D, E, and F and correlating these two residuals. Table 9.3 presents the partial correlations for the six-item example with task complexity and instruction difficulty that we have been dealing with.

Figure 9.6 presents the resulting network plot.

Still, there are no non-zero edges and hence S = 0. Luckily, we are dealing with several hundreds of participants in this example and E = 15 only, but in practice samples are often smaller and/or E is quite a bit bigger. To deal with that problem, the *least absolute shrinkage and selection operator* (LASSO; Santosa & Symes, 1986; Tibshirani, 1996, 2011). Succinctly put, this technique works such that edges that are close enough to zero *shrink to exactly 0* and thus do not need to be estimated. Consequently, S increases. LASSO uses a so-called *tuning parameter* to control the degree to which shrinkage takes place, which can be selected by minimising the *Extended BIC* (EBIC; Chen & Chen, 2008). This combination of EBIC and LASSO, that is used on partial correlations, has been called EBICglasso

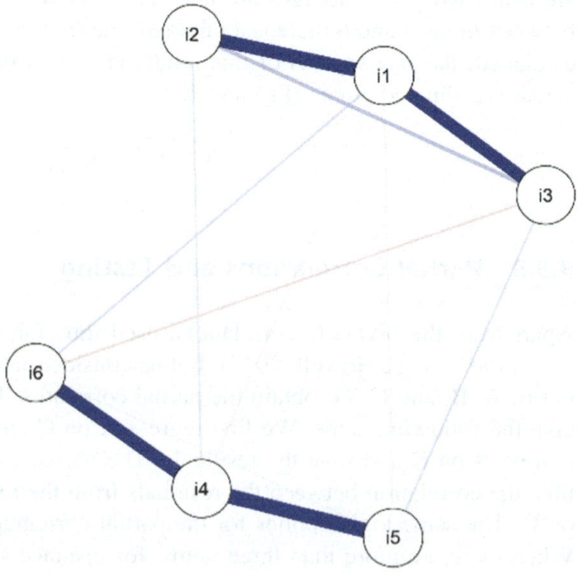

Fig. 9.6 Network plot for the six items using partial correlations (JASP)

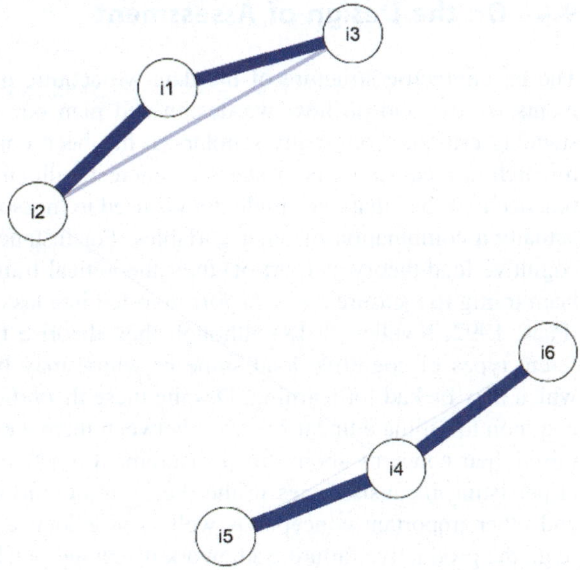

Fig. 9.7 Network plot for the six items using EBICglasso (*JASP*)

(e.g., Epskamp et al., 2018; Golino & Epskamp, 2017) and is incorporated amongst others in *JASP*. Figure 9.7 presents the resulting network plot for the example at hand.

Using EBICglasso, $E_E = 8$ (i1–i2, i1–i3, i2–i3, i4–i5, i4–i6, i5–i6, i2–i4, and i2–i6), and hence $S = 1 - (8/15) \approx 0.467$. The two cliques of items are still recognisable, but most of the connections between cliques—which were almost zero anyway—have now disappeared and that is in line with the two-factor model that estimated the correlation between factors to be only 0.069.

This example, as well as the other examples with EBICglasso in this book, uses the *default* option in *JASP* of a *tuning parameter* of 0.5. The tuning parameter typically varies between 0 and 0.5, where values closer to 0 tend to increase false positive rates while values closer to 0.5 are more cautious or conservative and tend to result in somewhat higher false negative rates (Epskamp & Fried, 2018). Even when false negative rates go up, fairly strong relations will normally still be visible unless sample sizes are too small for the size of the network we are dealing with or for network analysis in the first place, and given the usually moderate sample sizes in educational research and practice, using a good protection against high false positive rates is recommended. As becomes clear in later examples, the main goal of the network approach proposed in this book is to acquire useful visuals of basic structures: the most important relations between series of variables of interest should be visible, and less sizeable relations are often less important for educational research and practice anyway.

9.4 On the Design of Assessment

The psychometric structure of the data we acquire greatly depends on the instruments we use and on how we design and plan our measurements. Despite longstanding critique from many scholars, it has been common practice in educational research to measure traits or states of interest with single items. In some cases, the practice is so bad that *one* single item is used to measure a variable of interest that is actually a combination of other variables. For instance, many researchers who use cognitive load theory as (part of) their theoretical framework in their research have been trying to measure *mental effort* invested in a task with a single self-report item (Paas, 1992; Sweller, 2018) although they theorise that mental effort reflects different types of cognitive load some of which may be good for learning some of which may be bad for learning. Despite these theoretical considerations, it has been common to estimate linear relations between mental effort and learning. Many have raised their concerns about this measurement practice, and also many have pointed at persisting inconsistencies in the theory in definitions of types of cognitive load and other important concepts as well as at evidence from competing frameworks (e.g., the productive failure framework discussed in Chap. 1) that flies in the face of what cognitive load theory would predict.

These are reasons why I decided to abandon cognitive load theory a while ago (Leppink, 2019a) and are very well documented in a recent *Nature Scientific Reports* article by Solhjoo et al. (2019). In this article, the authors describe a study with $N = 15$ medical students on correlations between heart rate and heart variability on the one hand and clinical reasoning performance and self-reported measures of cognitive load on the other hand. The authors conclude (Solhjoo et al., 2019, p. 1): "*Despite the low number of participants, strong positive correlations were found between measures of intrinsic cognitive load and heart rate variability. Performance was negatively correlated with mean heart rate, as well as single-item cognitive load measures. Our data signify a possible role for using physiologic monitoring for identifying individuals experiencing high cognitive load and those at risk for performing poorly during clinical reasoning tasks.*" Red flags here are *single-item cognitive load measures*, the use of *mean heart rate* as one of many variables that could be correlated given how heart rate was measured (i.e., more than 24 h of measurement), in a sample of size 15 as stated in the abstract but being reduced to $N = 10$ because partial missing on 5 out of the 15 participants made the authors decide to just delete those five cases and use the 10 complete cases only. No information on the kind of missingness is provided (which is exemplar for how findings are reported altogether; some steps and outcomes are impossible to assess given the lack of information), and we know that this way of dealing with missing data is not to be recommended to say the least (see Chap. 3). Besides, for some correlations, the authors committed a classic and well-documented multiplication error: they multiplied the number of subjects in what they call 'final sample' by the number of clinical reasoning videos (performance tasks) to obtain a sample of '$N = 30$' and compute Pearson's correlations on that sample. The dangers of this multiplication approach are very well documented: positive correlations can appear negative and vice versa, even if sign (positive, negative) does not change substantial distortions in magnitude of correlations are likely, and CIs and *p*-values are not to be trusted (e.g., Leppink, 2015, 2019c; Leppink & Van Merriënboer, 2015; Picho & Artino, 2016; Snijders & Bosker, 2012; Tan, 2010). Given that some of the co-authors in the study by Solhjoo et al. (2019) also co-authored some of the works where the dangers of this multiplication approach are discussed, it is beyond me why this analytic approach was chosen in the study at hand. Finally, given that *Nature* is supposed to be one of the 'best' journals on our planet, it is difficult to understand how this piece of work got published there.

That said, the problem of single-item self-report measurement is not unique to cognitive load theory. Likewise, in research on *judgement of learning* (e.g., Kornell & Metcalfe, 2006; Metcalfe & Kornell, 2005; Thiede, Anderson, & Therriault, 2003; Thiede & Dunlosky, 1999), learners are asked to self-rate single items of which we hardly if at all know if learners can reflect on these questions, partly because they can refer to a multitude of things at once for different respondents so we will never know which factors contribute to scores and differences therein under what circumstances. Nevertheless, researchers perpetuate single-item measurement practices where they do not make sense as if no one ever raised them; progress in educational research and practice happens fairly slowly.

Of course, there are situations where the use of single items is defendable, and examples include *how old are you, how many units of alcohol do you drink per week,* and *are you married* (Schmidt, 2018). However, Schmidt (2018, p. 1) summarizes the core of the problem: "*sufficient reliability of an instrument is a precondition for it to be valid*" (remember from Chap. 3 in this book: reliability is a necessary though not sufficient condition for validity) and "*In particular, in true experiments, researchers do not worry much about reliability issues*". While 'researchers do not worry about' is way overgeneralised (there certainly is a critical mass of experimental researchers who are aware of the issues and have been trying hard to increase wider awareness), still quite many researchers do not understand that low reliability is a key contributor to low likelihood of independent experiments on the same phenomenon yielding similar results (i.e., replicability of findings). Single-item self-report measurements on mental effort, cognitive load or judgement of learning are incredibly noisy, and that noise can be greatly reduced by using more items. Although the concepts of item information and TIF in Chap. 5 are discussed in the context of dichotomous items, they also apply to other types of items; individual items come with high *SEM* and therefore low reliability. Even if we assume SEM = 0 (i.e., perfect reliability), the probability that two independent experiments with a power of 0.80 both yield a statistically significant outcome is 0.8 * 0.8 = 0.64; the higher SEM, the more that probability is pushed down (e.g., Leppink, 2019a).

9.4.1 Pseudoscience in Educational Measurement

Knowing this, it is easy to understand why none of the three solutions that Schmidt (2018) propose to defend the use of single items for complex variables like mental effort, cognitive load, and judgement of learning can be expected to work in educational research. The first of three 'solutions' proposed by Schmidt (2018) is to correlate the single item with a test that is purported to measure the same construct and from that point forward only to use the single item if we find a correlation of around 0.80 between the single item and the other test. Problem is that this should not happen, because single items are as noisy as they are and can never help us to tell which of a multitude of factors contributed to scores and differences therein on a single item (e.g., Leppink, 2019a), and where it happens it is probably due to the single question being presented together with the other questions, meaning that the response to the single item question is likely influenced by seeing the other questions. This is not only a reliability issue but a validity issue as well; a single item of mental effort cannot be expected to help us understand how good and bad cognitive load, which are together supposed to add up to mental effort, contribute to mental effort in a given situation. This is exactly why so many researchers use mental effort ratings in combination with performance and explain differences in mental effort ex post facto (i.e., after the fact) by explaining better performance as 'it must have been good load' and explaining poorer performance as 'it must have been bad load'. This has nothing to do with science; it is pseudoscience at best.

The second solution proposed by Schmidt (2018) is to compare two groups that are known to be different in terms of the construct measured on how they rate the individual item; if the difference is statistically significant, the single item can be considered to have sufficient discriminant validity. This solution just flies in the face of about everything we know about metacognition and how it develops, and of course still ignores the issues of low reliability and severely limited validity. Being novice in a topic often goes hand in hand with inaccurate self-assessments and poor metacognitive skills otherwise. Yet, expert-novice comparisons are the default way of studying this kind of discriminant validity question. Experts may self-report low or high confidence for different reasons than novices; the response scale will likely be very different for these groups. For these and other reasons, expert-novice comparisons have been known to add little to the validity argument: "*The major flaw is the problem of confounding: there are multiple plausible explanations for any observed between-group differences. The absence of hypothesized differences would suggest a serious flaw in the validity argument, but the confirmation of such differences add little*" (Cook, 2015, p. 829).

The third solution proposed by Schmidt (2018, p. 1) has to do with within-respondent differences: "*If such learning event is supposed to change the construct of interest, this change should be reflected in single-item measures taken before and after the event.*" This solution is problematic for a number of reasons. To start, while the conditions of Mill (1843) for causality—covariation, temporal order, and absence of alternative explanations—can be demonstrated to hold for *between-subjects* differences (e.g., randomised controlled experiments; Leppink,

2019a; Rosnow & Rosenthal, 2005), they raise serious questions when applied to *within-subject* differences, not in the last place because they require us to assume that the model for between-subjects differences is the same as the model for differences at the level of the individual, and we know that this is not the case. Besides, the temporal order is violated because there is an outcome variable measurement not only *after* but also *before* the event that is supposed to result in change, and that *before*-measurement constitutes one of a variety of sources that can provide alternative explanations for a change or absence of change. Although counterbalancing (e.g., Gravetter & Forzano, 2006; Rosnow & Rosenthal, 2005) and Latin square designs (Richardson, 2018) may help to reduce the impact of some of the confounding factors that resonate in pre-event post-event change, we will never fully get rid of it. One of the main confounding factors that we cannot get rid of is what in Chap. 1 in this book is defined as *recalibration* of the response scale; as we learn, self-report scales on effort, complexity, difficulty, and confidence are likely to undergo some *change* in meaning. Take a counterintuitive and seemingly absurdly simple probability problem like the *Monty Hall problem* (e.g., Selvin, 1975a, 1975b). In this problem, a respondent is asked by a quizmaster to choose which one of three doors should be opened, after being told that behind one of the doors is an expensive new car while behind the other two doors there is a goat. After expressing that choice, the quizmaster (who knows which door leads to the car) opens another door that does not have the car and gives the respondent the following choice: to stick with the initial choice or to switch doors. Most people would say that regardless of the decision in the latter, the probability of winning is 1/3. However, applying the complement rule, if the probability of winning by sticking with the initial choice is 1/3, given that there are only two options after the quizmaster has opened one door that for sure does *not* lead to the car, the probability of winning by switching doors is 2/3. Before the door was opened, we had a Uniform prior distribution: 1/3 chance of winning for each door. The quizmaster opening one of the losing doors not chosen by the participant resulted in a posterior distribution with 1/3 chance of winning for the door chosen by the participant, 0 chance for the door opened by the quizmaster, and 2/3 chance of winning for the door the participant could choose to switch to. Of course, it is still possible to lose by switching; that probability is 1/3, but we double the probability of winning by switching. Over an infinite number of games, sticking with the initial choice will result in winning in *one third* of the cases, while switching will result in winning in *two thirds* of the cases. People who have never seen this problem before commonly perceive this problem as *easy*, which would likely result in low effort, low complexity, low difficulty, and high confidence self-ratings. However, once we know the solution, most of us recognise the problem is not as easy as it seemed, and if we were confronted with another probability problem that is not the same as the Monty Hall problem but requires us to approach it with the same thinking as would be required in the Monty Hall problem, we may well perceive that second problem as requiring more effort, being more complex, being more difficult, and we may be less confident in our solution to that second problem.

Schmidt's (2018) 'central message' (p. 1) to "*Freely use single-item questionnaires because they are as effective as multi-item tests and far more time-efficient. But pay attention to the validity issue*" summarises brilliantly the perspective of many educational researchers who use these single-item tools and underlines some of the problems in educational measurement across the board. The unsubstantiated claim that single items are as effective as multi-item tools is diametrically opposed to all that we know about item information and TIF (e.g., Chap. 5 in this book). Instead, the gain in efficiency comes at the cost of a serious loss of information, high SEM, poor reliability, and very limited validity. While high reliability is not a sufficient condition for an instrument's validity, low reliability cannot be expected to result in substantial validity. Besides, for complex, multifaceted traits and states like cognitive load (e.g., which type[s] of cognitive load vary in what ways?), judgement of learning (*what* is supposed to be learned and *what* perhaps not, and is all of that captured in a single self-report item rating?), and constructs alike, there is no such thing as *la question pure* that can somehow cover the entire content of what is intended to be asked to respondents (Leppink & Pérez-Fuster, 2017).

9.4.2 Weak Design Bad Psychometrics

Unfortunately, this bad one-item practice is not limited to educational research but is omnipresent in educational practice as well. For instance, in the OSCE (see Chap. 2), medical students see a range of (simulated) patients also referred to as *stations* and receive, for each station, a single-item rating that reflects the student's 'overall' performance on that station, despite the fact that this 'overall' performance always has multiple facets or domains, including both procedure (e.g., questions, instructions, sequences of moves, making good use of time, structured session) and content (e.g., demonstrating empathy, listening actively, clinical reasoning). In terms of focus, stations may be as diverse as the human bowel system, the knee, the shoulder, the hip, the spine, cardiovascular issues, and many things more. Nevertheless, grades of all these different stations are commonly summed to obtain an overall score, and Cronbach's α is computed which is often terrible, partly because the fundamental assumption of unidimensionality is of course severely violated. The psychometric structure of this kind of OSCE data often is something like this. A cohort of $N = 233$ Year 2 students in Medical School X complete eight stations on a variety of topics and receive an integer performance rating ranging from 0 (minimum) to 5 (maximum) for each of these stations, and the sum of these eight station scores results in an overall exam score ranging from 0 (minimum) to 40 (maximum). For each of the stations, ratings are more or less symmetrically and unimodally distributed, and Table 9.4 presents M and SD as well as standardised factor loading λ for each station in a one-factor model and r for each pair of stations.

Cronbach's $\alpha = 0.510$, and since differences in SD across stations and differences in r across station pairs are relatively small, α is not much different from

Table 9.4 *M*, *SD*, and λ per station and *r* per pair of stations in the OSCE (*Jamovi*)

Item	1	2	3	4	5	6	7	8
M	2.670	2.416	2.579	2.253	2.622	2.562	2.597	2.258
SD	0.747	0.665	0.672	0.743	0.703	0.735	0.695	0.678
λ	0.360	0.182	0.351	0.266	0.340	0.380	0.467	0.385
2	0.139							
3	0.074	0.037						
4	0.113	−0.014	0.067					
5	0.081	0.015	0.155	0.085				
6	0.128	0.092	0.140	0.141	0.154			
7	0.182	0.141	0.143	0.099	0.154	0.193		
8	0.169	0.010	0.201	0.135	0.142	0.072	0.167	

McDonald's ω: $\omega = 0.514$. This happens because every station focusses on a different type of problem and single items are, as we know, very noisy. Exam score has $M = 19.957$ and $SD = 2.681$. However, from Chap. 5, we know that:

$$\rho = 1 - \text{SEM}^2, \text{ and therefore}$$
$$\text{SEM} = \sqrt{}(1 - \rho).$$

With $\rho = 0.510$, we find SEM = 0.700, and with $\rho = 0.514$, we find SEM = 0.697. When we multiply SEM by the *SD* of exam score, we obtain an estimate of SEM on the scale of the exam (0–40), so we find 1.877 using α and 1.869 using ω. While it is common practice to interpret differences of 1 point on the scale of 0–40 as one student (e.g., sum score 27) being better than another student (e.g., sum score 26), that difference falls within the SEM. We can use the SEM to obtain a 90 or 95% CI around *M*. However, as we saw in Chap. 5, items that provide good information around average performance are usually less informative towards the extremes of the performance distribution, meaning that the further we move away from *M* in either direction we are likely dealing with larger SEMs. Finally, Fig. 9.8 presents the network plot for the OSCE using EBICglasso.

The partial correlations between stations are so small that, when we use EBICglasso, they all shrink to zero, resulting in a network with S = 1 (100% sparsity). Note that this is likely due to a combination of fairly weak correlations to start with and a for network analysis only moderate sample size. Although the sample size of 233 is around the rule of thumb of around $N = 250$ for good performance in networks of 'moderate' size (networks of around 25 nodes count as 'moderate', e.g., Dalege, Borsboom, Harreveld, et al., 2017, so with only eight nodes we are dealing with a rather small network), penalties are applied for both parameters added and smaller sample size, making networks with zero edges estimated more likely.

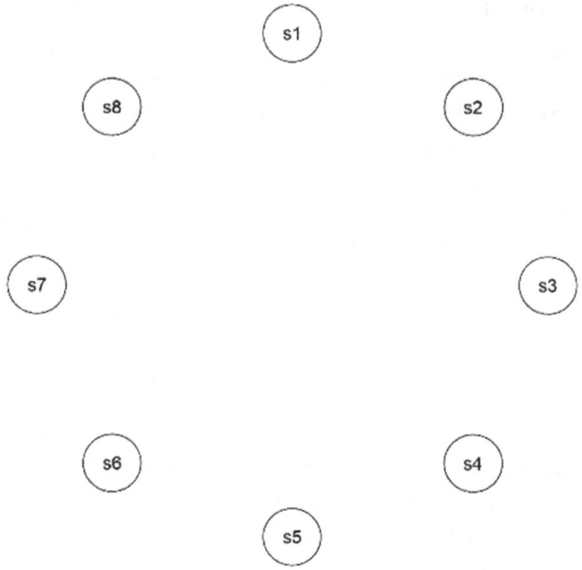

Fig. 9.8 Network plot for the eight stations (s1–s8) in the OSCE using EBICglasso (*JASP*)

9.4.3 Strong Design Good Psychometrics

Luckily, some medical schools moved away from this practice to a multi-item (also called: multi-domain, for instance: gathering medical information, explaining a diagnosis, managing a problem, empathic behaviour) instead of single-item (i.e., 'global' or 'overall' rating per station) assessment per station. This way, we can obtain much more reliable measurement with the same number of stations and, as long as there are no stringent validity issues, we may use fewer stations and still obtain better psychometrics. Therefore, in the final example of this chapter, we have $N = 233$ students (cf. previous example) complete four stations (instead of eight), but a student's performance on a given station is rated on three items or domains (e.g., questions, active listening, procedural steps; could be other domains as well, but they are the same across stations) on an integer scale from 0 (minimum) to 5 (maximum). Table 9.5 presents M and SD for each station and r for each pair of stations.

Although r is positive across item pairs, the station-specific item sets stand out. In line with assessment design, the best fitting confirmatory factor model is a four-factor model (i.e., one factor per station). The outcomes of this model are presented in Table 9.6.

Given that within station, the items have more or less the same SD and r is very similar across item pairs, α and ω yield almost the same outcomes, and these outcomes are much better than what we saw in the previous example. Using single items, reliability estimates hardly exceeded 0.5 for a series of eight stations, while

Table 9.5 *M* and *SD* per station and *r* per pair of stations in the multiple-domain scoring OSCE: items p1a–c are from station (patient) 1, items p2a–c are from station (patient) 2, items p3a–c are from station (patient) 3, and items p4a–c are from station (patient) 4 (*Jamovi*)

Item	p1a	p1b	p1c	p2a	p2b	p2c	p3a	p3b	p3c	p4a	p4b	p4c
M	2.691	2.704	2.798	2.712	2.815	2.764	2.708	2.678	2.635	2.794	2.730	2.760
SD	0.825	0.816	0.803	0.730	0.698	0.701	0.760	0.796	0.766	0.783	0.830	0.767
p1b	0.645											
p1c	0.667	0.691										
p2a	0.281	0.290	0.312									
p2b	0.290	0.305	0.241	0.572								
p2c	0.224	0.254	0.260	0.515	0.457							
p3a	0.254	0.277	0.214	0.182	0.231	0.177						
p3b	0.255	0.277	0.229	0.204	0.180	0.180	0.571					
p3c	0.244	0.282	0.265	0.243	0.277	0.208	0.586	0.606				
p4a	0.248	0.140	0.187	0.152	0.159	0.202	0.268	0.163	0.248			
p4b	0.198	0.187	0.215	0.255	0.233	0.245	0.298	0.220	0.298	0.604		
p4c	0.264	0.230	0.299	0.153	0.263	0.183	0.323	0.240	0.312	0.614	0.635	

Table 9.6 Confirmatory four-factor model outcomes in the multiple-domain OSCE (*Jamovi*): standardised loadings (λ), Cronbach's α, and McDonald's ω per factor, and *r* per factor pair

Factor (station)	F1	F2	F3	F4
λ item 1	0.792	0.783	0.749	0.752
λ item 2	0.820	0.727	0.751	0.793
λ item 3	0.840	0.649	0.799	0.812
Cronbach's α	0.858	0.761	0.810	0.828
McDonald's ω	0.858	0.764	0.811	0.829
F2 *r*	0.463			
F3 *r*	0.405	0.380		
F4 *r*	0.344	0.355	0.443	

here reliability estimates are above 0.76 for every single station. If we were to compute α and ω for all items together—which is somewhat odd given the four-factor structure but let us do it to compare the outcomes with the previous example—we would find $\alpha = 0.828$ and $\omega = 0.829$. In short, much better than the previous example, while we have only *half* the number of stations (!). Besides, doing this odd exercise of computing α and ω on *all* items demonstrates that α and ω do not necessary increase if we add items; these items actually need to have particular correlations with other items included in the computation. For the first station, α and ω are highest (0.858), because that is the station where *r* across item pairs is highest.

Finally, Fig. 9.9 presents the network plot for this final example using EBICglasso.

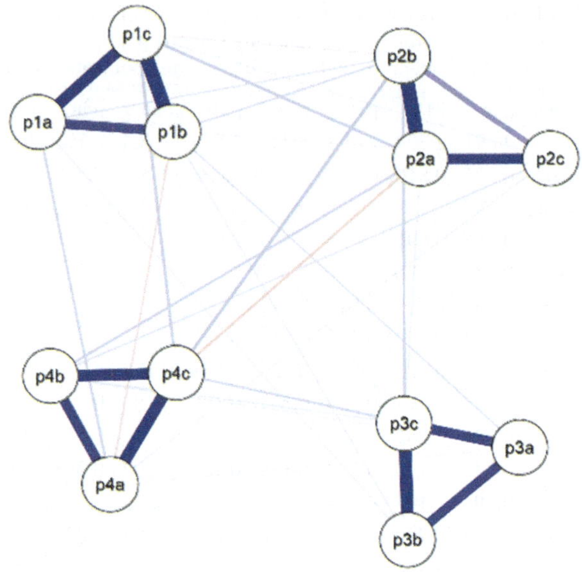

Fig. 9.9 Network plot for the multiple-domain OSCE using EBICglasso (JASP)

In this network, E = 66 and E_E = 42, hence S = 1 − (42/66) ≈ 0.364. The psychometric structure of this multiple-domain OSCE is reflected clearly in this network, even though we have a sample of 'only' N = 233.

9.5 A Pragmatic Network Approach

Whether we deal with multi-item questionnaires or multiple-domain assessments, we have a variety of methods available to help us understand if or to what extent questionnaire or assessment design actually resulted in the intended data structure. Although network analysis does not require thinking in terms of latent variables, latent variable models and network models can surely be used complementary to make sense of the psychometric structure of our instruments. Besides, both manifest grouping variables and latent profile analysis may help us to examine to what extent factor or network structures differ across groups. Therefore, it is not about 'either-or' but a matter of how we can combine different methods to develop a good understanding of the psychometrics of the instruments we use, be it in research or in educational practice. We can first examine if a sample at hand can be treated as one group or of a combination of groups, provided that the sample size allows for doing so; whenever a single-group approach makes sense, we perform confirmatory factor analysis and network analysis on the full sample, and if there are different groups to be distinguished, we can perform confirmatory factor analysis and network analysis for each of these groups (i.e., multi-group confirmatory factor analysis, and multi-group network analysis). For latent profile analysis, reporting the entropy and classifications is important, and to understand the outcomes of confirmatory factor analysis and network analysis, presenting a matrix of bivariate correlations is recommended (e.g., partial correlations can be computed from there). Finally, network analysis can also easily be combined with mixed-effects regression models that can account for residual covariance structures and item and group differences (and group-by-item interactions) simultaneously.

References

Borsboom, D., & Cramer, A. O. J. (2013). Network analysis: An integrative approach to the structure of psychopathology. *Annuals Reviews of Clinical Psychology, 9,* 91–121. https://doi.org/10.1146/annurev-clinpsy-050212-185608.

Chen, J., & Chen, Z. (2008). Extended Bayesian information criteria for model selection with large model spaces. *Biometrika, 95*(3), 759–771. https://doi.org/10.1093/biomet/asn034.

Cook, D. A. (2015). Much ado about differences: Why expert-novice comparisons add little to the validity argument. *Advances in Health Sciences Education, 20*(3), 829–834. https://doi.org/10.1007/s10459-014-9551-3.

Cramer, A. O. J., Waldorp, L. J., Van der Maas, H. L. J., & Borsboom, D. (2010). Comorbidity: A network perspective. *Behavioral and Brain Sciences, 33*(2–3), 137–150. https://doi.org/10.1017/S0140525X09991567.

Crutzen, R., & Peters, G. J. Y. (2017). Scale quality: Alpha is an inadequate estimate and factor-analytic evidence is needed first of all. *Health Psychology Review, 11*(3), 242–247. https://doi.org/10.1080/17437199.2015.1124240.

Dalege, J., Borsboom, D., Van Harreveld, F., & Van der Maas, H. L. J. (2017). Network analysis on attitudes: A brief tutorial. *Social Psychological and Personality Science, 8*(5), 528–537. https://doi.org/10.1177/1948550617709827.

Ding, C. S. (2018). *Fundamentals of applied multidimensional scaling for educational and psychological research.* New York: Springer. https://doi.org/10.1007/978-3-319-78172-3.

Dunn, T. J., Baguley, T., & Brunsden, V. (2014). From alpha to omega: A practical solution to the pervasive problem of internal consistency estimation. *British Journal of Psychology, 105*(3), 399–412. https://doi.org/10.1111/bjop.12046.

Epskamp, S., Borsboom, D., & Fried, E. I. (2018). Estimating psychological networks and their accuracy: A tutorial paper. *Behavior Research Methods, 50*(1), 195–212. https://doi.org/10.3758/s13428-017-0862-1.

Epskamp, S., & Fried, E. I. (2018). A tutorial on regularized partial correlation networks. *Psychological Methods, 23*(4), 617–634. https://doi.org/10.1037/met0000167.

Eyduran, E., & Akbaş, Y. (2010). Comparison of different covariance structure used for experimental design with repeated measurement. *The Journal of Animal & Plant Sciences, 20*(1), 44–51.

Golino, H. F., & Epskamp, S. (2017). Exploratory graph analysis: A new approach for estimating the number of dimensions in psychological research. *PLoS ONE, 12*(6), e0174035. https://doi.org/10.1371/journal.pone.0174035.

Gravetter, F. J., & Forzano, L. A. B. (2006). *Research methods for the behavioral sciences* (2nd ed.). London: Thomson Wadsworth.

Hagenaars, J. A., & McCutcheon, A. L. (2002). *Applied latent class analysis.* Cambridge: Cambridge University Press.

Howell, D. C. (2017). *Statistical methods for psychology* (8th ed.). Boston: Cengage.

Huynh, H., & Feldt, L. S. (1970). Conditions under which mean square ratios in repeated measurements designs have exact F-distributions. *Journal of the American Statistician, 65*(332), 1582–1589. https://doi.org/10.1080/01621459.1970.10481187.

Huynh, H., & Feldt, L. S. (1976). Estimation of the box correction for degrees of freedom from sample data in randomized block and split-plot designs. *Journal of Educational and Behavioral Statistics, 1*(1), 69–82. https://doi.org/10.3102/10769986001001069.

Iramaneerat, C., Smith Jr., E. V., & Smith, R. M. (2010). An introduction to Rasch measurement. In J. W. Osborne (Ed.), *Best practices in quantitative methods* (Chap. 4, pp. 50–70). London: Sage.

Kornell, N., & Metcalfe, J. (2006). Study efficacy and the region of proximal learning framework. *Journal of Experimental Psychology. Learning, Memory, and Cognition, 32*(3), 609–622. https://doi.org/10.1037/0278-7393.32.3.609.

Leppink, J. (2015). Data analysis in medical education research: A multilevel perspective. *Perspectives on Medical Education, 4*(1), 14–24. https://doi.org/10.1007/s40037-015-0160-5.

Leppink, J. (2019a). *Statistical methods for experimental research in education and psychology*. Cham: Springer. https://doi.org/10.1007/978-3-030-21241-4.

Leppink, J. (2019b). How we underestimate reliability and overestimate resources needed: Revisiting our psychometric practice. *Health Professions Education, 5*(2), 91–92. https://doi.org/10.1016/j.hpe.2019.05.003.

Leppink, J. (2019c). When negative turns positive and vice versa: The case of repeated measurements. *Health Professions Education, 5*(1), 76–81. https://doi.org/10.1016/j.hpe.2017.03.004.

Leppink, J., & Hanham, J. (2019). Human cognitive architecture through the lens of cognitive load theory. In C. B. Lee, J. Hanham, & J. Leppink (Eds.), *Instructional design principles for high-stakes problem-solving environments*. Singapore: Springer. https://doi.org/10.1007/978-981-13-2808-4_2.

Leppink, J., & Pérez-Fuster, P. (2017). We need more replication research—A case for test-retest reliability. *Perspectives on Medical Education, 6*(3), 158–164. https://doi.org/10.1007/s40037-017-0347-z.

Leppink, J., & Van Merriënboer, J. J. G. (2015). The beast of aggregating cognitive load measures in technology-based learning. *Journal of Educational Technology & Society, 18*(4), 230–245. https://www.jstor.org/stable/jeductechsoci.18.4.230.

Lu, K., & Mehrotra, D. V. (2009). Specification of covariance structure in longitudinal data analysis for randomized clinical trials. *Statistics in Medicine, 29*(4), 474–488. https://doi.org/10.1002/sim.3820.

McCutcheon, A. L. (1987). *Latent class analysis*. London: Sage.

Metcalfe, J., & Kornell, N. (2005). A region of proximal learning model of study time allocation. *Journal of Memory and Language, 52*(4), 463–477. https://doi.org/10.1016/j.jml.2004.12.001.

Mill, J. S. (1843). *A system of logic, ratiocinative and inductive being a connected view of the principles of evidence, and the methods of scientific investigation*. London: Harrison and co.

Paas, F. (1992). Training strategies for attaining transfer of problem-solving skills in statistics: A cognitive-load approach. *Journal of Educational Psychology, 84*(4), 429–434.

Peters, G. J. Y. (2014). The alpha and the omega of scale reliability and validity: Why and how to abandon Cronbach's alpha and the route towards more comprehensive assessment of scale quality. *European Health Psychologist, 16*(2), 56–69.

Picho, K., & Artino, A. R., Jr. (2016). 7 deadly sins in educational research. *Journal of Graduate Medical Education, 8*(4), 483–487. https://doi.org/10.4300/JGME-D-16-00332.1.

Revelle, W., & Zinbarg, R. E. (2009). Coefficients alpha, beta, omega, and the glb: Comments on Sijtsma. *Psychometrika, 74,* 145–154. https://doi.org/10.1007/s11336-008-9102-z.

Richardson, J. T. E. (2018). The use of Latin-square designs in educational and psychological research. *Educational Research Review, 24,* 84–97. https://doi.org/10.1016/j.edurev.2018.03.003.

Rosnow, R. L., & Rosenthal, R. (2005). *Beginning behavioral research: A conceptual primer* (5th ed.). London: Pearson Prentice-Hall.

Santosa, P., & Symes, W. W. (1986). Linear inversion of band-limited reflection seismograms. *SIAM Journal on Scientific and Statistical Computing, 7*(4), 1307–1330. https://doi.org/10.1137/0907087.

Schmidt, H. G. (2018). The single-item questionnaire. *Health Professions Education, 4*(1), 1–2. https://doi.org/10.1016/j.hpe.2018.02.001.

Selvin, S. (1975a). A problem in probability. *American Statistician, 29*(1), 67. https://www.jstor.org/stable/2683689.

Selvin, S. (1975b). On the Monty Hall problem. *American Statistician, 29*(3), 134. https://www.jstor.org/stable/2683443.

Snijders, T. A. B., & Bosker, R. J. (2012). *Multilevel analysis: An introduction to basic and advanced multilevel modelling* (2nd ed.). London: Sage.

Solhjoo, S., Haigney, M. C., McBee, E., Van Merriënboer, J. J. G., Schuwirth, L. W. T., Artino, A. R., Jr., et al. (2019). Heart rate and heart rate variability correlate with clinical reasoning performance and self-reported measures of cognitive load. *Nature: Scientific Reports, 9* (14668), 1–9. https://doi.org/10.1038/s41598-019-50280-3.

Sweller, J. (2018). Measuring cognitive load. *Perspectives on Medical Education, 7*(1), 1–2. https://doi.org/10.1007/s40037-017-0395-4.

Tan, F. E. S. (2010). Best practices in analysis of longitudinal data: A multilevel approach. In J. W. Osborne (Ed.), *Best practices in quantitative methods* (Chap. 30, pp. 451–470). London: Sage.

Thiede, K. W., Anderson, M. C. M., & Therriault, D. (2003). Accuracy of metacognitive monitoring affects learning of texts. *Journal of Educational Psychology, 95*(1), 66–73. https://doi.org/10.1037/0022-0663.95.1.66.

Thiede, K. W., & Dunlosky, J. (1999). Toward a general model of self-regulated study: An analysis of selection of items for study and self-paced study time. *Journal of Experimental Psychology. Learning, Memory, and Cognition, 25*(4), 1024–1037. https://doi.org/10.1037/0278-7393.25.4.1024.

Tibshirani, R. (1996). Regression shrinkage and selection via the lasso. *Journal of the Royal Statistical Society: Series B (Methodological), 58*(1), 267–288. https://doi.org/10.1111/j.2517-6161.1996.tb02080.x.

Tibshirani, R. (2011). Regression shrinkage and selection via the lasso: A retrospective. *Journal of the Royal Statistical Society: Series B (Methodological), 73*(3), 273–282. https://doi.org/10.1111/j.1467-9868.2011.00771.x.

Van der Maas, H. L., Dolan, C. V., Grasman, R. P., Wicherts, J. M., Huizenga, H. M., & Raijmakers, M. E. (2006). A dynamic model of general intelligence: The positive manifold of intelligence by mutualism. *Psychological Review, 113*(4), 842–861. https://doi.org/10.1037/0033-295X.113.4.842.

Cross-Instrument Communication 10

Abstract
Where Chap. 9 focusses on measures derived from single instruments, in this chapter, the psychometric approach discussed in Chap. 9 is extended to the study of interrelations between measures from different instruments. Possible advantages of as well as key issues in this endeavour of combining different measurement instrument instruments are discussed. This chapter helps to consolidate and practice with concepts and methods discussed in Chap. 9 and enables a smooth introduction to the concepts and methods discussed in Chaps. 11 and 12.

10.1 Introduction

In quite some situations in educational research and practice, we either deal with one single instrument or use several instruments but do not really look at how these instruments are interrelated. In educational practice, where we do have a variety of assessments from the same learners, we rarely use all that data to its full potential. Likewise, in randomised controlled experiments, where the interest lies in differences between conditions in terms of one or several outcome variables measured with one or several instruments, we often do not take a closer look at how measures obtained from different instruments relate to one another. This is unfortunate, because different (types of) measures may have quite a bit of explanatory or predictive power for each other, without having to engage in any kind of causal inference. In this chapter, we look at two types of situations: one in which two measures of interest are collected in a single sequence of activities, and one in which there are two different sequences of activities.

J. Leppink, *The Art of Modelling the Learning Process*, Springer Texts in Education,
https://doi.org/10.1007/978-3-030-43082-5_10

10.2 Example 1: Task Performance and Time Needed

In this first example, we take an innovative intervention aimed at reducing bullying behaviour. Bullying is a serious problem, and I am one of many people who suffered it for many years. In fact, I grew up without any real friends and without anyone believing in me. Before I entered university, no one gave five cents for my capacities or opportunities. I was 'stupid', 'lazy', 'useless', and even 'should never have been born'. Common responses to my decision to study Psychology were 'why not study something real' and 'are you doing this to help yourself?' No one ever thought I would get anything done in life, and the worst thing is that, for a moment, I believed that myself. But then came a time when insecurity and depression turned into anger, I turned from a Harry Potter profile into someone no longer to mess with, and just wanted to throw my punches onto and into the body of the next person whose leg kick bruised my leg, and whose punch made me sick in the stomach or made my nose bleed. Luckily, I never did so, even though I certainly could have. But I decided to get up and prove the bullies and trolls wrong, not so much for them but in the first place for myself. I worked as if there was no end, took multiple jobs to pay my studies at the expense of quality social life, and just continued until I saw some form of meaningful outcome and my life finally started to make sense. I travelled the world, spent substantial time in several countries, and saw and did things I would have never imagined. I used to be ashamed of my past and of myself, but I no longer am. On the long run, all the bullies and aggressors have achieved exactly the opposite of what they wanted: I have grown and do not mind going against a crowd that do not share my core values. I used to have massive stage freight, but now I only feel excitement in every opportunity to speak in public. I used to be too insecure to even put a full sentence on paper and was told I could never be an author, but by now I have published dozens and dozens of peer-reviewed works including three books.

That said, bullying—physical, emotional, or both—has had horrible consequences for too many people. If we tolerate this, let this happen—either by joining or by doing nothing about it—something is not right. We can do better than that. And if you are bullied (or were bullied but struggle to deal with it), do not believe your bullies; instead, stand up, fight your battle (which, as you have read, does not mean showing the same aggression), because you will see it is worth it.

Given the scale at which bullying takes place, in families, at schools, at workplaces, in other places, it is important to raise awareness of this problem as well as of ways to reduce the problem. Suppose, a group of social psychologists are interested in developing a new intervention against bullying aimed at kids of age 7–8. Part of that intervention is a series of videos of 2–3 min each in which professional actors simulate a series of simple scenarios, each of which demonstrates a particular type of bullying that kids of this age can identify with. This part of the intervention is programmed in an online learning environment as follows. First, the kids get to read a short introduction on the structure of the session. After that introduction, the first video is presented. Once that video is finished, by hitting the

'Enter' key or a mouse click brings, the user is asked to choose the one out of five alternatives (i.e., MCQ) that best represents what happened in the video just finished. Once the user has answered, hitting the 'Enter' key or a mouse click makes the next video appear on the screen. This process is repeated until nine videos with corresponding question have been completed. One of the five alternatives that is presented in all cases is 'there is no problem'; this is an incorrect response but allows the researchers to examine what proportions of students do not identify situations that we would agree demonstrate a specific form of bullying. More broadly, this setup enables researchers to see to what extent kids can accurately identify what is happening in a range of situations, and also allows researchers to keep track of how much time the individual user takes from the moment the question appears on the screen to the moment that the next video is presented (i.e., time in seconds from enter/mouse click hit to enter/mouse click hit).

10.2.1 Item Response

In total $N = 307$ kids participate. For each of the cases, the proportion of correct response is somewhere between 53.7 and 59.6% and the sum score is fairly symmetrically and unimodally distributed with $M = 5.098$ and $SD = 1.945$ (skewness = −0.219 and kurtosis = −0.644). With dichotomous variables, Pearson's r, Spearman's ρ, the Kendall's τ-coefficients, and Cramér's V yield the same point estimate for the strength of an association (albeit that V does not distinguish between positive and negative). Table 10.1 presents these point estimates for the nine scenarios in this intervention part.

Using *Stata*, we find −2LL = 3714.425 for the 1PL model and −2LL = 3706.377 for the 2PL model. The resulting LR test yields: $\chi^2_8 = 8.048$, $p = 0.429$. In short, no reason to move beyond 1 PL. In 1 PL, the difficulty estimates range from about −0.252 for scenarios 4 and 6 (where the proportion of correct response is 53.7%) to about −0.653 for scenario 9 (where the proportion of correct response is 59.6%). Figure 10.1 presents the TIF.

Table 10.1 Pearson's r estimates of the strength of association per scenario pair (*Jamovi*)

Scenario	1	2	3	4	5	6	7	8
2	0.055							
3	0.068	0.096						
4	0.051	0.101	0.026					
5	0.072	0.034	0.060	−0.035				
6	0.091	0.114	0.131	0.043	0.150			
7	0.001	0.082	0.149	0.052	0.100	0.118		
8	0.091	0.040	0.040	0.090	0.137	0.103	0.173	
9	0.060	0.078	0.116	0.168	0.133	0.155	0.170	0.071

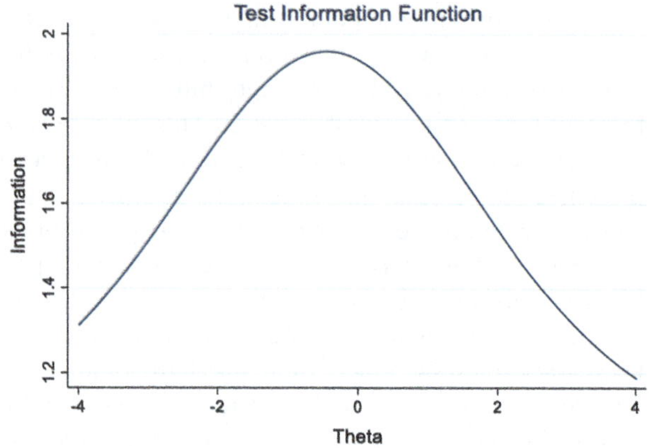

Fig. 10.1 TIF for scenarios 1–9 in the intervention against bullying (Stata)

The peak of the curve is at 1.960, which corresponds with a reliability of about 0.490 and a SEM of about 0.714 as per formulae in Chap. 5.

10.2.2 Response Time

Across scenarios, response time is more or less symmetrically and unimodally distributed with *M*s ranging from 50.880 (scenario 9) to 54.031 (scenario 6) seconds and *SD*s ranging from 10.367 (scenario 5) to 11.207 (scenario 8) seconds. Table 10.2 presents Pearson's *r* for each pair of scenarios.

For each of the scenarios, the researchers observe that the response time is on average lower when a correct response is provided than when an incorrect response is provided, as presented in Table 10.3.

These differences between incorrect and correct response are fairly substantial.

Table 10.2 Pearson's *r* for response times per scenario pair (Jamovi)

Scenario	1	2	3	4	5	6	7	8
2	0.043							
3	0.058	0.068						
4	0.068	−0.050	−0.054					
5	0.095	0.036	0.117	−0.041				
6	0.082	0.114	0.181	0.092	0.021			
7	0.091	0.133	0.125	−0.019	0.026	0.080		
8	0.045	0.028	0.018	−0.006	0.085	0.108	−0.009	
9	0.088	0.096	0.106	0.019	0.106	0.056	0.040	0.077

Table 10.3 *M* and *SD* response time for correct and incorrect response time and Cohen's d of difference per scenario (*JASP*): response time is on average shorter for correct than for incorrect response

Scenario	Incorrect: *M* (*SD*)	Correct: *M* (*SD*)	Cohen's *d*
1	55.659 (9.678)	49.247 (10.481)	−0.632
2	56.566 (11.340)	49.414 (9.778)	−0.680
3	55.744 (10.404)	47.304 (10.276)	−0.817
4	55.168 (9.392)	47.609 (9.944)	−0.780
5	55.949 (9.601)	49.024 (9.944)	−0.707
6	57.759 (10.125)	50.822 (9.512)	−0.708
7	55.739 (10.278)	50.766 (10.116)	−0.488
8	56.291 (9.881)	48.204 (10.902)	−0.771
9	54.415 (9.909)	48.485 (10.176)	−0.589

10.2.3 Performance-Time Relations

If we were to express the difference between incorrect and correct response in Pearson's *r*, we would find −0.299 for scenario 1, −0.322 for scenario 2, −0.376 for scenario 3, −0.363 for scenario 4, −0.330 for scenario 5, −0.334 for scenario 6, −0.236 for scenario 7, −0.356 for scenario 8, and −0.278 for scenario 9. These correlations are stronger than the ones in Tables 10.1 and 10.2; the correlations between two different measures within scenario are stronger than the within-measure between-scenario correlations. This is not to be interpreted as some kind of general pattern but can certainly occur in some studies. Figure 10.2 presents the network plot based on the correlations reported in this first example thus far.

The thick red lines connecting item response of a given case and its response time (e.g., for scenario 4: c4 and t4) represent the negative correlations associated with the differences between correct and incorrect response in average response time (i.e., incorrect responses on average seeing longer response times than correct responses). There are many blue lines as well, because most of the within-measure between-scenario correlations (i.e., Tables 10.1 and 10.2) are positive.

Finally, it is possible to test for response-by-scenario interaction in the analysis of differences in response time between correct and incorrect responses, that is: whether, or the extent to which, the difference in average response between correct and incorrect response varies across scenarios. We can do this using a two-level mixed-effects linear regression model. In one of the examples in Chap. 9, we compare five different residual covariance structures: CS, CSH, HF, AD1, and UN. We can also use these in the current example, and we introduce two types of residual covariance structures not yet discussed but which are sometimes useful: first-order factor-analytic (i.e., FA1) and its more flexible alternative that allows for varying V_{RES} (i.e., FA1H) (e.g., De Los Campos & Gianola, 2007; Zapata-Valenzuela, 2012). In HF, λ is a constant factor and V_{RES} is allowed to vary across scenarios. In FA1, V_{RES} is treated as constant but λ is allowed to vary across scenarios (i.e., each scenario has its own loading in a one-factor model), and in FA1H, both λ and V_{RES} are allowed to vary across scenario. Finally, given the low

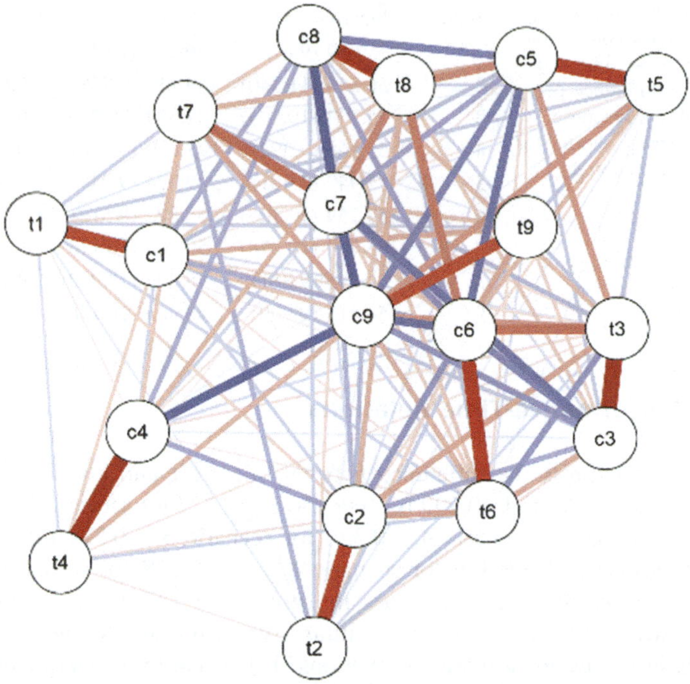

Fig. 10.2 Network plot using bivariate correlations in the intervention against bullying (*JASP*): c1–c9 are item responses (correct vs. incorrect), while t1–t9 are the response times

correlations of response times between scenarios, some readers may wonder if we need to account for that correlation at all. For that reason, we enter two other residual covariance structures in the comparison: *independence* (ID) and *diagonal* (DI). Both ID and DI assume uncorrelated residuals, but V_{RES} is allowed to vary in DI while it is treated as constant in ID.

Table 10.4 presents the -2RLL for the nine residual covariance structures just mentioned and LR testing outcomes of all comparisons between UN and the other eight structures which can all in some way be seen as nested or simplified versions of UN.

In other words, none of the models appear to perform significantly worse than UN. How can this happen? Well, although UN is the most flexible model, it also comes at the cost of needing a large number of *df*, because we estimate 36 r_{RES}s and 9 V_{RES}s. However, to decide which residual covariance structure to select, we can do a number of other comparisons using the -2RLL values in Table 10.4. For example, ID is a special case of all other structures, including CS. For the difference in -2RLL between CS and ID, we find: $\chi^2_1 = 6.714$, $p = 0.010$. In other words, CS is significantly better than ID. The next comparison is CS and CSH, for which we find: $\chi^2_8 = 4.262$, $p = 0.833$. This outcome is similar to what we would obtain in a

Table 10.4 Comparison of nine residual covariance structures in the intervention against bullying: UN, ID, DI, CS, CSH, HF, AD1, FA1, and FA1H (SPSS)

Structure	*df*	-2RLL	LR test χ^2_{df}	LR test *p*-value
UN	45	20542.095	–	–
ID	1	20586.352	$\chi^2_{44} = 44.257$	0.461
DI	9	20582.005	$\chi^2_{36} = 39.91$	0.300
CS	2	20579.638	$\chi^2_{43} = 37.543$	0.706
CSH	10	20575.376	$\chi^2_{35} = 33.281$	0.551
HF	10	20570.504	$\chi^2_{35} = 28.409$	0.777
AD1	17	20575.113	$\chi^2_{28} = 33.018$	0.235
FA1	10	20568.971	$\chi^2_{35} = 26.876$	0.836
FA1H	18	20564.906	$\chi^2_{27} = 22.811$	0.695

comparison between FA1 and FA1H, indicating insufficient evidence for a need to account for varying V_{RES}. Finally, CS can be considered a special case of FA1; the constant r_{RES} in CS would translate in a constant instead of in a varying λ. For the comparison of CS and FA1, we find: $\chi^2_8 = 10.667$, $p = 0.221$. In other words, a CS model will do.

Now that we have decided on the random part of our mixed-effects model, we turn to the fixed part (i.e., we switch from REML to FIML). Table 10.5 presents marginal R^2 (i.e., R^2_M), AIC, and BIC for each of five competing models.

AIC prefers Model 3, whereas BIC prefers Model 2 and it is easy to understand why. For item differences, though statistically significant (main effect: $p = 0.003$), we need $df = 8$ for the main effect of item (and, given $df = 1$ for correct vs. incorrect response, $df = 8$ for the interaction term as well), and the added value in R^2_M is only 0.007 or 0.008 (i.e., $r_M \approx 0.084$ or $r_M \approx 0.089$). For BIC, such an increase in *df* for only a small increase in R^2_M cannot be justified. However, R^2_M associated with correct vs. incorrect response is 0.099 or 0.100, quite a different order of magnitude (i.e., $r_M \approx 0.315$ or $r_M \approx 0.316$).

So, what is this R^2_M about? This is the equivalent of R^2 in an ordinary, single-level linear regression model (i.e., ID). Under CS and other models that assume *correlated* residuals, we can distinguish between variance of fixed effects (V_{FIXED}) and variance of random effects (V_{RANDOM}). Consequently, we can distinguish between three different R^2-statistics, one for fixed effects (R^2_M), one for random effects (R^2_R), and one

Table 10.5 R^2_M, AIC, and BIC for each of five competing models (*Jamovi*)

Model	R^2_M	AIC	BIC
0: *null model*	0.000	20921.906	20939.678
1: *item*	0.008	20912.950	20978.115
2: *response*	0.100	20644.501	20668.198
3: *item + response*	0.107	20636.772	20707.861
4: *full*	0.109	20645.483	20763.964

for fixed and random effects combined (R^2_C) (Nakagawa, Johnson, & Schielzeth, 2017; Nakagawa & Schielzeth, 2013):

$$R^2_M = V_{FIXED}/(V_{FIXED} + V_{RANDOM} + V_{RES}),$$
$$R^2_R = V_{RANDOM}/(V_{FIXED} + V_{RANDOM} + V_{RES}), \text{ and}$$
$$R^2_C = R^2_M + R^2_R = (V_{FIXED} + V_{RANDOM})/(V_{FIXED} + V_{RANDOM} + V_{RES}).$$

Under ID, no random effects (other than a constant V_{RES}) are estimated, meaning that $V_{RANDOM} = 0$, and therefore $R^2_R = 0$ and:

$$R^2_M = R^2_C = R^2 = V_{FIXED}/(V_{FIXED} + V_{RES}).$$

Further, in situations where there are no fixed effects to be estimated, $V_{FIXED} = 0$, and therefore $R^2_M = 0$ and:

$$R^2_R = R^2_C = V_{RANDOM}/(V_{RANDOM} + V_{RES}).$$

10.3 Example 2: Two Exams

In Chap. 9, we discuss an example of a multiple-domain OSCE. In many medical schools that use OSCEs, students face OSCEs more than once in their curriculum. To extend the example from Chap. 9, suppose we have data from a cohort of $N = 380$ students on their Year 2 and Year 3 OSCE, each of which follow the same structure as the multiple-domain OSCE discussed in Chap. 9, except that for each station, each domain is rated on an integer scale from 1 (minimum) to 9 (maximum).

10.3.1 Exams as Separate Occasions

The data of both exams are similar to the example exam in Chap. 9 (i.e., comparable *M*s and *SD*s across stations and similar bivariate correlation matrices), and we therefore proceed with network analysis. Figures 10.3 and 10.4 present the network plot of the Year 2 exam and Year 3 exam, respectively, using the bivariate correlations.

Next, Figs. 10.5 and 10.6 present the network plot of the Year 2 exam and Year 3 exam, respectively, using EBICglasso.

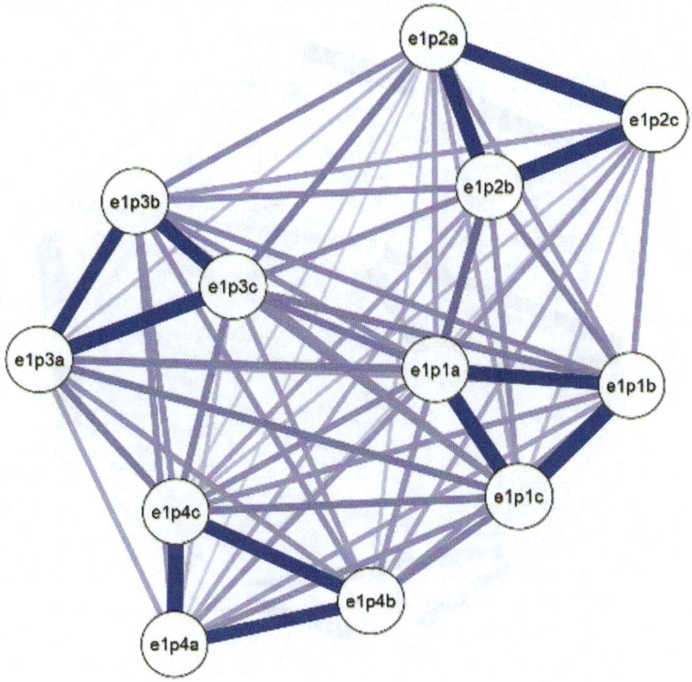

Fig. 10.3 Network plot using bivariate correlations in year 2 exam (*JASP*)

In the Year 2 exam, $E_E = 45$ and hence $S \approx 0.318$, and in the Year 3 exam, $E_E = 47$ and hence $S \approx 0.288$. In both exams, the assessment structure is well reflected in the data.

10.3.2 Exams as Repeated or Extended Assessments

Thus far, we have learned how different items within each exam can be clustered (i.e., four clusters of three domains, one cluster per station). However, can we somehow link the scores from the two exams as well (i.e., do they have some explanatory or predictive power for each other)? There are different ways of addressing this question. An easy way is to correlate composite scores of the eight stations: each station results in one composite score, which is in practice often the sum or average of the station-specific domain scores; let us use the average, to stay

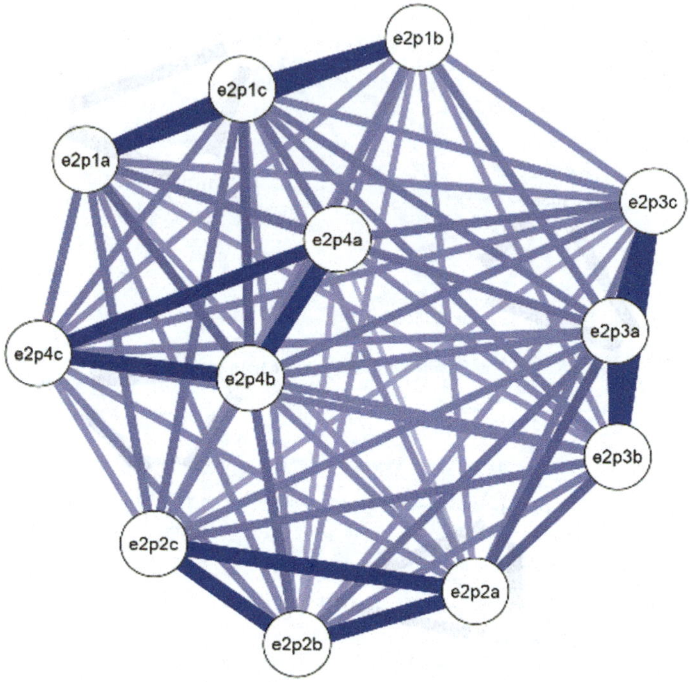

Fig. 10.4 Network plot using bivariate correlations in year 3 exam (JASP)

on the 1–9 scale. Table 10.6 presents *M* and *SD* for each of the eight stations and *r* for each station pair.

Although the correlations between stations in the Year 3 exam are slightly higher than the other correlations, the correlations between stations in the Year 2 exam and cross-exam correlations are of a similar magnitude. Figure 10.7 presents the network plot of the eight station (composite) scores using EBICglasso.

In this network, $E = 28$ and $E_E = 25$, hence $S \approx 0.107$. The eight stations are quite interrelated. Finally, we can also go a level deeper and take the domain scores instead of the composite scores as input. Figure 10.8 presents the resulting network plot using EBICglasso.

In this network, $E = 276$, $E_E = 131$, and hence $S \approx 0.525$.

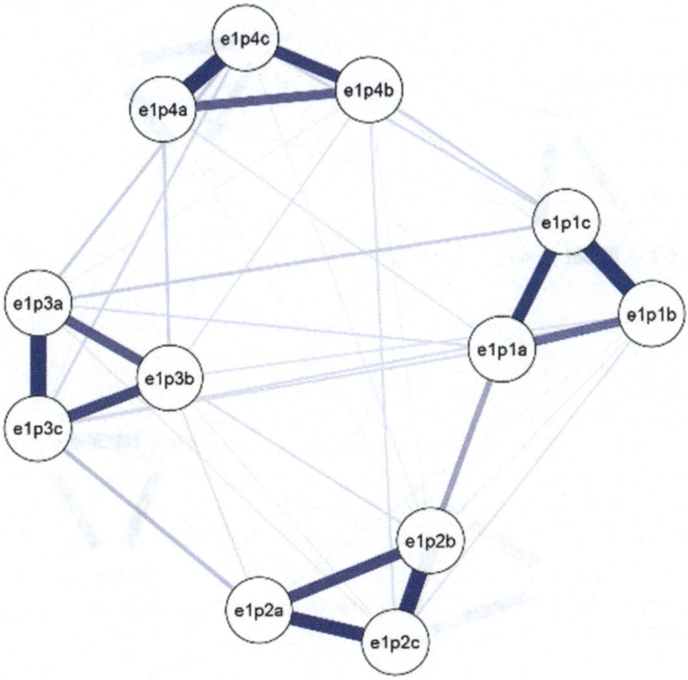

Fig. 10.5 Network plot in year 2 exam (*JASP*) using EBICglasso

10.4 A Note of Caution

While network analysis provides an attractive method to visualise the psychometric structure of an instrument (Chap. 9) and to visualise relations between measures of different instruments (this chapter), it is important to keep in mind that adding more nodes (i.e., variables) to a network, like any model becoming more complex, puts higher demands on the sample size. In very large sample networks (e.g., $N > 10000$), even very small correlations may be visible, whereas in sample sizes of 200–250 small though not very small correlations will likely not be visible at all and we may sometimes end up with an empty network (i.e., S = 1, see Chap. 9 for an example). In short, the more parameters we add and/or the smaller the sample

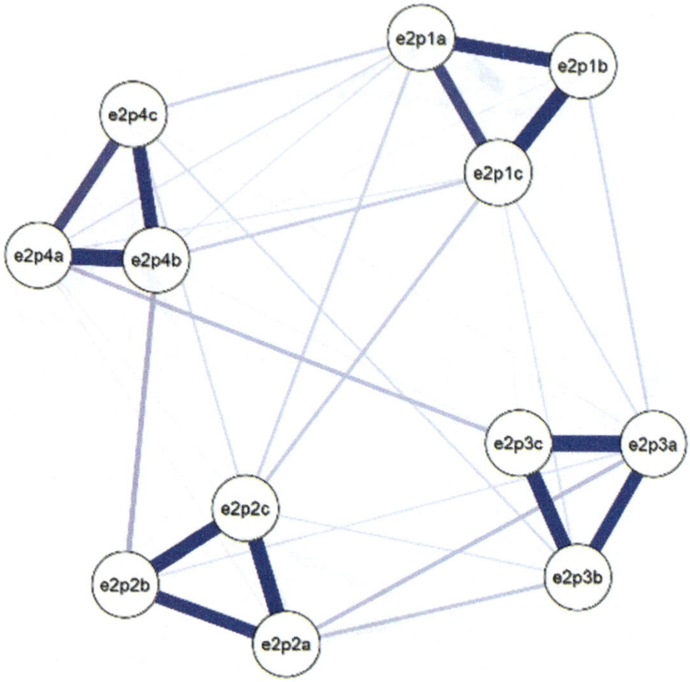

Fig. 10.6 Network plot in year 3 exam (JASP) using EBICglasso

Table 10.6 Pearson's r for each station pair in the year 2 (e1p1–e1p4) and year 3 (e2p1–e2p4) OSCE (JASP)

Station	e1p1	e1p2	e1p3	e1p4	e2p1	e2p2	e2p3	e2p4
M	4.995	5.006	5.004	5.003	4.972	4.983	5.003	5.057
SD	0.908	0.867	0.812	0.837	1.039	1.059	1.131	1.074
e1p2	0.284							
e1p3	0.343	0.261						
e1p4	0.318	0.193	0.303					
e2p1	0.287	0.291	0.269	0.298				
e2p2	0.272	0.261	0.181	0.190	0.383			
e2p3	0.268	0.296	0.207	0.213	0.410	0.434		
e2p4	0.190	0.328	0.251	0.268	0.456	0.375	0.424	

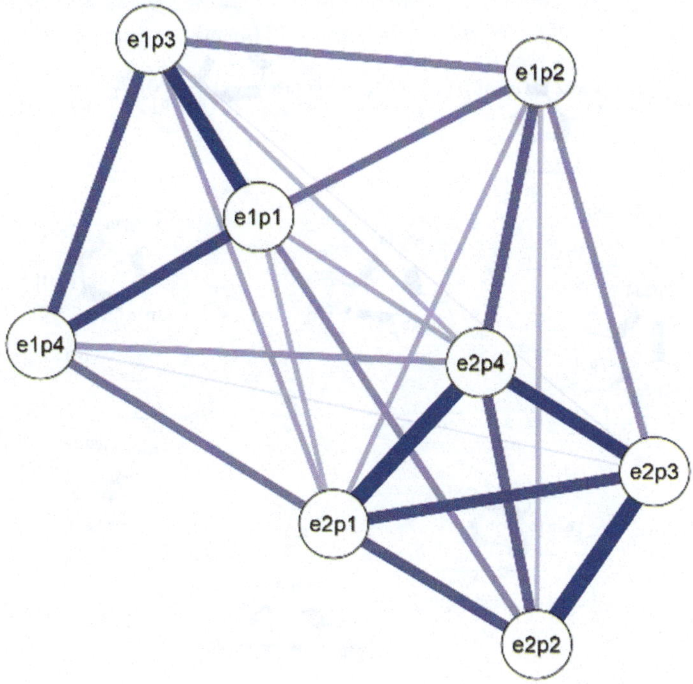

Fig. 10.7 Network plot of the eight composite scores using EBICglasso (*JASP*)

size, the stronger the penalty applied. In the example in Fig. 10.8, we deal with a sample size of $N = 380$ students and a network of 24 nodes, which meets the recommendation of at least $N = 250$ for a network of around 25 nodes. If we try to merge so many measures from different instruments that we end up with a considerably larger number of nodes, but we do not increase our sample size accordingly, there is a real chance that meaningful connections are missed.

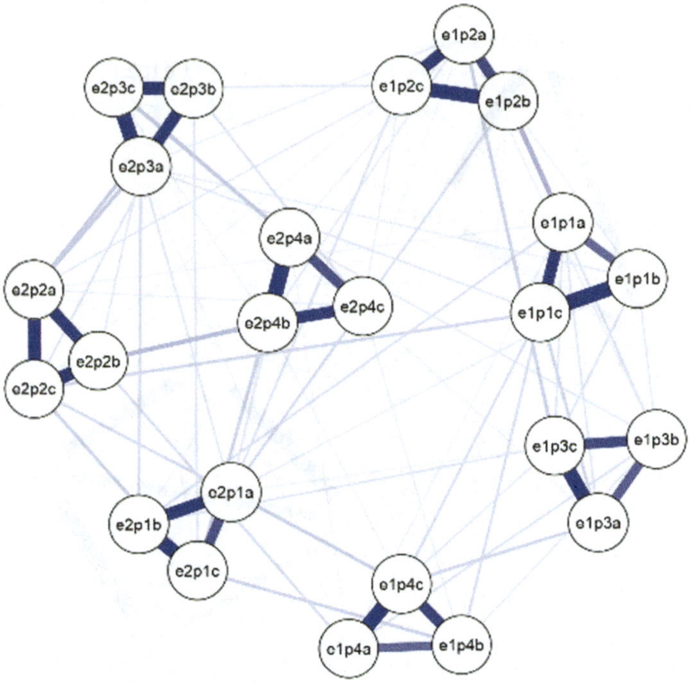

Fig. 10.8 Network plot of the domain scores of the year 2 and year 3 exams using EBICglasso (*JASP*)

References

De Los Campos, G., & Gianola, D. (2007). Factor analysis models for structuring covariance matrices of additive genetic effects: A Bayesian implementation. *Genetics Selection Evolution, 39,* 481–494. https://doi.org/10.1186/1297-9686-39-5-481.

Nakagawa, S., & Schielzeth, H. (2013). A general and simple method for obtaining R^2 from generalized linear mixed-effects models. *Methods in Ecology and Evolution, 4,* 133–142. https://doi.org/10.1111/j.2041-210x.2012.00261.x.

Nakagawa, S., Johnson, P. C. D., & Schielzeth, H. (2017). The coefficient of determination R^2 and intra-class correlation coefficient from generalized linear mixed-effects models revisited and expanded. *Journal of the Royal Society Interface, 14*(134), 1–11. https://doi.org/10.1098/rsif.2017.0213.

Zapata-Valenzuela, J. (2012). Use of analytic factor structure to increase heritability of clonal progeny tests of Pinus taeda L. *Chilean Journal of Agricultural Research, 72*(3), 309–315.

Temporal Structures 11

Abstract

In this chapter, the longitudinal component from Chaps. 1–8 (and one example in Chap. 10) is introduced again, but now in the context of the mixed-effects variable network approach discussed in Chaps. 9 and 10 as a way to study autocorrelation and cross-correlation in longitudinal studies. This facilitates the discussion of residual covariance, RI and random slope (RS), auto-regressive correlation, and other concepts that are key for Chaps. 12–16, among others through the use of powerful visuals (i.e., networks). Individual variable series and series of correlated variables are discussed.

11.1 Introduction

The kind of communication between measures discussed in Chap. 10 does not require a longitudinal or repeated-measures component. However, in some settings, the same measures are used repeatedly, either in a series of occasions in a limited time interval or over a longer, longitudinal path. When dealing with this kind of different waves of data collected in a particular temporal order, we have quite a variety of different options for modelling the residual covariance structure (i.e., the random part of a mixed-effects model), including many of the options discussed in Chaps. 9 and 10. For the fixed part of the model, things are not much different from previous chapters. Therefore, most of this chapter focusses on options for the random part.

J. Leppink, *The Art of Modelling the Learning Process*, Springer Texts in Education,
https://doi.org/10.1007/978-3-030-43082-5_11

11.2 Random Effects

In one of the examples in Chap. 10, we compare nine types of residual covariance structures: UN, ID, DI, CS, CSH, HF, AD1, FA1, and FA1H. In practice, apart from situations where residual correlations are very close to zero (i.e., smaller than 0.01, especially when samples are on the smaller side) or (almost entirely) different groups instead of (largely) the same groups of respondents are measured at subsequent time points, ID and DI are rarely if ever useful when dealing with repeated-measures or longitudinal data. Besides, in repeated-measures or longitudinal studies, FA1 and FA1H are generally unlikely candidates as well.

CS, which is effectively a RI model, is attractive in that regardless of the number of measurement occasions $df = 2$ (i.e., one for r_{RES}, one for V_{RES}) and it is less sample size demanding than its more flexible alternatives. CSH is an easy alternative to CS that does not need many *df* more if the number of measurement occasions is fairly limited; when there are only two measurement occasions, CSH and UN are the same. While UN is often useful when the number of measurement occasions is fairly small (e.g., up to four or five measurement occasions), with increasing numbers of measurement occasions some of the less *df*-consuming alternatives such as HF or AD1—or similar fairly low *df*-consuming RI-RS combinations (e.g., Leppink, 2019)—are more likely to be preferred.

Given k measurement occasions, UN can be understood as follows: RI, $k - 1$ RS, and the covariances of all RI-RS and RS-RS pairs. In fact, *all* residual covariance structures can be conceived in terms of more or less complex structures of RI (i.e., CS), RS, combinations of RI and RS, and eventually more or fewer covariance terms between RI-RS and/or RS-RS combinations. Common software programmes are really flexible in this sense: we can start with a UN model and remove RI, RS and/or covariance terms one by one to obtain a model that is to be preferred using information criteria and/or LR testing.

11.2.1 Equidistant Versus Non-equidistant Measurement Occasions

The structures discussed thus far have in common that measurement occasions need not be equidistant in time. However, in some repeated-measures and longitudinal studies, we deal with equidistant measurement occasions: the distance between any pair of adjacent measurements is the same. If so, the variety of options to choose from for modelling the residual covariance structure increases.

One type of residual covariance structure that is quite common in longitudinal studies is *first-order autoregressive* (i.e., AR1) structure (e.g., Lu & Mehrotra, 2009; Tan, 2010). In AR1, r_{RES} is not constant but follows a simple mathematical function:

$$r_{RES} = r^{k+1}.$$

In this formula, k is the number of items in between a given set of two items: $k = 0$ for adjacent items (e.g., items 1 and 2, items 5 and 6), $k = 1$ for having one item in between (e.g., items 1 and 3, items 4 and 6), $k = 2$ for having two items in between (e.g., items 1 and 4), etcetera. Thus, r_{RES} holds for the pair of occasions 1 and 2 as well as for the pair of occasions 2 and 3 and for the pair of occasions 3 and 4, while for the pair of occasions 1 and 3 and the pair of occasions 2 and 4 we have r_{RES}^2, and for the pair of occasions 1 and 4 we have r_{RES}^3. This logic extends to larger sequences of measurement occasions. This is an attractive option in that it uses as few *df* as CS but allows r_{RES} to differ, and an easy extension of AR1 for varying V_{RES} is found in AR1H.

Although AR1 at first appears flexible, it falls short when the difference in r_{RES} between adjacent and non-adjacent pairs does not follow this simple function. A slightly more flexible structure in that respect is found in a covariance structure named after the German mathematician Otto Toeplitz (1881–1940): the *Toeplitz* (TP) covariance structure (e.g., Bareiss, 1969; Littell, Pendergast, & Natarajan, 2000; Lu & Mehrotra, 2009). In this covariance structure there is *one* r_{RES} for adjacent pairs, *one* r_{RES} for the next distance (e.g., occasions 1 and 3, occasions 2 and 4), *one* r_{RES} for the next distance (e.g., occasions 1 and 4), and so forth. In comparison to AR1, TP requires more *df* but is also more flexible. An extension of TP for varying V_{RES} is found in TPH.

There are plenty more structures one can think of, some of which are discussed in the final chapters of this book, but the ones discussed this far are common candidates in longitudinal studies. AR1, TP, and their extensions to account for varying V_{RES} are potentially useful when measurement occasions are equidistant; the further we move away from that characteristic, the less these structures make sense.

11.2.2 Network and Model Comparisons

Let us have a look at an example that allows us to compare all structures discussed thus far. Suppose, we have four equidistant measurement occasions at which we measure two outcome variables, *A* and *B* (could be test scores, could be questionnaire scale scores), in a sample of $N = 347$, on an integer scale from 0 to 100. At each occasion, these variables are more or less symmetrically and unimodally distributed, and *M*s and *SD*s per variable and *r* per variable pair are as reported in Table 11.1.

From Table 11.1, a few things become clear. To start, for both variables, *SD* increases with time. Further, within measure, there is a decline in *r* as the distance between occasions increases, which is normal in many repeated-measures and longitudinal studies. Finally, the correlation between measures also decreases with time (i.e., $r = 0.472$ at occasion 1, $r = 0.300$ at occasion 2, $r = 0.185$ at occasion 3, and $r = 0.112$ at occasion 4). Figure 11.1 presents the corresponding network plot using EBICglasso.

Table 11.1 *M* and *SD* per variable per occasion and *r* for each variable pair (A_1–A_4: variable *A* at occasions 1–4; B_1–B_4: variable *B* at occasions 1–4) (*Jamovi*)

Variable	A_1	A_2	A_3	A_4	B_1	B_2	B_3	B_4
M	58.795	57.481	56.885	56.009	59.752	58.352	57.948	56.942
SD	5.923	8.333	10.233	10.929	5.668	8.865	10.423	11.285
A_2	0.657							
A_3	0.506	0.761						
A_4	0.417	0.623	0.816					
B_1	0.472	0.349	0.258	0.216				
B_2	0.343	0.300	0.247	0.209	0.681			
B_3	0.240	0.211	0.185	0.170	0.524	0.772		
B_4	0.126	0.156	0.133	0.112	0.376	0.638	0.807	

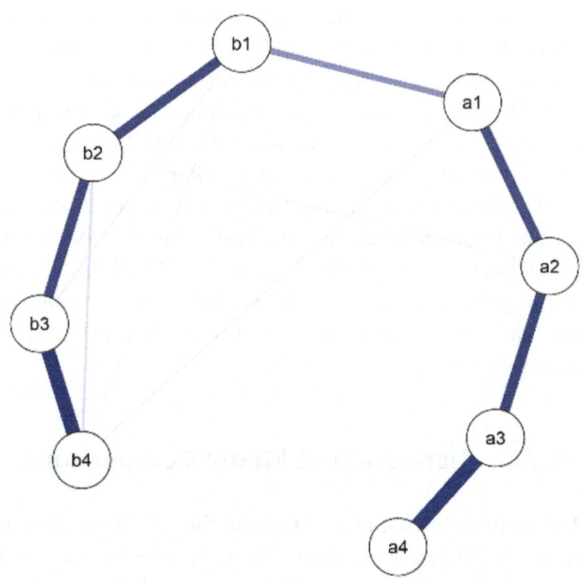

Fig. 11.1 Network plot of variables *A* and *B* each measured at four occasions (*JASP*) using EBICglasso

In this network, E = 28, E_E = 18, hence S ≈ 0.357. Leaving the correlation between A and B at different occasions aside for a moment, the picture we see for both *A* and *B* (i.e., strong link mainly between adjacent occasions) is pretty common in repeated-measures and longitudinal studies. With regard to correlations between measures and changes therein with time, the pattern to be expected really depends on what variables we are measuring. Tables 11.2 and 11.3 present a comparison of residual covariance structures for the data at hand, for variables *A* and *B* respectively, in terms of −2RLL and outcomes of LR testing of each structure against UN (i.e., the most complex structure, in which all other structures are nested). In these comparisons, RS_3 is a RS from occasion 1 to occasion 3 (to account for the increase

Table 11.2 Comparison of residual covariance structures in terms of −2RLL and LR test outcomes (*SPSS*) for variable *A*

Structure	*df*	−2RLL	LR test χ^2_{df}	LR test *p*-value
UN	10	9038.669	–	–
RI-RS_3-RS_4 C	7	9166.902	$\chi^2_3 = 128.233$	<0.001
RI-RS_3-RS_4	4	9364.166	$\chi^2_6 = 325.497$	<0.001
RI-RS_4 C	4	9356.589	$\chi^2_6 = 317.920$	<0.001
RI-RS_4	3	9384.057	$\chi^2_7 = 345.388$	<0.001
CS	2	9424.636	$\chi^2_8 = 385.967$	<0.001
CSH	5	9242.830	$\chi^2_5 = 204.161$	<0.001
HF	5	9241.146	$\chi^2_5 = 202.477$	<0.001
AD1	7	9038.745	$\chi^2_3 = 0.076$	0.995
AR1	2	9193.763	$\chi^2_8 = 155.094$	<0.001
AR1H	5	9065.368	$\chi^2_5 = 26.699$	<0.001
TP	4	9189.138	$\chi^2_6 = 150.469$	<0.001
TPH	7	9065.336	$\chi^2_3 = 26.667$	<0.001

Table 11.3 Comparison of residual covariance structures in terms of −2RLL and LR test outcomes (*SPSS*) for variable *B*

Structure	*df*	−2RLL	LR test χ^2_{df}	LR test *p*-value
UN	10	9060.067	–	–
RI-RS_3-RS_4 C	7	9247.612	$\chi^2_3 = 187.545$	<0.001
RI-RS_3-RS_4	4	9432.549	$\chi^2_6 = 372.482$	<0.001
RI-RS_4 C	4	9425.772	$\chi^2_6 = 365.705$	<0.001
RI-RS_4	3	9448.765	$\chi^2_7 = 388.698$	<0.001
CS	2	9499.958	$\chi^2_8 = 439.891$	<0.001
CSH	5	9281.909	$\chi^2_5 = 221.842$	<0.001
HF	5	9258.249	$\chi^2_5 = 198.182$	<0.001
AD1	7	9066.810	$\chi^2_3 = 6.743$	0.081
AR1	2	9264.524	$\chi^2_8 = 204.457$	<0.001
AR1H	5	9084.829	$\chi^2_5 = 24.762$	<0.001
TP	4	9247.662	$\chi^2_6 = 187.595$	<0.001
TPH	7	9077.594	$\chi^2_3 = 17.527$	0.001

in V_{RES}), RS_4 is a RS from occasion 1 to occasion 4 (to account for the increase in V_{RES}), and C in the RI-RS combinations indicates that all covariances between these terms are estimated as well (i.e., where C is not mentioned, these covariances are fixed to 0). Although one can think of many more options of residual covariance structures (e.g., RS_3 and/or RS_4 without RI), the structures in Tables 11.2 and 11.3 are the most likely candidates.

For *A*, AD1 and UN yield almost the same −2RLL, indicating that we lose almost nothing in the simplification from UN to AD1. For *B*, some may argue in favour of AD1 and others may favour UN, depending on whether we test at $\alpha = 0.05$ or $\alpha = 0.10$. Testing at the $\alpha = 0.10$ can be defended, because we already know the direction of the difference between UN and AD1: the latter is always a reduction of the former and can therefore never result in a reduction of −2RLL relative to the most flexible model. When in doubt, it is always an option to present fixed effects of interest under both structures. For the example at hand, we present the outcomes for both variables under AD1.

11.3 Fixed Effects

Given equidistant measurement occasions, we have a number of options for the fixed part, and which ones we consider is partly a matter of which hypotheses, if any, we formulated prior to the study. The most flexible way of treating differences between occasions in average score is to treat each occasion as having its own *M*; given four occasions, this comes down to $df = 3$. However, we can also test linear ($df = 1$) and quadratic polynomials ($df = 2$), which are less flexible (i.e., the $df = 3$ model can be conceived as a cubic polynomial) but may be preferred if they describe the change in score over time well enough. Table 11.4 presents AIC and BIC for each of four competing models: no differences across occasions (Model 0: null model), linear polynomial (Model 1), quadratic polynomial (Model 2), all different (Model 3: cubic) for each of the two variables measured.

Both AIC and BIC prefer Model 1: although the difference in *M* from occasion to occasion are not *exactly* linear, going beyond linear does not result in an improvement in the explanation of differences to such an extent that AIC or BIC is convinced that we need a more complex model. Of course, if we were not dealing with equidistant occasions, linear or quadratic interpretations would make no sense (although for instance ordinal hypotheses may still be considered and tested, see for example: Leppink, 2019), just like considering any of AR1, TP or their extensions for unequal V_{RES} would not make sense. However, now that we do have equidistant occasions, it makes sense to consider linear and quadratic polynomials as more parsimonious alternatives to the 'all are different' model.

Table 11.4 AIC and BIC of four competing models in the four-occasions study (*SPSS*)

	Variable *A*		Variable *B*	
Model	AIC	BIC	AIC	BIC
0: *null model*	9081.852	9123.737	9110.931	9152.816
1: *linear*	9057.461	9104.582	9087.208	9134.329
2: *quadratic*	9058.631	9110.987	9088.584	9140.941
3: *cubic*	9059.397	9116.989	9087.544	9145.135

References

Bareiss, E. H. (1969). Numerical solution of linear equations with Toeplitz and Vector Toeplitz matrices. *Numerische Mathematik, 13*(5), 404–424. https://doi.org/10.1007/BF02163269.

Leppink, J. (2019). *Statistical methods for experimental research in education and psychology*. Cham: Springer. https://doi.org/10.1007/978-3-030-21241-4.

Littell, R. C., Pendergast, J., & Natarajan, R. (2000). Modelling covariance structure in the analysis of repeated measures data. *Statistics in Medicine, 19*, 1793–1819. https://doi.org/10.1002/(SICI)1097-0258(19961015)15:19<1987::AID-SIM318>3.0.CO;2-Q.

Lu, K., & Mehrotra, D. V. (2009). Specification of covariance structure in longitudinal data analysis for randomized clinical trials. *Statistics in Medicine, 29*(4), 474–488. https://doi.org/10.1002/sim.3820.

Tan, F. E. S. (2010). Best practices in analysis of longitudinal data: A multilevel approach. In J. W. Osborne (Ed.), *Best practices in quantitative methods* (Chap. 30, pp. 451–470). London: Sage.

References

Longitudinal Assessment Networks 12

Abstract

Different assessments in a curriculum (e.g., a Bachelor's or Master's programme) can shed light on somewhat different aspects of learning. Simultaneously, there is some intercorrelation between assessments that at first may have little to do with each other. For instance, although high performance on a multiple-choice exam does not imply you can also do a good physical examination, correlations in the 0.3–0.5 range between multiple-choice exams and physical examination assessments are quite common. This chapter demonstrates how the mixed-effects variable network approach discussed in Chaps. 9–11 can help to visualise and understand the interdependence of assessment components in a curriculum or programme.

12.1 Introduction

In Medical School Z, the five-year Bachelor of Medicine Bachelor of Surgery (MBBS) programme has a wide variety of carefully planned assessments. While some of these assessments pertain to elective modules and special interest projects taken by small groups or even individual students, most of the assessments are taken by all students and form a coherent assessment programme as follows. At the end of each of Years 1–4 of the programme, students have a 200-item MCQ exam on *Applied Life Sciences* (ALS) and a 200-item MCQ exam on *Health and Society* (H&S) in the same week in the first half of June. A week later, students have a multi-station multiple-domain assessment OSCE (see Chaps. 9 and 10 for examples), and there is another OSCE in the same period at the end of Year 5. Finally, three times a year—mid-September, mid-January, and mid-May—all students from all years sit a 200-item progress test (see also Chaps. 1, 2, and 8), the items of which are sampled from a very large item bank (i.e., 12,000+ items and

J. Leppink, *The Art of Modelling the Learning Process*, Springer Texts in Education,
https://doi.org/10.1007/978-3-030-43082-5_12

growing; items sampled in one test will not appear in a test for at least three years) such that a total of over twenty content areas agreed by an international progress testing consortium is covered with fixed numbers of items. For the ease of the example, all these exams result in a score from 0 (minimum) to 100% (maximum) for each of $N = 300$ students in Cohort X that is now graduating from Year 5, results in fairly symmetrically and unimodally distributed scores for each exam, and we take a look at how these exams are interrelated, using the first sit (i.e., not re-sit exam) results of all students.

12.2 Knowledge

M and *SD* of each of the four ALS exams (ALS_1–ALS_4) and for each of the four H&S exams ($H\&S_1$–$H\&S_4$) are provided in Table 12.1 along with *r* for each pair of these in total eight exams.

Within both ALS and H&S, correlations between adjacent exams are higher than correlations between non-adjacent exams. The within-year correlation between ALS and H&S is highest in Year 4 and lowest in Year 1, but even the within-year correlation between ALS and H&S in Year 4 is substantially lower than the correlation between two adjacent exams on the same topic. For adjacent exams within topic, the proportion of variance in one exam explained by the other exam is between 15.9% (ALS_1 and ALS_2) and 28.0% (ALS_3 and ALS_4; for the H&S exams, we find values between these two percentages). Figure 12.1 presents the network plot of the series of eight ALS and H&S exams using EBICglasso.

In this network, $E = 28$, $E_E = 12$, and therefore $S \approx 0.571$. In line with Table 12.1, the best variable to explain exam performance in a given topic at time point *t* (e.g., *t* = Year 3) is the performance on that same topic at time point '*t* minus 1' (e.g., Year 2 being '*t* minus 1').

Table 12.1 *M* and *SD* of exam performance and *r* per exam pair for the series of ALS and H&S exams (*Jamovi*)

Exam	ALS_1	ALS_2	ALS_3	ALS_4	$H\&S_1$	$H\&S_2$	$H\&S_3$	$H\&S_4$
M	49.599	50.863	54.197	59.053	49.082	50.818	53.883	59.229
SD	8.531	11.148	10.620	11.082	9.111	10.440	10.671	11.230
ALS_2	0.398							
ALS_3	0.146	0.529						
ALS_4	0.128	0.324	0.508					
$H\&S_1$	0.043	0.016	0.020	0.029				
$H\&S_2$	0.017	0.178	0.104	0.139	0.455			
$H\&S_3$	0.130	0.135	0.183	0.156	0.064	0.408		
$H\&S_4$	0.030	0.148	0.179	0.259	0.018	0.255	0.465	

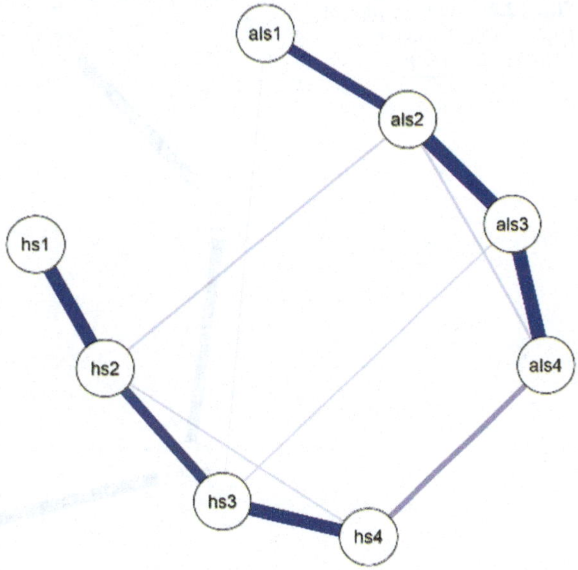

Fig. 12.1 Network plot of ALS_1–ALS_4 and $H\&S_1$–$H\&S_4$ using EBICglasso (*JASP*)

12.3 Technique and Skill

Where the ALS and H&S exams assess different types of knowledge, OSCEs are intended to assess a set of techniques and skills that are essential in clinical examination. Table 12.2 presents *M* and *SD* per OSCE and *r* per pair of OSCEs.

We see a pattern for the OSCEs that is quite similar to that of ALS and H&S: adjacent exams are moderately correlated, but non-adjacent exams not so much. Figure 12.2 presents the resulting network plot using EBICglasso.

Only four edges (E_E) of ten possible edges (E) are estimated, making this a fairly sparse network (S = 0.600). Figure 12.3 presents the network plot for all ALS, H&S, and OSCEs using bivariate correlations.

Within year, and especially in Years 2, 3, and 4, the OSCE is somewhat correlated with ALS and H&S, although these correlations are not as high as correlations between adjacent OSCEs are stronger. Table 12.3 presents within-year

Table 12.2 *M* and *SD* of OSCE performance in each of the five years ($OSCE_1$–$OSCE_5$) and r per OSCE pair (*Jamovi*)

Exam	$OSCE_1$	$OSCE_2$	$OSCE_3$	$OSCE_4$	$OSCE_5$
M	51.220	53.618	56.902	53.847	55.472
SD	9.162	10.779	11.480	10.824	10.166
$OSCE_2$	0.382				
$OSCE_3$	0.109	0.356			
$OSCE_4$	0.063	0.160	0.384		
$OSCE_5$	−0.008	0.012	0.095	0.403	

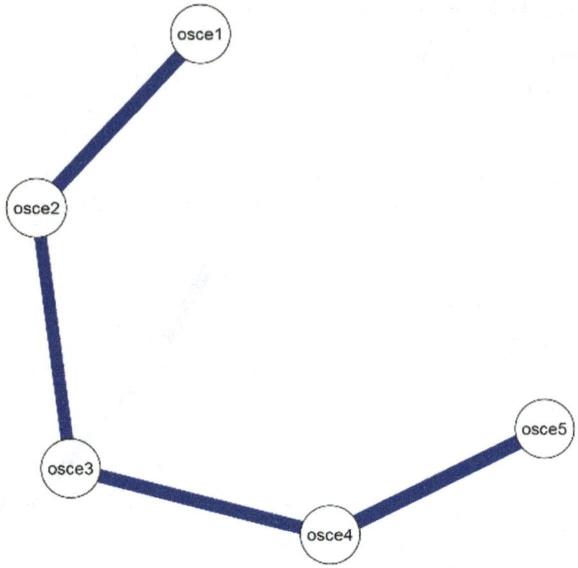

Fig. 12.2 Network plot of $OSCE_1$–$OSCE_5$ using EBICglasso (*JASP*)

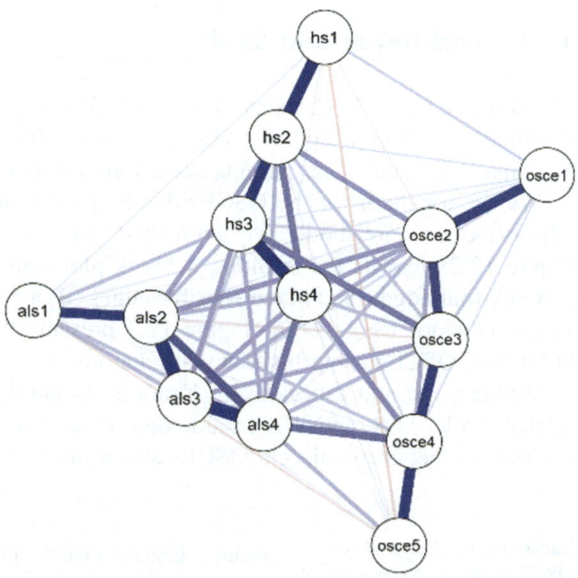

Fig. 12.3 Network plot of ALS_1–ALS_4, H&S_1–H&S_4, and $OSCE_1$–$OSCE_5$ using bivariate correlations (*JASP*)

OSCE-ALS and OSCE-H&S correlations as well as how much of the variance in OSCE performance in a given year can be explained by the combination of ALS and H&S.

Table 12.3 Pearson's r of within-year OSCE-ALS and OSCE-H&S and proportion of explained variance in OSCE performance using ALS and H&S (R^2) (*Jamovi*)

Year	r OSCE-ALS	r OSCE-H&S	R^2 OSCE
1	0.046	0.095	0.011
2	0.200	0.201	0.068
3	0.170	0.253	0.080
4	0.287	0.218	0.105

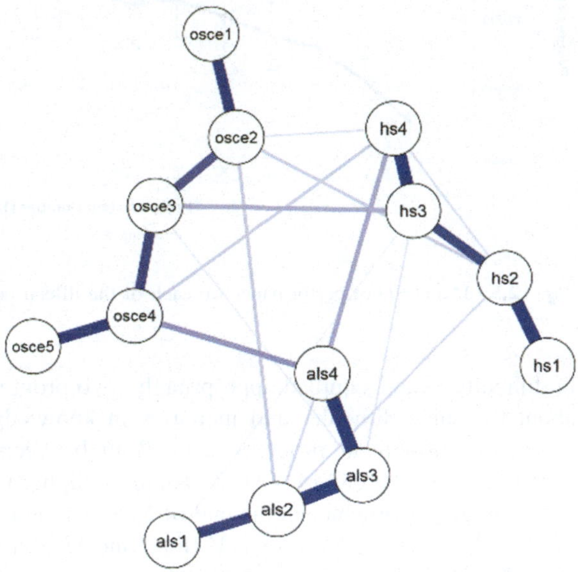

Fig. 12.4 Network plot of ALS_1–ALS_4, $H\&S_1$–$H\&S_4$, and $OSCE_1$–$OSCE_5$ using EBICglasso (*JASP*)

OSCE Year 5 only correlates substantially with OSCE Year 4 ($r = 0.403$, Table 12.2) and to some extent with ALS Year 4 ($r = 0.147$), but all other correlations are within the [−0.1; 0.1] range. Figure 12.4 presents the network plot for all ALS, H&S, and OSCEs using EBICglasso.

In this network, E = 78, $E_E = 23$, hence S ≈ 0.705. OSCE Year 4 is well connected with both OSCE Year 3 and OSCE Year 5 and to some extent also with ALS Year 4 and H&S Year 4. Together, OSCE Year 3, ALS Year 4, and H&S Year 4 explain 21.6% of the variance in OSCE Year 4.

12.4 Progress

Given that more difficult items are used in subsequent ALS and H&S exams and more difficult stations are used in subsequent OSCEs, an increase in knowledge or skill does not necessarily result in higher individual or M scores in subsequent years. However, with progress tests, that is different; although individual items vary

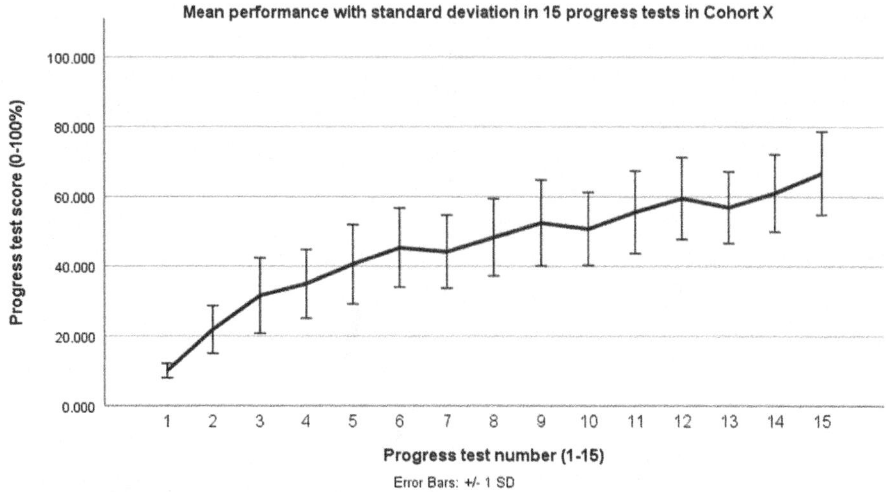

Fig. 12.5 *M* and *SD* of performance on each of the fifteen progress tests in Cohort X (*SPSS*)

in difficulty, when sampled appropriately, two progress tests should all in all be of about the same difficulty and increases in knowledge should translate in higher scores on subsequent progress tests. Both between and within cohort, average performance at the end of Year 2 should be higher than that at the end of Year 1, and average performance at the end of Year 3 should be higher than that at the end of Year 2. Figure 12.5 presents *M* (line) and *SD* (bars around line) of performance on each of the fifteen progress tests taken in the five years (i.e., three tests per year).

Figure 12.5 demonstrates that average performance increases from test to test, although there is a slight drop from Test 6 (last test in Year 2) to Test 7 (first test in Year 3), a slight drop from Test 9 (last test in Year 3) to Test 10 (first test in Year 4), and a slight drop from Test 12 (last test in Year 4) to Test 13 (first test in Year 5), probably at least partly between the exams in June and the start of the new academic year in September there is not much activity. The low *M* and small *SD* on the first test reflect a pattern to be expected at the very start of Year 1. We could now present the entire correlation matrix for all fifteen progress tests but will suffice with the network plot using bivariate correlations presented in Fig. 12.6.

This plot reveals a pattern that is similar to what we have seen for each of the other exam types: correlations are strongest between adjacent tests and weakest when the distance between exams is largest. The only case where the correlation between adjacent tests is somewhat weaker is between the first two tests in Year 1 ($r = 0.251$), but that is likely at least to some extent due to severe restriction of range in the first test of Year 1. Table 12.4 presents the within-year correlations between each of the progress tests with each of ALS, H&S, and OSCE.

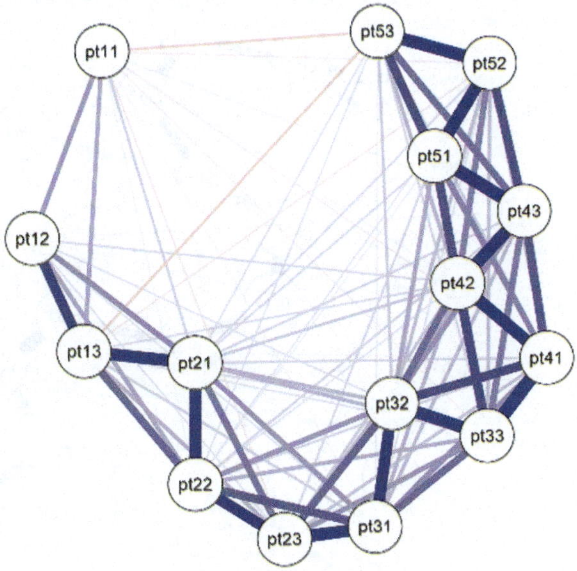

Fig. 12.6 Network plot of the progress tests in Year 1 (pt11–pt13), Year 2 (pt21–pt23), Year 3 (pt31–pt33), Year 4 (pt41–p43), and Year 5 (pt51–pt53), using bivariate correlations (*JASP*)

Table 12.4 Within-year *r* for each progress test (September, January, May) with ALS, H&S, and OSCE (*Jamovi*)

Year	Exam	September	January	May
1	ALS	0.123	0.222	0.204
	H&S	0.119	0.284	0.120
	OSCE	0.007	0.189	0.132
2	ALS	0.280	0.467	0.326
	H&S	0.284	0.413	0.254
	OSCE	0.341	0.445	0.252
3	ALS	0.266	0.398	0.309
	H&S	0.337	0.445	0.407
	OSCE	0.331	0.506	0.333
4	ALS	0.364	0.496	0.331
	H&S	0.369	0.444	0.360
	OSCE	0.309	0.447	0.343
5	OSCE	0.349	0.460	0.299

Although we see somewhat weaker correlations in Year 1, from Year 2 onward, the correlations are mostly in the [0.3; 0.5] range, and especially the January progress test helps to explain performance on each of the other exams. Figure 12.7 presents the network plot for the four ALS exams (ALS_1–ALS_4), the four H&S exams ($H\&S_1$–$H\&S_4$), the five OSCEs ($OSCE_1$–$OSCE_5$), and the progress tests in Year 1 (pt_{11}–pt_{13}), in Year 2 (pt_{21}–pt_{23}), in Year 3 (pt_{31}–pt_{33}), in Year 4 (pt_{41}–pt_{43}), and in Year 5 (pt_{51}–pt_{53}), using EBICglasso.

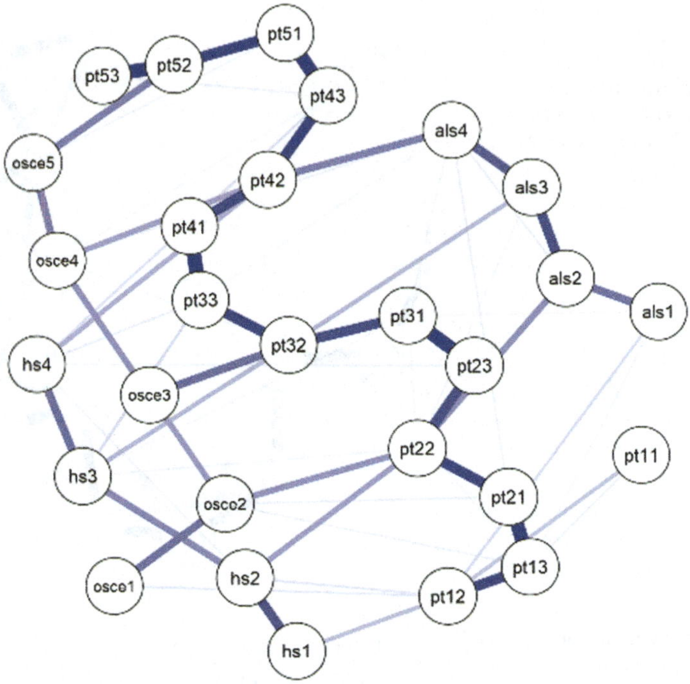

Fig. 12.7 Network plot for the all exams in Cohort X (*JASP*)

This is a relatively sparse network (E = 378, $E_E = 83$, S ≈ 0.780). As can be expected from Table 12.4, especially the second progress test in each year (i.e., pt_{12}, pt_{22}, pt_{32}, pt_{42}, and pt_{52}) is well connected with other exams taken in the same year. Whether we take the OSCE, the ALS, or the H&S exam in year *t*, we can reasonably predict performance on that exam using performance in year '*t* minus 1' on the OSCE, ALS or H&S, respectively, and the January progress test from year *t*; adding the latter, we no longer need to use other same-year exams (e.g., we no longer need to use ALS_4 to predict $H\&S_4$ or vice versa) but obtain better R^2-values. Table 12.5 presents the resulting R^2-values of that model per exam per year (Year 1 excluded, because there is no Year 0).

These are pretty good values. As a comparison, in the randomised controlled experiments done in educational research, we often deal with R^2-values in the [0; 0.05] range, occasionally encounter R^2-values around 0.1, and rarely find R^2-values above 0.15. Yet, randomised controlled experiments are used to make recommendations for educational practice. In assessment programmes such as in Medicine, R^2-values in the [0.3; 0.4] range are not uncommon.

Table 12.5 Predicting OSCE, ALS, and H&S performance in year *t* using the January progress test in year *t* and OSCE, ALS, or H&S performance in year '*t* minus 1', respectively (*Jamovi*): R^2-value per exam for Year 2, Year 3, Year 4, and Year 5

Year	OSCE	ALS	H&S
2	0.319	0.352	0.365
3	0.330	0.381	0.334
4	0.299	0.438	0.362
5	0.334	–	–

12.5 The Big Picture

The networks in this chapter build forth on concepts discussed in Chaps. 9–11 and provide a good picture of how different types of exams in an assessment programme are interrelated, and which exams we can use to reasonably predict performance at later occasions. Where we can reasonably predict poor future performance, we can consider ways of early intervention and remediation, providing students with opportunities to improve in areas of weakness. While in approaches like programmatic assessment "*information about a student's strengths and weaknesses is collected across different assessment methods rather than within*" (Uijtdehaage & Schuwirth, 2018, p. 350), true longitudinal assessment is about using *both between- and within*-method information. Correlations between adjacent exams of the same type in the [0.3–0.6] range are common and in some cases these correlations even exceed that range. Repeated assessments on the same topic (e.g., ALS, H&S, and OSCEs in subsequent years) shed light on a particular competence at different points in time. Simultaneously, different methods to some extent shed light on different aspects of competence. However, even methods that at first appear to have little if anything in common do tend to correlate to some extent, at least when administered in similar time periods (e.g., ALS, H&S, and OSCE in the same period in the same academic year). Even if a combination of knowledge tests only explains 7–10% of the variance in OSCE performance, this overlap is useful and makes sense when we realise that, although having knowledge does not imply one can do a good clinical examination, having no knowledge whatsoever should be very unlikely to result in a good clinical examination. Correlations between knowledge tests and OSCEs in the [0.3; 0.5] range are not uncommon, even if those knowledge tests cover a range of topics (e.g., progress test) and the OSCE includes different types of stations that are at best moderately correlated. Top performing students are usually not top performers in just a few exams and average or low performers in other exams, and struggling students often demonstrate poor performance at multiple occasions. This contributes to the intercorrelation of exams of the same type (e.g., correlations between progress tests) and exams of different types administered in a given period (e.g., correlation between the OSCE in Year 4 and progress tests in that year). Even if insufficiently competent students manage to pass the standard in a particular exam, the chance of doing so in a series of exams is unlikely. As far as the progress test is concerned, even if we use it only formatively until the final (i.e., third) test in Year 5, it is unlikely that a student who fails to demonstrate progress until Year 5 all of a sudden grows to the standard set for the end of Year 5.

As discussed in Chap. 11, in longitudinal studies (of which longitudinal assessment programmes can be seen as examples), it is normal to have higher correlations for adjacent occasions than for non-adjacent occasions, and that the correlation drops further with increasing distance between occasions. Even if in a three-occasion assessment context, there is substantial correlation between the first and third occasion, the partial correlation between these two occasions (i.e., the correlation between the residuals of the first occasion regressed on second occasion and the residuals of the third occasion regressed on the second occasion) may well be zero or close to zero. While we could reasonably predict performance on the third occasion by performance on the first occasion, using the second occasion as predictor probably results in a better model and the first occasion may then no longer be of added value.

Some may wonder if we could not obtain more accurate predictions by using scores on specific content areas within the progress test instead of using scores of the whole progress test, since the latter covers over twenty content areas. The answer to this question depends among others on how reliable our measurement is of each of the content areas as well as of specific stations in the OSCE or other exams. If we have a sufficiently reliable measurement of students' knowledge of the anatomy of the human shoulder (e.g., items in a progress test on that matter) and we have a sufficiently reliable measurement of students' performance on an OSCE station on a particular shoulder problem, we might well be able to fairly accurately explain differences between students in performance on an OSCE station on that shoulder problem using the sufficiently reliable knowledge assessment. However, in practice we often do not have such a reliable measurement. Besides, even if we have sufficiently reliable measurements at the level of such subscales, adding more variables to our models comes with increased demands on sample size. The network in Fig. 12.7 is already one with 28 nodes (and therefore E = 378), and we need our sample size of $N = 300$ for that.

That said, the network approach presented in this chapter can help to examine to what extent interrelations between different assessment components differ across cohorts or change as a result of a change in the assessment programme. For instance, before a particular medical school introduces progress testing, its longitudinal assessment network may be something like in Fig. 12.4, while after introduction of progress testing, we see something similar to Fig. 12.7. Similarly, if the board of a given MBBS programme decide to get rid of the Year 1 OSCE and replace it by something else, or to move one of the ALS or H&S exams in a given year to a few months earlier in the year, we will likely see some changes in the network. Even people who prefer to take more of what they would call a 'qualitative' approach rather than compute correlations could use networks like the ones presented in this chapter to think in a holistic manner about their assessment programme and if the interrelations between different components in the programme are more or less in line with the programme they envisioned.

Whether we think directly in terms of correlations or more 'holistically', longitudinal assessment networks provide easy visuals of the phenomenon that differences between students in competence—even if that competence has many aspects or facets—tend to translate into related differences on: (1) adjacent exams of the same type; and to some extent also (2) on two somewhat different exams which do have some common component (e.g., some knowledge being needed to be able to do a good clinical examination) and are administered in more or less the same time period.

Reference

Uijtdehaage, S., & Schuwirth, L. W. T. (2018). Assuring the quality of programmatic assessment: Moving beyond psychometrics. *Perspectives on Medical Education, 7*(6), 350–351. https://doi.org/10.1007/s40037-018-0485-y.

Part IV
Time Series

Randomised Controlled Experiments 13

Abstract

Although many randomised controlled experiments in Education are about comparing learning outcomes between conditions right after study or practice, there are experiments that involve repeated measurements as well. This chapter focusses on experiments that involve series of repeated measurements, some of which may occur prior to treatment. Besides, since there is evidence that assessment can itself influence learning, this chapter also discusses experimental designs with time series that allow for testing and estimating the impact of assessment on learning outcomes at a later time.

13.1 Introduction

In recent years, we have seen an increased interest in the accuracy of self-assessment, task selection, and other skills associated with metacognition and SRL. Suppose, a group of educational researchers have developed a new simple checklist that may support self-assessment of learning task performance among high school students who are learning geometry. They decide to study the effect of this checklist on self-assessment, on actual learning task performance, and on the difference between self-assessment and actual learning task performance. The rationale behind this interest is as follows. We know that newcomers in a topic are generally not that good at self-assessing their own performance, and if we want learners to make their own study activity choices, inaccurate self-assessment can be a problem. Underestimation will likely result in too easy learning tasks being chosen, whereas overestimation can be expected to result in too complex learning tasks being chosen by a learner. In environments where learners can freely choose learning tasks from a range of complexity levels and we are able to monitor both task selection and performance on any given task selected, we can quantify

J. Leppink, *The Art of Modelling the Learning Process*, Springer Texts in Education,
https://doi.org/10.1007/978-3-030-43082-5_13

tendencies of under- and overestimation or under- and overchallenge. Consider a learning environment on probability calculus tasks that have two possible outcomes: correct or incorrect performance. One would not want to see learners aim for increasingly complex tasks if the tasks they are choosing are being performed incorrectly. Likewise, it is undesirable to see learners for increasingly simple tasks while the tasks they are choosing are performed correctly. The former would be a tendency towards *overchallenge*, while the latter is a tendency towards *underchallenge*. Both tendencies move away from the concept of *zone of proximal development* (see Chap. 1), where learning is expected to take place, and can be quantified for the individual learner on an underchallenge-overchallenge dimension ranging from −1 or 100% underchallenge to 1 or 100% overchallenge (i.e., values closer to 0 being better; Leppink, Paas, Van Gog, and Van Merriënboer, 2019). Besides, another type of undesirable behaviour is to switch between underchallenge and overchallenge; this kind of fluctuation may indicate either uncertainty or random choice behaviour and can be quantified for the individual learner into a [0; 1] variability statistic as well (i.e., values closer to 0 being better; Leppink et al., 2019).

In environments where learners are not given a choice with regard to what learning task to do next, it can still be useful to measure self-assessment of learning task performance and compare that to actual task performance, as the group of educational researchers who have developed the new simple checklist want to do. Consistent over- and underestimation are likely to result in over- and underchallenge if learners are given the choice and going back and forth between over- and underestimation may well result in fluctuation on the over- and underchallenge dimension in a sequence of learning tasks where learners have the choice. Inaccurate self-assessment, whichever direction, is unlikely to result in accurate learning task selection (i.e., tasks within the learner's zone of proximal development). Besides, the researchers wonder if the checklist might not only affect self-assessment but actual learning task performance as well. They decide to set up an experiment to investigate this further. They develop a series of six geometry learning tasks that are of more or less the same complexity level and are typically used early on in geometry coursework. Each of the six learning tasks requires the learner to complete nine steps, each of which is scored as incorrect (0) or correct (1) resulting in a task score on a scale of 0 (minimum) to 9 (maximum). Each of the steps is of very similar complexity. At the end of each task, learners are asked to self-assess their performance of the task just completed on that 0–9 scale. The correct answers are provided only after the completion of the sixth task with self-assessment. The only thing the researchers still wonder about is how to set up the different conditions of the experiment, that is: *where* and *how* the checklist is used.

13.2 Different Options

The researchers have a number of options available. A first option is to randomly allocate the full sample (*N*) to either of two conditions: one in which participants receive the checklist all along, and one in which participants do not receive the checklist at all. This setup can be useful for instance when effects of checklist use are small and/or only become visible after some tasks (i.e., condition-by-time interaction effect).

A second option is to present the checklist to both groups, but for instance in one group for the first three tasks and in the other group for the last three tasks. This allows to give all participants the treatment for an equal number of tasks and allows for studying condition-by-time interaction as well. One type of interaction pattern that may occur is that in the group where the checklist is presented in the first three tasks, performance is superior to that in the other group for the first three tasks but no longer for the last three tasks.

A third option would combine the first two options in a 2-by-2 setup: receive checklist in the first three tasks (yes or no) and receive checklist in the last three tasks (yes or no). If the checklist has an immediate positive effect that does not easily fade, this could result in the group not receiving the checklist at all performing worst and the other three groups performing more or less the same (i.e., interaction effect).

13.2.1 Three Groups

There are many other options (e.g., Leppink, 2019), including the following. We randomly divide the total sample in three groups. In the first group, participants do not get to use the checklist. In the second group, participants use the checklist for the fifth and sixth task, and in the third group, participants use the checklist for the third, fourth, fifth, and sixth task. In other words, the first two tasks are the same in all three groups: no checklist is used for the first or second task in any of the three groups. In other words, contrary to the first three options discussed, no one starts off with checklist; we have at least two 'control' (i.e., no checklist) measurements for every participant. If the checklist has an immediate effect, we should see a difference in trajectory in at least one of the outcome variables from the second to the third task between the group that starts to use the checklist in the third task and the other two groups, and we should see a similar difference from the fourth to the fifth task between the group that starts to use the checklist in the fifth task and the group that does not use the checklist at all. However, if there is an effect but one that occurs less immediately or needs some time to become noticeable, it is possible we will see any kind of difference in trajectory only somewhere towards the end of the sequence between the group that starts to use the checklist in the third task and the other two groups.

13.2.2 Baseline Measurements

In this design with three groups, the first two measurements are *baseline* measurements for which the three groups can be considered as one sample from one population. In a quasi-experiment, where no random allocation to groups or conditions occurs, it is usually safer to consider different groups as coming from different populations and regressing to their own M, but in the case of randomised controlled experiments, *prior to any treatment* there is regression to a *common M* and we should account for that in our statistical models (e.g., Leppink, 2019; Twisk et al., 2018; Van Breukelen, 2006). Another way to look at this is as three groups that can be distinguished in terms of when they switch from control to treatment condition: *early* (i.e., third task), *late* (i.e., fifth task) or *never* (i.e., remain in control condition).

In a statistical model that treats the groups as different for each of the six tasks, such as repeated-measures analysis of variance (e.g., Field, 2018), we use a total of 18 *df* for intercept ($df = 1$), task main effect ($df = 5$), group main effect ($df = 2$), and group-by-task interaction effect ($df = 10$). However, in a statistical model that correctly accounts for the design (i.e., different switch from control to treatment for different groups), we only need 12 *df* for that fixed part because 6 *df* are no longer needed: we save 4 *df* for the difference between *late* and *never* and we save 2 *df* for the difference between *early* and the other two groups. The resulting regression equation for the score on a response variable of interest Y for participant j in task i is as follows:

$$\begin{aligned} Y_{ij} = B_{0j} &+ [B_1 * \text{task } 2_{ij}] + [B_2 * \text{task } 3_{ij}] + [B_3 * \text{task } 4_{ij}] + [B_4 * \text{task } 5_{ij}] + [B_5 * \text{task } 6_{ij}] \\ &+ [B_6 * \text{early} * \text{task } 3_{ij}] + [B_7 * \text{early} * \text{task } 4_{ij}] + [B_8 * \text{early} * \text{task } 5_{ij}] + [B_9 * \text{early} * \text{task } 6_{ij}] \\ &+ [B_{10} * \text{late} * \text{task } 5_{ij}] + [B_{11} * \text{late} * \text{task } 6_{ij}] + \text{residual}_{ij}. \end{aligned}$$

This is a regression model that estimates the twelve parameters of the fixed part (i.e., all of B_0–B_{11}), six of which pertain to a difference in trajectory between two groups (i.e., B_6–B_{11}), and subscript j in B_0 represents the RI. In other words, this is a RI (i.e., CS) model. Depending on our sample size, we may also add one or a few RS terms, which may or may not correlate with each other and/or with the RI term. An easy RI-RS combination is found in including RS for task 6:

$$\begin{aligned} Y_{ij} = B_{0j} &+ [B_1 * \text{task } 2_{ij}] + [B_2 * \text{task } 3_{ij}] + [B_3 * \text{task } 4_{ij}] + [B_4 * \text{task } 5_{ij}] + [B_{5j} * \text{task } 6_{ij}] \\ &+ [B_6 * \text{early} * \text{task } 3_{ij}] + [B_7 * \text{early} * \text{task } 4_{ij}] + [B_8 * \text{early} * \text{task } 5_{ij}] + [B_9 * \text{early} * \text{task } 6_{ij}] \\ &+ [B_{10} * \text{late} * \text{task } 5_{ij}] + [B_{11} * \text{late} * \text{task } 6_{ij}] + \text{residual}_{ij}. \end{aligned}$$

The only difference between this equation and the previous one is that we have now added a 'j' to B_5: we estimate the variance in the trajectory from task 1 to task 6. When we allow the RI and RS term to correlate, we need 3 *df* for the random part of our model: one for the RI variance, one for the RS variance, and one for their covariance.

The above models can be used for each response variable in the experiment: self-assessment, actual performance, and the difference between these two (i.e., self-assessment minus actual performance). However, even if self-assessment in this experiment turns out to be somewhat poor, self-assessment of learning task performance and actual learning task performance are likely going to be correlated to some extent. Given that self-assessment and task performance are measured on the same 0–9 scale and learners provide their self-assessment without knowing their actual performance, we can consider self-assessment and task performance as two scores on the same task that will often not be the same, and the difference between self-assessment and task performance for any given task will likely differ between participants. There is a way to model all this simultaneously in a three-level model, with participant as upper level (*k*), task as middle level (*j*), and rater (self-assessment vs. actual task performance) as lowest level (*i*), in which we include RI at the participant level (*k*), RI at the task level (*j*), RS for the difference between self-assessment and actual performance at the task level (*j*), and the covariance between the RI and RS at the task level. With this model, in which we use only 4 *df* for the random part, we can estimate all fixed and random effects simultaneously leaving residual_{ijk} at 0:

$$
\begin{aligned}
Y_{ijk} = B_{0jk} &+ \left[B_1 * \text{task}\,2_{jk}\right] + \left[B_2 * \text{task}\,3_{jk}\right] + \left[B_3 * \text{task}\,4_{jk}\right] + \left[B_4 * \text{task}\,5_{jk}\right] + \left[B_5 * \text{task}\,6_{jk}\right] \\
&+ \left[B_{6j} * \text{self}_{ijk}\right] + \left[B_7 * \text{task}\,2 * \text{self}_{ijk}\right] + \left[B_8 * \text{task}\,3 * \text{self}_{ijk}\right] + \left[B_9 * \text{task}\,4 * \text{self}_{ijk}\right] \\
&+ \left[B_{10} * \text{task}\,5 * \text{self}_{ijk}\right] + \left[B_{11} * \text{task}\,6 * \text{self}_{ijk}\right] + \left[B_{12} * \text{task}\,3 * \text{early}_{jk}\right] + \left[B_{13} * \text{task}\,4 * \text{early}_{jk}\right] \\
&+ \left[B_{14} * \text{task}\,5 * \text{early}_{jk}\right] + \left[B_{15} * \text{task}\,6 * \text{early}_{jk}\right] + \left[B_{16} * \text{task}\,5 * \text{late}_{jk}\right] + \left[B_{17} * \text{task}\,6 * \text{late}_{jk}\right] \\
&+ \left[B_{18} * \text{task}\,3 * \text{early} * \text{self}_{ijk}\right] + \left[B_{19} * \text{task}\,4 * \text{early} * \text{self}_{ijk}\right] + \left[B_{20} * \text{task}\,5 * \text{early} * \text{self}_{ijk}\right] \\
&+ \left[B_{21} * \text{task}\,6 * \text{early} * \text{self}_{ijk}\right] + \left[B_{22} * \text{task}\,5 * \text{late} * \text{self}_{ijk}\right] + \left[B_{23} * \text{task}\,6 * \text{late} * \text{self}_{ijk}\right].
\end{aligned}
$$

In this model, B_{0jk} expresses the RI terms at levels *j* and *k* and B_{6j} expresses the RS term at level *j*, we need 24 *df* for the fixed part (i.e., all of B_0–B_{23}) of which 12 are related to differences between groups (i.e., B_{12}–B_{23}). The aforementioned models, which use only 12 *df* can be used for each outcome variable when samples are on the smaller side, for instance $N = 120$ spread out over three groups of $n = 40$. However, in an experiment where we deal with larger samples, for example $N = 300$ spread out over three groups of $n = 100$, the latter model allows to model all three outcome variables—self-assessment, actual performance, and the difference between the two—all at once. Let us have a look at both options.

13.3 Each Outcome Variable Separately

The educational researchers have logistic means for a random sample of $N = 300$ and divide that into three groups of $n = 100$ each. No severe departures from symmetric and unimodal distributions are encountered in any of the groups for any of the outcome variables of interest. Table 13.1 presents *M* and *SD* of each outcome variable per group per task.

Table 13.1 *M* and *SD* of self-assessment, actual learning task performance, and the difference between the two (self-assessment minus actual learning task performance) per group per task (*Jamovi*)

Group	Task	Self-assess (0–9)	Perform (0–9)	Difference (0–9)
		M (*SD*)	*M* (*SD*)	*M* (*SD*)
1 (*early*)	1	4.830 (1.378)	4.080 (1.098)	0.750 (1.038)
	2	5.020 (1.400)	4.220 (1.079)	0.800 (1.005)
	3	4.370 (1.152)	4.200 (0.910)	0.170 (0.829)
	4	4.590 (1.371)	4.240 (0.976)	0.350 (1.067)
	5	4.420 (1.499)	4.290 (0.935)	0.130 (1.186)
	6	4.300 (1.352)	4.100 (0.823)	0.200 (1.181)
2 (*late*)	1	5.130 (1.561)	4.100 (1.000)	1.030 (1.077)
	2	5.020 (1.223)	4.100 (1.068)	0.920 (0.971)
	3	5.170 (1.303)	4.220 (1.088)	0.950 (0.892)
	4	5.150 (1.403)	4.290 (1.028)	0.860 (1.005)
	5	4.900 (1.283)	4.330 (0.954)	0.570 (0.967)
	6	4.670 (1.264)	4.400 (0.985)	0.270 (0.897)
3 (*never*)	1	5.110 (1.262)	3.910 (1.045)	1.200 (0.899)
	2	4.860 (1.511)	4.010 (1.141)	0.850 (0.999)
	3	4.950 (1.303)	4.120 (1.066)	0.830 (0.975)
	4	5.060 (1.403)	4.200 (1.025)	0.860 (0.975)
	5	4.950 (1.283)	4.220 (1.031)	0.730 (1.014)
	6	5.070 (1.264)	4.230 (1.014)	0.840 (0.982)

From Table 13.1, it appears that the intervention does not seem to have any noticeable effect on actual learning task performance but does appear to have a somewhat beneficial effect on the accuracy of self-assessment: self-assessment is on average more in line with actual learning task performance starting the third task in the *early* group and starting fifth or sixth task in the *late* group.

13.3.1 Random Effects

There are quite a few options for modelling the random part, the most flexible of which is UN, where we need: $df = 21$ (i.e., fifteen r_{RES} and six V_{RES}, or: one for the RI, five for the RSs for the difference between task1 and any of the other five tasks, and fifteen for the RI-RS and RS-RS covariances; either way, we have $residual_{ij} = 0$). We can also consider several other structures discussed in Chap. 11: CS (i.e., RI), CSH, HF, AD1, and if we can treat the tasks as equidistant, AR1, ARH1, TP, and TPH. A variant of AR1 that may also be considered for this kind of data is AR1 with first-order moving average (MA1): ARMA(1,1) or ARIMA (1,0,1), where ARIMA stands for *autoregressive integrated moving average* (e.g., Box, Jenkins, & Reinsel, 1994; Brockwell & Davis, 2009; Hannan, 1970; Whittle,

1951). In ARIMA terms, AR1 is ARIMA(1,0,0), and when we add MA1, we obtain ARIMA(1,0,1). The third parameter in the ARIMA model, which is '0' in ARIMA (1,0,1) is discussed in Chap. 16 in this book.

ARMA(1,1) can be useful for so-called *stationary* time series: while scores on an outcome variable of interest may change over time, the *way* in which it changes does not really change (e.g., change more or less following a linear function). For performance, for example, we see fairly small changes over time (Table 13.1) and *SD* does not vary much from task to task. For self-assessment and the difference between self-assessment and performance, we see some group-specific changes as a function of treatment but, like differences in performance, we can account for those in the fixed part of our model. In the ARMA(1,1) model, the AR1 states that a score of individual j in task i is partly a function of the score of that individual j in task 'i minus 1', and the MA1 component adds that the score of individual j in task i is also partly a function of residual in task i and residual in task 'i minus 1'. In more complex models, we would go back further in time. For instance, AR2 and MA2 would involve the score (AR2) and error (MA2) in task 'i minus 2' as well. However, as discussed in examples in Chaps. 11 and 12, it is in practice frequently sufficient to just consider the previous task or occasion, meaning there is no need to go two or even more tasks or occasions back. ARMA(1,1) requires only 3 *df*: one for AR1, one for MA1, and one for V_{RES}.

Table 13.2 presents the estimates of all r_{RES} and V_{RES} in the UN model, accounting for the fixed part of the design (i.e., all of B_0–B_{11} in the first equation in this chapter), for self-assessment.

Table 13.3 presents the estimates of all r_{RES} and V_{RES} in the UN model, accounting for the fixed part of the design (i.e., all of B_0–B_{11} in the first equation in this chapter), for actual learning task performance.

Table 13.2 UN for self-assessment: 15 r_{RES} and 6 V_{RES} estimates (<u>*SPSS*</u>)

	Task 1	Task 2	Task 3	Task 4	Task 5	Task 6
V_{RES}	1.983	1.905	1.779	1.795	1.892	1.756
Task 2	0.456					
Task 3	0.405	0.516				
Task 4	0.355	0.345	0.401			
Task 5	0.299	0.276	0.295	0.428		
Task 6	0.190	0.209	0.356	0.299	0.302	

Table 13.3 UN for actual learning task performance: 15 r_{RES} and 6 V_{RES} estimates (<u>*SPSS*</u>)

	Task 1	Task 2	Task 3	Task 4	Task 5	Task 6
V_{RES}	1.099	1.202	1.048	1.018	0.948	0.891
Task 2	0.774					
Task 3	0.688	0.795				
Task 4	0.605	0.702	0.763			
Task 5	0.496	0.602	0.595	0.722		
Task 6	0.389	0.448	0.492	0.584	0.677	

Table 13.4 UN for self-assessment minus performance: 15 r_{RES} and 6 V_{RES} estimates (*SPSS*)

	Task 1	Task 2	Task 3	Task 4	Task 5	Task 6
V_{RES}	1.043	0.979	0.811	1.030	1.123	1.054
Task 2	−0.090					
Task 3	−0.064	0.052				
Task 4	0.040	−0.010	−0.004			
Task 5	0.051	−0.009	−0.067	−0.001		
Task 6	−0.015	−0.014	0.034	−0.060	−0.075	

Table 13.4 presents the estimates of all r_{RES} and V_{RES} in the UN model, accounting for the fixed part of the design (i.e., all of B_0–B_{11} in the first equation in this chapter), for the difference between self-assessment and actual task performance (i.e., self-assessment minus performance).

Clearly, autocorrelation is strongest for performance and weakest for the difference between self-assessment and performance. The latter is quite normal: subtracting scores from two correlated variables may well result in an outcome variable with residual correlations fairly close to zero.

Finally, Table 13.5 presents -2RLL values of each of a range of residual covariance structures for each outcome variable.

For self-assessment, only three structures appear to perform reasonably well compared to UN: ARMA(1,1), TP, and TPH. For ARMA, the resulting LR test yields: $\chi^2_{18} = 25.557$, $p = 0.110$. For TP, we find: $\chi^2_{15} = 20.708$, $p = 0.146$, and for TPH, we find: $\chi^2_{10} = 18.473$, $p = 0.047$. Compared to TP, TPH comes at only a very minor reduction in -2RLL at the cost of 5 *df* more. We cannot do any LR testing comparing ARMA(1,1) with TP or TPH, since ARMA(1,1) is not nested in either of these two. Some might argue in favour of TP because it is slightly more flexible, whereas others might argue that both ARMA(1,1) and TP can be considered valid simplifications of UN and ARMA(1,1) can be defended as the most

Table 13.5 Comparison of residual covariance structures for self-assessment (SA), performance (PF), and the difference between self-assessment and performance (DIF) (*SPSS*)

Structure	*df*	SA -2RLL	PF -2RLL	DIF -2RLL
UN	21	5850.983	3898.838	5126.081
ID	1	6235.087	5194.040	5144.953
DI	6	6233.402	5185.659	5135.922
CS	2	5907.950	4159.439	5143.759
CSH	7	5905.143	4150.637	5134.772
HF	7	5901.255	4131.147	5141.415
AD1	7	5929.916	3952.655	5130.973
AR1	2	5943.437	3968.622	5143.923
AR1H	7	5940.789	3965.079	5135.088
ARMA(1,1)	3	5876.540	3926.669	5142.806
TP	6	5871.691	3922.762	5140.507
TPH	11	5869.456	3920.050	5131.593

parsimonious option. In ARMA(1,1), we find the following estimates: 0.852 ($p < 0.001$) for AR1, 0.416 ($p < 0.001$) for MA1, and 1.852 for V_{RES}.

For performance, the same three structures stand out as possible alternatives to UN. For ARMA(1,1), we find: $\chi^2_{18} = 27.831$, $p = 0.065$. For TP, we find: $\chi^2_{15} = 23.924$, $p = 0.066$. For TPH, we find: $\chi^2_{10} = 21.212$, $p = 0.020$. Testing two-sided, both ARMA(1,1) and TP appear defendable, while testing one-sided (i.e., simplifications always mean we explain less) would result in preferring UN. If we take the same structure as for self-assessment, ARMA(1,1), we find the following estimates: 0.856 ($p < 0.001$) for AR1, 0.744 ($p < 0.001$) for MA, and 1.023 for V_{RES}.

For the difference between self-assessment and performance, all alternatives to UN can be considered valid simplifications of UN. In line with the comparisons of Tables 13.2, 13.3, and 13.4, ID and DI now appear to perform quite well. For the difference between ID and DI, we find: $\chi^2_5 = 9.031$, $p = 0.108$. We also see that ID and CS yield more or less the same -2RLL and DI and CSH do so as well. The only structure that performs significantly better than ID is AD1: $\chi^2_6 = 13.980$, $p = 0.003$. Thus, for this difference outcome variable, we opt for AD1.

13.3.2 Fixed Effects

Since UN is also discussed in Chaps. 9–11 but ARMA(1,1) only for the first time in this book in this chapter, and the latter does not perform much worse than UN for self-assessment and performance, Table 13.6 presents the outcomes of the fixed effects for self-assessment and performance under ARMA(1,1) and the outcomes of the fixed effects for the difference between self-assessment and performance under AD1.

Table 13.6 Fixed effect estimates with SE for each of the outcome variables (*SPSS*)

Term	SA: *B* (*SE*)	PF: *B* (*SE*)	DIF: *B* (*SE*)
B_0 (fixed intercept)	5.023 (0.078)	4.030 (0.058)	0.993 (0.059)
B_1 (task 2)	−0.057 (0.085)	0.080 (0.042)	−0.137 (0.086)
B_2 (task 3)	0.024 (0.102)	0.178 (0.056)	−0.105 (0.087)
B_3 (task 4)	0.071 (0.106)	0.248 (0.064)	−0.133 (0.093)
B_4 (task 5)	−0.042 (0.138)	0.256 (0.083)	−0.263 (0.121)
B_5 (task 6)	0.073 (0.142)	0.256 (0.091)	−0.153 (0.118)
B_6 (early * task 3)	−0.652 (0.147)	−0.084 (0.081)	−0.716 (0.110)
B_7 (early * task 4)	−0.483 (0.153)	−0.103 (0.094)	−0.510 (0.124)
B_8 (early * task 5)	−0.543 (0.178)	−0.051 (0.113)	−0.600 (0.149)
B_9 (early * task 6)	−0.781 (0.182)	−0.234 (0.122)	−0.640 (0.144)
B_{10} (late * task 5)	−0.131 (0.169)	0.035 (0.093)	−0.160 (0.149)
B_{11} (late * task 6)	−0.469 (0.175)	0.105 (0.109)	−0.570 (0.144)

For both self-assessment and the difference between self-assessment and performance, all interaction terms are statistically significant at $\alpha = 0.01$ (two-sided) except for B_{10} (self-assessment: $p = 0.439$; performance: $p = 0.284$). For performance, none of the interaction terms are statistically significant at $\alpha = 0.05$ (two-sided). In sum, it appears that we have insufficient evidence to assume any kind of effect of checklist use on actual performance but do see some beneficial effect of checklist use on self-assessment (i.e., a reduced M tendency of overestimation).

13.4 All Outcome Variables Simultaneously

With the more extensive model, where we double *df* for the fixed part because we treat self-assessment and actual performance as correlated variables—correlations between these two variables are in the [0.499; 0.770] range within each of six tasks in each group—but need only 4 *df* for the random part, we obtain almost the same outcomes for the fixed part. That said, while it is still possible to run this model in *SPSS*, more powerful packages like *Stata* and *MLwiN* will do the job better and much faster. *SPSS* is usually a good option for two-level models with not too many fixed effects and not too large samples (e.g., not $N = 10{,}000$). When the sample size, complexity of the fixed part and/or number of levels increase, *SPSS* is generally very slow (e.g., a fairly complex three-level of four-level model may take half an hour) and may suffer from serious convergence issues. However, in *Stata* and *MLwiN*, convergence is achieved within seconds for this kind of models.

As discussed in earlier chapters in this book, FIML is commonly used for the estimation of fixed effects in linear, binary logistic, multinomial logistic, and ordinal regression as well as in latent variable models such as confirmatory factor analysis. Is has in fact been around since the early 1950 (Fisher, 1950). For more complex data structures, FIML is an iterative process. In *MLwiN*, this process is done using *iterative generalised least squares* (IGLS; Goldstein, 1986, 1987), and the equivalent for REML (used for random effects) is *restricted iterative generalised least squares* (RIGLS; Goldstein, 1989). For a simple two-level RI model, *MLwiN* with RIGLS and *SPSS* with REML should yield the same estimates of the RI variance and its *SE*, *MLwiN* with IGLS and *SPSS* with (FI)ML should yield the same estimates of the fixed effects and the same -2LL for a given model.

Using RIGLS in *MLwiN*, we obtain the following random effects variance and covariance estimates in our example study: 0.646 ($SE = 0.058$) for the participant-level (i.e., *k*) RI variance, 0.389 ($SE = 0.014$) for the task-level (i.e., *j*) RI variance, 1.007 ($SE = 0.034$) for the task-level RS variance, and finally −0.095 ($SE = 0.016$) for the RI-RS covariance (and $V_{RES} = 0$). In short, it does not seem we can omit any of these random terms. Table 13.6 presents the outcomes of the fixed effects of this model under IGLS.

Table 13.7 Fixed effect estimates with SE for each of the outcome variables using IGLS in *MLwiN*

Term	*B* (*SE*)
B_0 (fixed intercept)	4.030 (0.059)
B_1 (task 2)	0.080 (0.051)
B_2 (task 3)	0.165 (0.059)
B_3 (task 4)	0.240 (0.059)
B_4 (task 5)	0.267 (0.076)
B_5 (task 6)	0.277 (0.076)
B_6 (self)	0.993 (0.058)
B_7 (task 2 * self)	−0.137 (0.082)
B_8 (task 3 * self)	−0.103 (0.091)
B_9 (task 4 * self)	−0.133 (0.091)
B_{10} (task 5 * self)	−0.263 (0.115)
B_{11} (task 6 * self)	−0.153 (0.115)
B_{12} (task 3 * early)	−0.046 (0.089)
B_{13} (task 4 * early)	−0.081 (0.089)
B_{14} (task 5 * early)	−0.058 (0.102)
B_{15} (task 6 * early)	−0.258 (0.102)
B_{16} (task 5 * late)	0.007 (0.097)
B_{17} (task 6 * late)	0.067 (0.097)
B_{18} (task 3 * early * self)	−0.720 (0.122)
B_{19} (task 4 * early * self)	−0.510 (0.122)
B_{20} (task 5 * early * self)	−0.600 (0.141)
B_{21} (task 6 * early * self)	−0.640 (0.141)
B_{22} (task 5 * late * self)	−0.160 (0.141)
B_{23} (task 6 * late * self)	−0.570 (0.141)

The estimates of B_0–B_5 in Table 13.7 are almost the same as the estimates of B_0–B_5 for task performance in Table 13.6, that the estimates of B_6–B_{11} in Table 13.7 are almost the same as the estimates of B_0–B_5 for the difference between self-assessment and task performance in Table 13.6, the estimates of B_{12}–B_{17} in Table 13.7 are similar to the estimates of B_6–B_{11} for task performance in Table 13.6, and the estimates of B_{18}–B_{23} in Table 13.7 are almost the same as the estimates of B_6–B_{11} for the difference between self-assessment and task performance in Table 13.6. There are some differences, because we use *more information* for our fixed part in this more complex model (Table 13.7) than we do in the simpler one-by-one outcome variable approach (Table 13.6) and the modelling of the random part is somewhat different, but the results are very similar.

13.5 Other Time Experiments

There are many other examples of experiments that involve a repeated-measures component, including experiments involving immediate and delayed testing (Chap. 2) or sequences of worked examples to be studied and problems to be solved (Leppink, 2019). While the latter are often compared in terms of average performance on a single post-test, the problems to be solved in the study phase that precedes the post-test can also be used as performance indicators. For instance, take the following eight sequences that constitute eight between-subjects conditions in a randomised controlled experiment in which there is a post-test immediately after these sequences:

Example-Example-Problem (and next: post-test)
Example-Problem-Problem (and next: post-test)
Problem-Example-Problem (and next: post-test)
Problem-Problem-Problem (and next: post-test)
Example-Example-Example (and next: post-test)
Example-Problem-Example (and next: post-test)
Problem-Example-Example (and next: post-test)
Problem-Problem-Example (and next: post-test).

The eight sequences (i.e., combinations of examples and problems) together can be conceived as a three-way design: first task (problem or example), second task (problem or example), and third task (problem or example). A three-way model can then be used to estimate the main effects and two- and three-way interaction effects on post-test performance. However, the third problem in the sequence in itself also constitutes a mini-post-test for a two-way comparison involving the first four conditions, and the second problem in the sequence can be treated as a mini-post-test for a one-way comparison of example and problem taken in the first round (i.e., the second, fourth, sixth, and eighth condition). All these comparisons help us to get more out of the data than the one-way comparisons of final post-test performance we usually see in this kind of experiments.

A similar logic applies to the type of design discussed in Chap. 2 involving a delayed post-test for all conditions but an immediate post-test only for half of the conditions. Under a positive testing effect, conditions undergoing an immediate post-test should demonstrate higher *M* delayed post-test performance compared to the conditions that are not offered the immediate post-test.

References

Box, G. E. P., Jenkins, G. M., & Reinsel, G. C. (1994). *Time series analysis: Forecasting and control* (3rd ed.). Upper Saddle River, NJ: Prentice Hall.

Brockwell, P. J., & Davis, R. A. (2009). *Time series: Theory and methods* (2nd ed.). New York: Springer.

Field, A. (2018). *Discovering statistics using IBM SPSS statistics* (5th ed.). London: Sage.

Fisher, R. A. (1950). *Contributions to mathematical statistics*. New York: Wiley.

Goldstein, H. (1986). Multilevel mixed linear model analysis using iterative generalized least squares. *Biometrika, 73,* 43–56. https://doi.org/10.1093/biomet/73.1.43.

Goldstein, H. (1987). Multilevel covariance component models. *Biometrika, 74,* 430–431. https://doi.org/10.1093/biomet/74.2.430.

Goldstein, H. (1989). Restricted unbiased iterative generalized least-squares estimation. *Biometrika, 76,* 622–623. https://doi.org/10.1093/biomet/76.3.622.

Hannan, E. J. (1970). *Multiple time series*. New York: Wiley.

Leppink, J. (2019). *Statistical methods for experimental research in education and psychology*. Cham: Springer. https://doi.org/10.1007/978-3-030-21241-4.

Leppink, J., Paas, F., Van Gog, T., & Van Merriënboer, J. J. G. (2019). How to measure effects of self-regulated learning with checklists on the acquisition of task selection skills. In S. Tindall-Ford, S. Agostinho, & J. Sweller (Eds.), *Advances in cognitive load theory: Rethinking teaching (Chap. 6)*. London: Routledge.

Twisk, J. W. R., Bosman, L., Hoekstra, T., Rijnhart, J., Welten, M., & Heymans, M. (2018). Different ways to estimate treatment effects in randomised controlled trials. *Contemporary Clinical Trials Communications, 10,* 80–85. https://doi.org/10.1016/j.conctc.2018.03.008.

Van Breukelen, G. J. P. (2006). ANCOVA versus change from baseline: More power in randomized studies, more bias in nonrandomized studies. *Journal of Clinical Epidemiology, 59* (9), 920–925. https://doi.org/10.1016/j.jclinepi.2006.02.007.

Whittle, P. (1951). *Hypothesis testing in time series analysis*. Uppsala, Almqvist & Wiksells.

14 Static and Dynamic Group Structures

Abstract

Much of our learning takes place through interaction with others. Careful study of social networks allows us to better understand who interact with each other and may therefore become more similar in their knowledge of particular content, development of a particular skill, or perspectives on specific questions, and why some individuals may learn more than others. Apart from whether or not people interact, social networks can be based on the frequency or intensity of interactions and may change with time or with the type of content we are considering. This chapter focusses on examples of static (i.e., non-changing) and dynamic (i.e., changing) social networks, and how these can inform our analytic approach in studies involving time series at different units of analysis: individuals, groups of individuals, or situations.

14.1 Introduction

Social networks can vary in size from only a few people to large groups of people, although in the case of the latter, a social network can often also be understood in terms of smaller networks that are connected through specific individuals. The extent to which we can account for network structures in our data analysis depends on a number of factors. A first important factor is sample size: keeping other factors constant, the required sample size increases as model complexity increases. A second factor, which is partly related to sample size as well, is the strength of connections between individuals in a network. In the variable networks discussed in Chaps. 9–12, weaker connections translate in weaker links and, in some cases (i.e., using EBICglasso in the presence of very weak links and/or in relatively 'small' samples), in no links at all. Likewise, relatively small gains in *ICC* due to weak interactions between individuals or due to relatively poor correlations between

J. Leppink, *The Art of Modelling the Learning Process*, Springer Texts in Education,
https://doi.org/10.1007/978-3-030-43082-5_14

repeated measurements may not always result in substantially better models. Finally, we often have only partial data on the networks we are interested in. For instance, in curricula where students are assigned to learning groups, the learning groups constitute a structure we have data on and that we can model, but cross-group interaction can be monitored only in particular circumstances—such as through online communication—and even then, often only to a certain degree. That said, where we do have data—through assigned groups, through online communication, and/or in other forms—we will do well to account for the network structure as well as we can. In this chapter, we look at examples of different types of network structures and how we can model them.

14.2 Study 1: Task Performance Ratings by Faculty, Self, and Peer

At Medical School X, a total of 160 Year-5 medical students who know they will be facing their oral exit exam later in the academic year take part in a mock oral exit exam, which attempts to simulate the real exit exam. In the real exit exam, two faculty members independently rate on a VAS from 0 (minimum) to 10 (maximum) the performance of the candidate in each of three cases. Each case takes 15 min. In the mock exam, the ratings are provided by one faculty member and a Year-5 student. The latter replaces one faculty member as a peer assessor. There are logistic facilities for 80 mock exams, and the same faculty member M (i.e., a very experienced oral exit examiner) rates in all 80 mock exams. The 160 students are randomly allocated to doing the exam (n = 80) and peer assessor (n = 80) and then paired randomly such that each exam consists of: faculty member M, one student performing the mock exam, and one student being the peer assessor. After each of three cases in an exam, all actors in a cluster of three independently rate the performance of the mock examinee: the student performing the mock exam (i.e., self-assessment), the other student in the cluster (i.e., peer assessment), and faculty member M (i.e., faculty rating). In other words, for each of 80 mock exams, we have a total of nine ratings: three for each of three tasks.

14.2.1 Network Structure

Based on the mock exam structure, a straightforward way to model the network structure is as 80 clusters, each of which consists of a different pair of students (i.e., the N = 160 students divided over 80 pairs), who are all connected to the same faculty member M (i.e., the one who appears in all mock exams). However, this network structure can also be viewed as a three-level structure: cluster (upper level), actor within cluster (middle level), and task (lowest level). This structure can be modelled as a three-level model with random effects at the level of cluster (RI and/or RS) and/or actor within cluster (RI and/or RS, or residual covariance structure otherwise), and treating task (main effect), role (main effect), and task-by-role (interaction effect) as fixed effects.

14.2.2 Random Effects

For each task, ratings are distributed fairly unimodally and symmetrically for each assessor, and we find $M = 5.457$ ($SD = 0.730$) for faculty, $M = 4.940$ ($SD = 0.718$) for self, and $M = 5.758$ ($SD = 0.634$) for peer in Task 1, $M = 5.537$ ($SD = 0.778$) for faculty, $M = 5.269$ ($SD = 0.739$) for self, and $M = 5.740$ ($SD = 0.653$) for peer in Task 2, and $M = 5.689$ ($SD = 0.774$) for faculty, $M = 5.378$ ($SD = 0.786$) for self, and $M = 5.755$ ($SD = 0.755$) for peer in Task 3. In other words, it appears that across tasks, peer ratings are on average slightly higher while self-ratings are on average slightly lower than the average faculty rating. The most flexible way to model the random part is through cluster-level RI in combination with UN for the combination of the lower two levels. For the data at hand, we find for the cluster-level RI variance: $V_{RI} = 0.076$ ($SE = 0.022$, $p < 0.001$). For the UN part, we find: $r_{RES} = 0.038$ for Tasks 1 and 2 ($p = 0.587$), $r_{RES} = -0.008$ for Tasks 1 and 3 ($p = 0.916$), and $r_{RES} = 0.079$ for Tasks 2 and 3 ($p = 0.255$), and we find $V_{RES} = 0.409$ for Task 1, $V_{RES} = 0.460$ for Task 2, and $V_{RES} = 0.506$ for Task 3. The −2RLL of this model is 1567.775. When we replace UN by a simpler residual covariance structure, we obtain −2RLL = 1570.074 for AR1 (4 *df* less than UN), −2RLL = 1570.045 for ARMA(1,1) (3 *df* less than UN), −2RLL = 1567.990 for AR1H (2 *df* less than UN), −2RLL = 1570.045 for TP (3 *df* less than UN), −2RLL = 1567.990 for TPH (1 *df* less than UN), −2RLL = 1568.652 for CSH (2 *df* less than UN), −2RLL = 1570.737 for CS (4 *df* less than UN), −2RLL = 1569.370 for DI (3 *df* less than UN), and −2RLL = 1571.426 under ID (5 *df* less than UN). In short, performing all LR tests as in previous chapters reveals that all alternatives to UN can be considered valid simplifications, including ID, and hence we are left with the cluster-level RI term only. Adding a cluster-level RS for Task 2 (i.e., the difference between Task 1 and Task 2) yields −2RLL = 1571.205, adding a cluster-level RS for Task 3 (i.e., the difference between Task 1 and Task 3) yields −2RLL = 1569.666, and adding both cluster-level RS for Task 2 and Task 3 yields −2RLL = 1569.280. In other words, for the random part of our model, a cluster-level RI term will do. In that model, we obtain for that RI term $V_{RI} = 0.081$, which corresponds with $ICC = 0.152$. Adding an actor-level RI term yields for that RI term $V_{RI} = 0.017$, which corresponds with $ICC = 0.036$ ($p = 0.406$). In substantially larger samples (e.g., several hundreds of clusters), $ICC = 0.036$ would result in alternatives to the ID structure to be preferred, but with only 80 clusters that is not the case.

14.2.3 Fixed Effects

Now that we have decided on the random part, we turn to the fixed part of the model. Figure 14.1 presents the effects plot, with the bold lines (with 95% CI) representing the fixed effects or role (1 = faculty, 2 = self, 3 = peer) and task (1, 2, 3) and the thin lines representing the random effect (i.e., cluster-level RI variance: the thin lines are parallel, because no RS is involved).

Figure 14.1 does not hint at a substantial interaction effect or substantial task main effect but does appear to reveal a substantial role effect. Table 14.1 presents R^2_M, −2LL, AIC, and BIC for each of five competing fixed-effects model parts (cf. examples in earlier chapters involving two main effects and an interaction effect).

From Table 14.1, we can infer that R^2_M of the interaction effect (i.e., Model 4 minus Model 3) is about 0.011, in short: small. The LR test of the interaction effect yields: $\chi^2_4 = 10.121$, $p = 0.038$. For this test, $df = 4$ because that is the product of role *df* (i.e., 3 − 1 = 2) and task *df* (i.e., 3 − 1 = 2). For the task main effect, R^2_M is about 0.014, which is small as well. For that reason, BIC prefers Model 2 even though LR testing and AIC result in a preference for Model 4. The difference between Model 2 and Model 4 in terms of *df* is 6, and the gain in R^2_M is only about 0.025. If the gain in R^2_M was smaller or the difference in *df* was much smaller (e.g., $df = 2$), BIC might also prefer Model 4 or at least the preference for Model 2 would not be as pronounced. The larger the difference in *df* between competing models, the larger the likelihood that AIC and BIC disagree in terms of which model is to be preferred. However, presenting Fig. 14.1 and Table 14.1, readers can understand how we arrived at our conclusions with regard to model selection and can decide for themselves if they had made the same choice or a different one. Besides, there are three pairs of roles, some of which differ more than others. There are quite a few possible approaches to multiple testing involving these pairs of roles, most of which assume the 'no difference' $\boldsymbol{H_0}$ to hold across pairs or fix the prior probability of that $\boldsymbol{H_0}$ to 0.50 (for a review of different approaches, see Leppink, 2019). In the case of a factor with three categories, five possible models can be identified: the null model

Fig. 14.1 Effects plot in Study 1: fixed effects of role (1 faculty, 2 self, 3 peer), task (1, 2, 3), and their interaction, and cluster-level RI as random effect (parallel thin lines) (*Jamovi*)

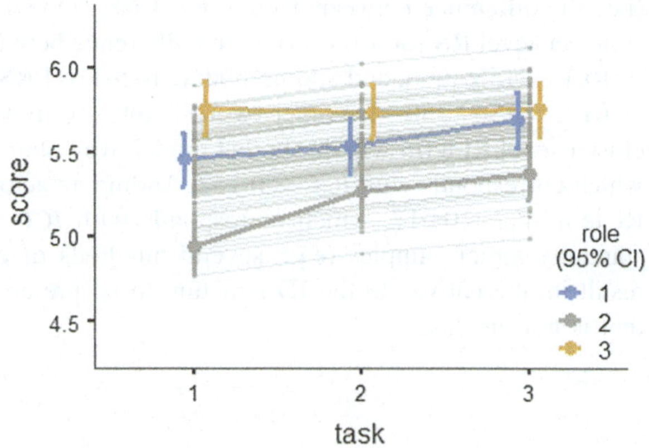

Table 14.1 Five competing fixed-effects parts in Study 1 in terms of R^2_{McF}, −2LL, AIC, and BIC (Jamovi)

Model	R^2_{M}	−2LL	AIC	BIC
0: *null*	0.000	1643.032	1649.032	1662.770
1: *task*	0.014	1631.500	1641.500	1664.396
2: *role*	0.089	1565.479	1575.479	1598.375
3: *task + role*	0.103	1552.445	1566.445	1598.500
4: *full*	0.114	1542.324	1564.324	1614.695

Table 14.2 Five competing post-hoc models for the role main effect in Study 1 in terms of R^2_{McF}, −2LL, AIC, and BIC (Jamovi)

Model	R^2_{M}	−2LL	AIC	BIC
0: *null*	0.000	1643.032	1649.032	1662.770
1: *peer differs*	0.052	1599.111	1607.111	1625.428
2: *self differs*	0.079	1574.754	1582.754	1601.071
3: *faculty differs*	0.003	1640.680	1648.680	1666.997
4: *all differ*	0.089	1565.479	1575.479	1598.375

(cf. Model 0 in Table 14.1), a model in which faculty and self are equal but differ from peer (Model 1), a model in which faculty and peer are equal but differ from self (Model 2), a model in which self and peer are equal but differ from faculty (Model 3), and a model in which all roles differ from each other (cf. Model 1 in Table 14.1, Model 4 for the current comparison). Table 14.2 presents R^2_{M}, −2LL, AIC, and BIC for each of these five competing models.

Although the difference between Model 2 and Model 4 in terms of R^2_{M} is only about 0.010, BIC prefers Model 4 because now the difference between the two models in terms of *df* is only 1. In cases where AIC and BIC disagree, AIC may be preferred in the presence of initial expectations of specific differences while BIC provides a more stringent threshold where no hypotheses are available (for more information, see Leppink, 2019).

14.3 Study 2: Free Online Interaction

Study 1 presents an example of a static network that is treated as a fixed number of clusters within which interaction takes place. In the second study, we take a look at a situation where a group of $N = 147$ students who are enrolled in a four-week online learning module can freely interact with each other using that online environment. Online activity is tracked, and for the sake of simplicity we focus only on the number of peers that students interact with (i.e., 0–146) and not on the content or intensity of these interactions. Suppose, we find that 5 students (3.4%) interact with 2 peers, 43 students (29.3%) interact with 3 peers, 63 students (42.9%) interact with 4 peers, 26 students (17.7%) interact with 5 peers, and 10 students (6.8%) interact with 6 peers. In social network jargon and software like SocNetV, this measure is also called the *degree centrality* (DC). In this case, DC varies from 2 to 6. Other useful measures provided by SocNetV include the *rescaled information centrality* (RIC, in SocNetV called *IC*') and the *rescaled eigenvector centrality* (REVC, in SocNetV called *EVC*').

Both the RIC and the REVC can be conceived as slightly more sophisticated extensions of the DC. The RIC measures the information flow for each student given the strengths of connections with peers (which in this example are '0' in the case of no interaction and '1' in the case of interaction) and distances between students in the network. To obtain a score on the scale of 0–1 (i.e., 0–100%), the individual student's score is divided by the sum of all students' scores. A student's REVC is a function of both the number of connections that student has with peers and the numbers of connections these other students have. Each student's score is divided by the highest observed score, such that the student with the highest REVC has REVC = 1.

Given how DC, RIC, and REVC are computed, the student with the highest DC is not necessarily the student with the highest RIC or highest REVC, and the student with the highest RIC does not necessarily have the highest REVC either. DC, RIC, and REVC are best considered as three related measures that all may shed some light on connectedness of individuals in a network and how that connectedness may relate to other variables of interest, and which measure is to be preferred will partly depend on the research question(s) at hand.

At the end of the module, all 147 students individually complete two tests: the first one a week after the module, and the second one a week after the first one. Both tests can be considered as parallel versions: although they comprise different items, they have the same numbers of items and can be considered equivalent in terms of content and difficulty.

14.3.1 Network Measures and Test Performance

Given that RIC and REVC use information that is used to compute DC but are not simple linear transformations of DC, these three measures are usually correlated but not perfectly. Figure 14.2 presents the scatterplot of the relation between DC and RIC.

As indicated in Fig. 14.2, although the relation between DC and RIC is not perfect, a linear model performs quite well. It is therefore not surprising that we find $R^2 = 0.760$ for a linear model and, only slightly higher, $R^2 = 0.770$ for a quadratic model. Figure 14.3 presents the scatterplot of the relation between DC and REVC.

Again, a linear model performs fairly well: we find $R^2 = 0.568$ for a linear model and, only slightly higher, $R^2 = 0.578$ for a quadratic model. However, Fig. 14.4 demonstrates that the relation between RIC and REVC appears to be better described as quadratic rather than as linear.

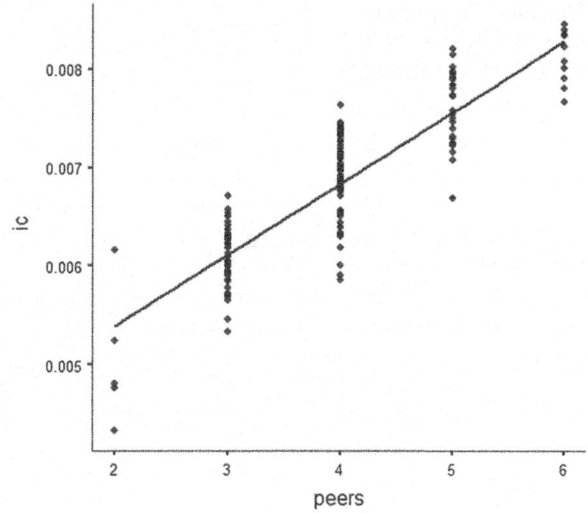

Fig. 14.2 The relation between DC (peers) and RIC (ic) in Study 2 (*Jamovi*)

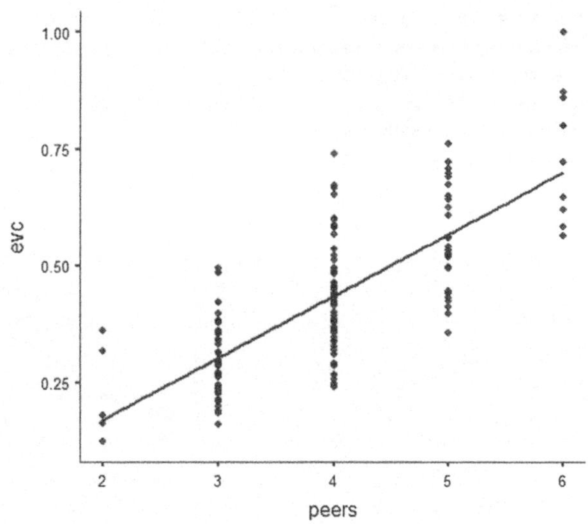

Fig. 14.3 The relation between DC (peers) and REVC (evc) in Study 2 (*Jamovi*)

We find R^2 = 0.605 for a linear model and R^2 = 0.637 for a quadratic model. Figure 14.5 presents the scatterplot for the relation between the two test scores.

We find R^2 = 0.582 for a linear model and R^2 = 0.586 for a quadratic model. Figure 14.6 presents the scatterplot for the relation between DC and the first test score (score0).

We find R^2 = 0.059 for a linear model and R^2 = 0.121 for a quadratic model. Without presenting all possible other scatterplots, Table 14.3 presents R^2-values for linear and quadratic models for the relation between DC and each test score, for the

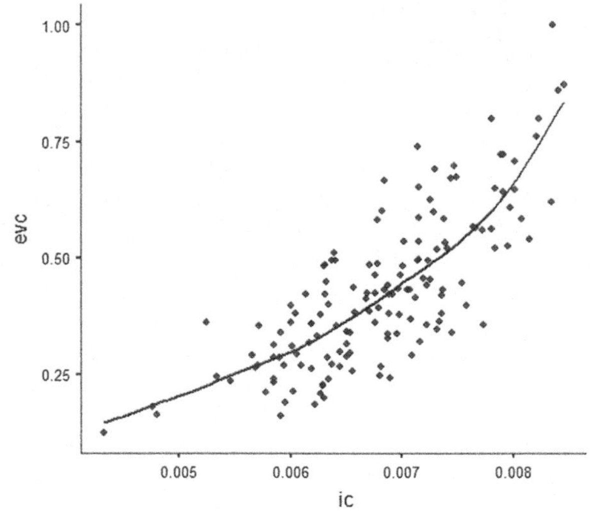

Fig. 14.4 The relation between RIC (ic) and REVC (evc) in Study 2 (Jamovi)

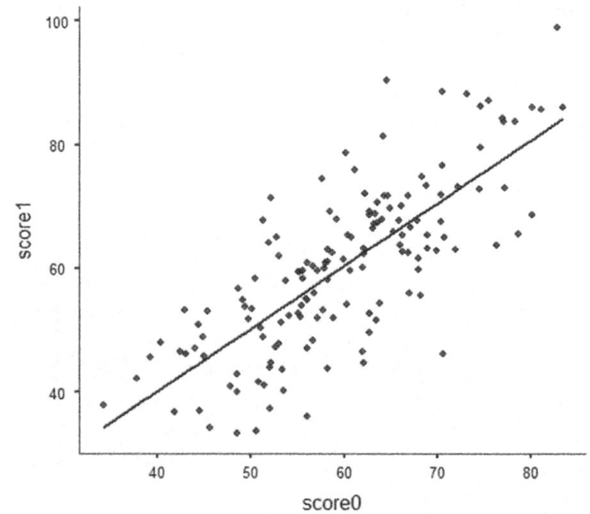

Fig. 14.5 The relation between the two test scores: one week (score0: 0–100%) and two weeks (score1: 0–100%) after module completion (Jamovi)

relation between RIC and each test score, and for the relation between REVC and each test score.

Table 14.3 illustrates that more complex measures do not always explain more variance in outcome variables of interest than simple measures: the single best predictor of score0 is DC in a quadratic model, and for score 1 the three measures perform about the same in a quadratic model. Therefore, let us use DC as predictor in the remainder of this study.

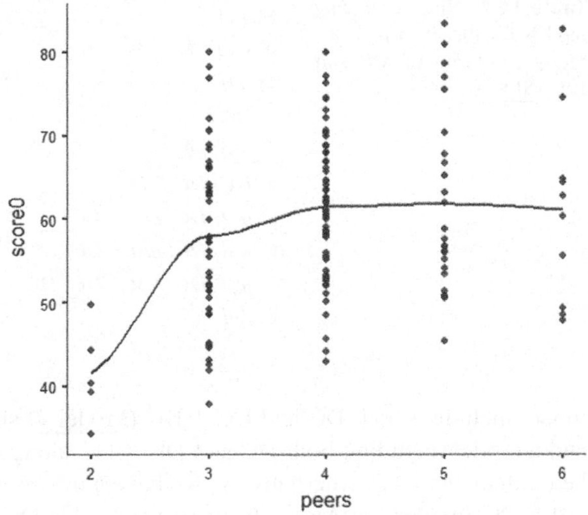

Fig. 14.6 The relation between DC and score0 (*Jamovi*)

Table 14.3 R^2-values for linear and quadratic models for the relation between social network metrics and test scores (*Jamovi*)

	First test (score0)		Second test (score1)	
	R^2 linear	R^2 quadratic	R^2 linear	R^2 quadratic
DC	0.059	0.121	0.020	0.035
RIC	0.093	0.107	0.040	0.040
REVC	0.055	0.055	0.033	0.039

14.3.2 Random Effects

Given two tasks and a quadratic relation between DC and test score, the following effects can form the fixed part of our model: test (linear term of test), DC (linear term of DC), DC * DC (quadratic term of DC), test * DC (linear test-by-DC interaction), and test * DC * DC (quadratic test-by-DC interaction). Given that DC is not a within-subject variable, but test is a within-subject variable with two categories (i.e., first and second test, which are well correlated), two candidates for the random part are CS and CSH. For CSH ($df = 3$), we find −2RLL = 2120.733, and for CS ($df = 2$), we find −2RLL = 2155.399. Clearly, CSH is to be preferred.

14.3.3 Fixed Effects

We use CSH for the random part. For the fixed part, we have several competing models. The model that has all the aforementioned main and interaction terms is the most complex one (Model 8), while the null model (Model 0) is the simplest one. Three possible main effects models are test (Model 1), DC (Model 2), and both main effects (Model 3). Expecting a quadratic relation between DC and test score, a

Table 14.4 Nine competing models for the fixed part in Study 2 in terms of AIC and BIC (SPSS)

Model	AIC	BIC
0: *null*	2158.029	2172.763
1: *test*	2159.659	2178.077
2: *DC*	2150.932	2169.350
3: *test, DC*	2152.562	2174.663
4: *DC, DC * DC*	2142.554	2164.655
5: *test, DC, DC * DC*	2144.184	2169.969
6: *test, DC, test * DC*	2153.987	2179.772
7: *test, DC, test * DC, DC * DC*	2145.609	2175.077
8: *full*	2146.043	2179.195

model including both DC and DC * DC (Model 4) should do better than Model 2, and a model including both DC and DC * DC along with test (Model 5) should to better than Model 3. Alternatively, we have a model with both main effects and the test * DC interaction (Model 6) or one that adds DC * DC along the terms in the latter (i.e., Model 7). Table 14.4 compares these models in terms of AIC and BIC.

Both AIC and BIC prefer Model 4. In the light of the two tests being parallel versions, this finding is not surprising.

14.4 Study 3: The Learning Group and Other Peers

In some situations, we have a combination of predefined learning groups or clusters alike on the one hand and data on communication outside these predefined learning groups on the other hand. For example, in a recent study with $N = 693$ students from a total of 132 groups across four modules at a business school in the United Kingdom, Rienties and Tempelaar (2018) found that students with more intergroup relative to intragroup learning relations demonstrated better performance on assessments than students with more intragroup learning relations. Where we can monitor which students communicate with each other, and have data on attendance and other variables that are likely to influence learning outcomes, we may detect students who are relatively isolated or who tend to be absent more than is normal at an early stage and we can seek to talk to them and see how we can help them.

Suppose, we have a group of $N = 500$ students who are enrolled in a ten-week module on research methods. The module consists of ten learning group meetings, five online lectures with a discussion board that provides facilities for 1-to-1 and small-group communication, and an end-of-module exam that results in a score from 0 (minimum) to 30 (maximum). The 500 students are randomly allocated to $k = 50$ learning groups, each of which meet 10 times during the module (i.e., once a week). Attendance of these group meetings is recommended though not mandatory. Of the 500 students, 179 (35.8%) do not miss any meeting, 200 (40.0%) miss one meeting, 84 (16.8%) miss two meetings, 29 (5.8%) miss three meetings, and the remaining 8 (1.6%) miss four meetings. There is somewhat more missing in some than in other learning groups: only on average 0.3 meetings are missed in the groups where least missing takes place, while in the group where most missing takes place on average 1.6 meetings are missed.

14.4.1 Network Measures

From the discussion board communications, we can count the number of peers outside one's own learning group that each student communicates with. In the learning group where least outgroup communication takes place, that number is on average 2.7, while in the learning group where most outgroup communication takes place, that number is on average 5.4. Looking at the level of the individual student, 8 students (1.6%) do not communicate outside their group, 27 students communicate with only one peer outside their group (5.4%), 84 students (16.8%) communicate with two peers outside their group, 102 students (20.4%) communicate with three peers outside their group, 90 students (18.0%) communicate with four peers outside their group, 80 students (16.0%) communicate with five peers outside their group, 57 students (11.4%) communicate with six peers outside their group, 23 students (4.6%) communicate with seven peers outside their group, 18 students (3.6%) communicate with eight peers outside their group, 10 students (2.0%) communicate with nine peers outside their group, and 1 student (0.2%) communicates with ten peers outside the own group. In other words, there is quite a range.

Figure 14.7 presents the distribution of the number of peers communicated with outside one's own learning group, for each number of learning group meetings missed.

Both variables are count variables. When we use the number of learning group meetings missed as a predictor of the number of peers communicated with outside one's own learning group, the latter constitutes the outcome variable, with $M = 4.016$ and a variance of 3.803. Using Poisson regression, we obtain an R^2-value of 0.012, and the LR test yields: $\chi_4^2 = 5.792$, $p = 0.215$. It is a χ^2-test at $df = 4$, because five categories for the predictor variable are observed (i.e., 0, 1, 2, 3, and 4). Some may wonder if we could not include the predictor variable as a covariate assuming a linear relation between predictor and outcome variable. Doing so with a Poisson model, we find an R^2-value of 0.002, and the corresponding LR test yields: $\chi_1^2 = 1.019$, $p = 0.313$. If the learning groups were substantially larger in size, we could do a two-level Poisson model treating learning group (upper level) and student (lower level) as hierarchical levels (e.g., in Stata), but sizes of only $n = 10$ per learning group are very small for two-level Poisson models. Even for two-level linear models, we may estimate the RI variance in a two-level model, but group sizes are too small to obtain meaningful RS variance estimates. In any case, in a two-level model that accounts for group nesting, p-values are larger and CIs smaller than in models that do not account for the group nesting, because the latter slightly overestimate the effective sample size. Failing to account for repeated

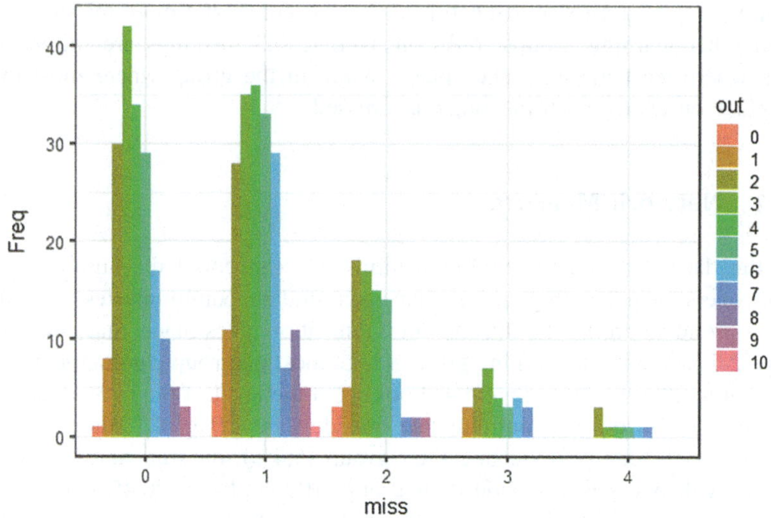

Fig. 14.7 Relation between the number of peers communicated with outside one's own learning group (i.e., 'out') and the number of learning group meetings missed (i.e., 'miss') (*Jamovi*)

measurements from the same participants (e.g., treating 20 students measured twice as having 40 students measured once) tends to result in overestimated *SE*s and hence too large *p*-values and too wide CIs for within-subject effects, while failing to account for group nesting (e.g., students within learning groups) tends to result in slightly underestimated *SE*s and hence too small *p*-values and too narrow CIs for between-subjects effects (e.g., the number of learning group meetings missed) (e.g., Leppink, 2015; Tan, 2010). In other words, even though we have too small groups to meaningfully account for group nesting, if our LR tests yield *p*-values of 0.215 and 0.313 without accounting for the group nesting indicates, these *p*-values would be larger (i.e., further away from 0.05) rather than smaller if we could account for the group nesting.

14.4.2 Predicting Exam Performance

Exam performance ranges from 11 to 30 with $M = 19.980$ and $SD = 3.118$, and a skewness of 0.133 and a kurtosis of −0.169. Figure 14.8 presents the histogram of the exam score distribution.

Figures 14.9 and 14.10 graphically depict the relation between exam score and number of learning group meetings missed and between exam score and number of peers outside one's own learning group communicated with, respectively.

Students who miss no meetings or at most one meeting on average perform somewhat better on the exam than students who miss more meetings. For outgroup

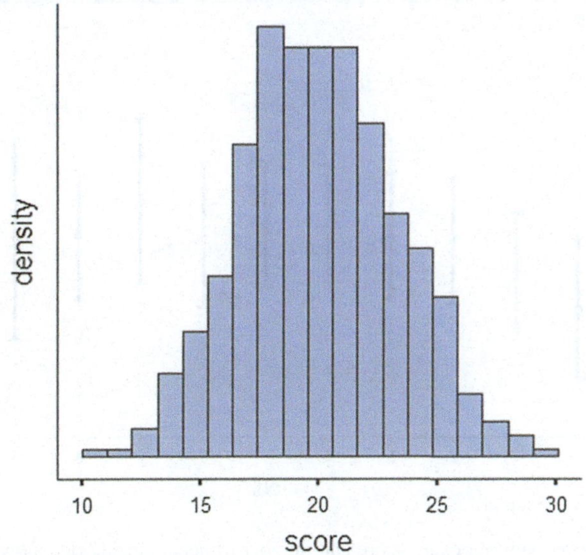

Fig. 14.8 Distribution of exam score in Study 3 (*Jamovi*)

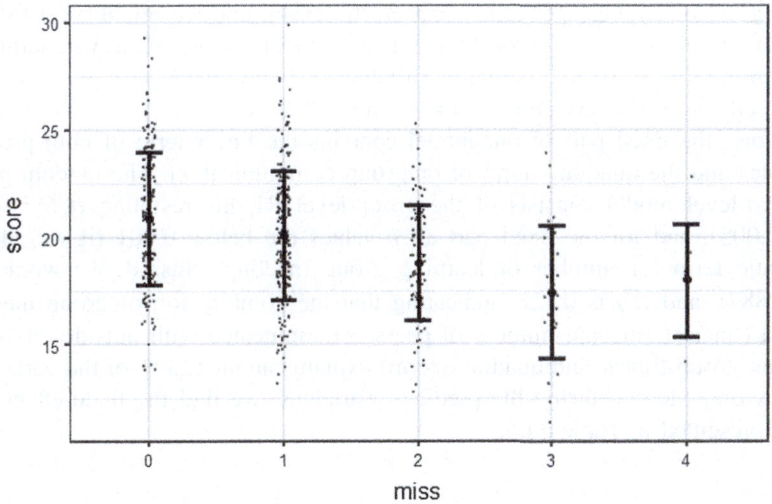

Fig. 14.9 Relation between exam score and number of learning group meetings missed in Study 3: bars indicate SD around M (*Jamovi*)

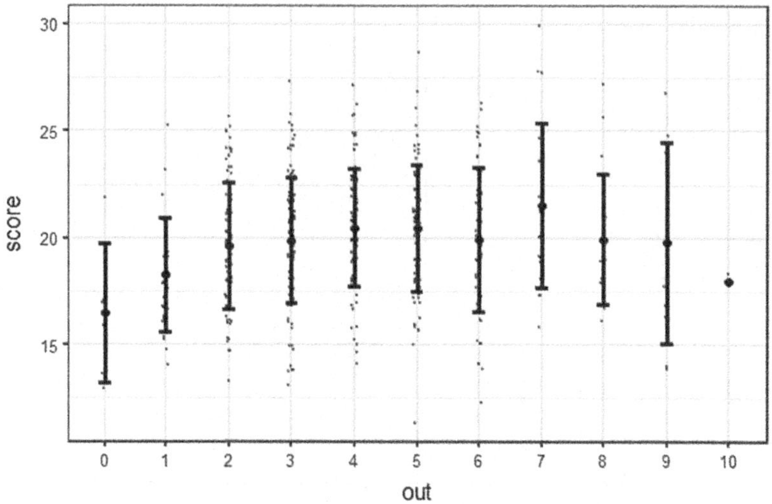

Fig. 14.10 Relation between exam score and number of peers outside one's own learning group communicated with missed in Study 3: bars indicate SD around M (*Jamovi*)

communication, it appears that students who do not communicate outside their own group at all on average perform worst on the exam, and we might want to add a quadratic term to our model for the prediction of exam score. However, adding the interaction term of the two predictor variables does not make sense here; there are many cells with 0 observations and also quite a few with only 1 or 2 observations. Therefore, the fixed part of our model contains the linear term of both predictor variables and the quadratic term of outgroup communication. The random part of our two-level model consists of the group-level RI; the resulting *ICC* is 0.070 ($p = 0.005$), and for the fixed part all *p*-values are below 0.001 (if we added a quadratic term for number of learning group meetings missed, we would find $p = 0.887$), and R^2_M is 0.128, indicating that the combination of group meetings missed (linear term) and number of peers communicated with outside one's own learning group (linear and quadratic term) explains about 12.8% of the variance in exam score. Mean centring the predictor variables, we find the fixed-effects estimates presented in Table 14.5.

Table 14.5 Predicting exam score by number of learning group meetings missed and number of peers communicated with outside one's own learning group: regression coefficients (b), SEs, and 90% CIs (*Jamovi*)

Term	*b*	*SE*	90% CI LB	90% CI UB
Intercept	19.980	0.165	19.709	20.251
Miss (linear)	−0.965	0.135	−1.187	−0.742
Out (linear)	1.003	0.244	0.601	1.405
Out (quadratic)	−0.092	0.026	−0.135	−0.048

From these estimates, it follows that students who do not miss any learning group meetings and communicate with 5 (or 6) peers outside their own learning group are predicted to do best on the exam.

14.5 Study 4: Different Learning Groups for Different Modules

We have seen some examples of situations where students are allocated to learning groups for a given module. In practice, the composition of these learning groups often changes throughout the year (e.g., from module to module or from semester to semester). Consider a situation where we have 625 students enrolled in a series of online modules that require students to complete a series of learning tasks in groups of 25 students, through the use of an online discussion board and communication media such as WhatsApp and Facebook. For module A, the 625 students are randomly allocated to 25 learning groups. For module B, which starts after completion of module A, students are randomly allocated to 25 learning groups that are different in composition from the learning groups for module A and such that no students are in the same learning group for the two modules. For both modules, all learning groups consist of $n = 25$ students.

In the study at hand, each student has one set of 24 peers in one's learning group for module A and another set of 24 peers in one's learning group for module B. This is the most extreme alternative to a situation where learning groups remain exactly the same for modules A and B. At the end of each module, there is an exam that results in a percentage score (i.e., 0–100%); completing the exam means completing the module. For the exam after module A, students from the same learning group for module A will likely be a bit more similar in their exam performance than random students from different learning groups. The same logic will likely apply to the exam after module B, but especially when the two modules are on similar content—for instance module A on research designs and module B on data analysis—the grouping structure from module A may still resonate to a smaller degree in module B exam performance as well.

14.5.1 Analysis Per Module

Both exams are fairly symmetrically and unimodally distributed with $M = 54.827$ and $SD = 11.848$ for module A and $M = 52.104$ and $SD = 10.520$ for module B. If we analyse the data per module and can reasonably treat the students as a random sample of possible students who could sign up for the module, we can estimate the RI variance associated with learning group for a given exam, but we do not have fixed effects to take into account unless there is an interest in specific variables such as encountered in Studies 1–3 in this chapter. Without such variables, for a given exam, we are dealing not with a mixed-effects but with a random-effects model.

Besides, given that the learning groups for the two modules are completely different and the learning-group structure of one module is not hierarchically higher or lower than that of the other module (i.e., we cannot treat these groupings as two separate levels), even if the grouping structure from module A still resonates to some extent in module B exam performance we cannot account for it if we want to account for the grouping structure from module A. Thus, for module B, we have to choose, and we can actually see which grouping structure explains more of the variance in exam performance by first running a random-effects model using the grouping structure from module A and then the same model using the grouping structure from module B.

For module A, we find *ICC* = 0.043 ($p = 0.004$), meaning R^2_C—which in this case equates R^2_R since R^2_M is now 0 (i.e., no fixed effects in the model)—is 0.043. For module B, we find *ICC* < 0.001 (i.e., $R^2_C < 0.001$) when using the grouping structure from module A, and we find *ICC* = 0.119 ($p < 0.001$) when using the grouping structure from module B. In other words, using the grouping structure from module B for the exam performance of module B will do.

14.5.2 Modules Together

A straightforward way to involve both exam scores in the analysis and appropriately account for the grouping structure with respect to the model response variable is to treat module B exam score as response variable, module A exam score as a predictor variable, and use the learning group structure from module B for the random part. Figure 14.11 presents the scatterplot for the relation between exam scores per module B learning group.

There is not much difference in slope across learning groups (i.e., low RS variance). It is therefore not surprising that, in a two-level model using module B exam score as response variable and module A exam score as fixed-effect predictor, we obtain $R^2_C = 0.418$ when including both RI and RS and $R^2_C = 0.416$ when including only RI (*Jamovi*). Turning to the fixed part, we find $R^2_M = 0.308$, which is in this case entirely attributed to module A exam score (i.e., the only fixed effect in the model). In other words, when we appropriately account for the grouping structure, we find that about 30.8% of the variance in module B exam score can be attributed to module A exam score another about 10.8% (i.e., 0.416 minus 0.308) can be attributed to the learning group structure in module B.

If modules A and B are on similar content and it makes sense to compare scores across modules (e.g., percentage scores based on large numbers of items), and the interest lies in estimating the difference in average performance between exams, an alternative way to analyse the results is to treat module A and module B as two correlated exams taken by the same students and include exam as the only fixed effect. The level structure is then as follows: the fifty learning groups (i.e., modules A and B together) constitute the upper level; the 625 students, each of whom appears in two of the fifty learning groups, form the middle level; and the lowest

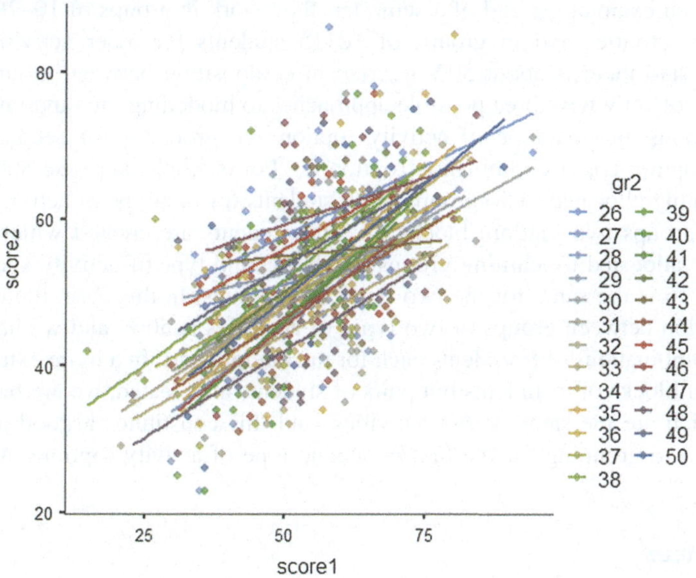

Fig. 14.11 Relation between exam scores (score1 = module A, score2 = module B) per module B learning group (gr2) in Study 4 (*Jamovi*)

level is formed by the two exams, which are stations to be passed by all students (who appeared in two learning groups, each). The random part of our model then consists of a group-level RI term, a student-level RI term, and either equal or unequal V_{RES} for the two exams (cf. CS vs. CSH for the combination of student and exam). Assuming equal V_{RES}, we find −2RLL = 9299.987, and under unequal V_{RES}, we find −2RLL = 9277.472 (*SPSS*). Given two exams, the difference in *df* between equal and unequal V_{RES} is 1; hence, varying V_{RES} is to be preferred. In this model, we obtain the following estimates for the random part: group-level V_{RI} = 7.927, student-level V_{RI} = 67.159, module A V_{RES} = 67.600, and module B V_{RES} = 30.949. For the exam fixed effect, we find a point estimate of 2.723 (i.e., given all learning groups of the same size and no missing data, the difference in *M* exam score between the two modules: 54.827–52.104) and *SE* = 0.872, which results in a 95% CI of [0.963; 4.484] and a 90% CI of [1.256; 4.191].

14.6 Other Structures

The structures discussed in this chapter are quite common, and very similar structures can often be modelled in similar ways. In other cases, we can use combinations of approaches discussed in this chapter and previous chapters. For instance, if we have somewhat larger numbers of students (e.g., 800, 1100, 1500) who face an exam at the end of a semester, they work in groups of 10–20 students for some activities and in groups of 10–15 students for other activities in the semester, and there is about 50% overlap in composition between groups for the two types of activities, three possible approaches to modelling the random part may be: grouping for first type of activity (option A), grouping for second type of activity (option B), or combination (option C). For example, suppose 800 students are randomly allocated to 50 groups of 16 students for first type of activity, of each of these groups two random blocks of eight students are created which are then randomly allocated to learning groups for the second type of activity such that no group of 16 is the same for the two types of activities. In this case, the overlap in composition between groups of two types of activities is 50%, and we have a total of 100 combinations of 8 students each for the random part. In a more extreme case, where not blocks of 8 students but pairs of students are created, we are back to 400 pairs which are the same across activities, and this constitutes a good alternative (option C) to grouping for the first or second type of activity (options A and B).

References

Leppink, J. (2015). Data analysis in medical education research: A multilevel perspective. *Perspectives on Medical Education, 4*(1), 14–24. https://doi.org/10.1007/s40037-015-0160-5.

Leppink, J. (2019). *Statistical methods for experimental research in education and psychology*. Cham: Springer. https://doi.org/10.1007/978-3-030-21241-4.

Rienties, B., & Tempelaar, D. (2018). Turning groups inside out: A social network perspective. *Journal of the Learning Sciences, 27*(4), 550–579. https://doi.org/10.1080/10508406.2017.1398652.

Tan, F. E. S. (2010). Best practices in analysis of longitudinal data: A multilevel approach. In J. W. Osborne (Ed.), *Best practices in quantitative methods* (Chap. 30, pp. 451–470). London: Sage.

Progress Testing in Larger Cohorts 15

Abstract

An assessment method in place in medical schools and some other schools in a few countries that involves larger series for all cohorts in a programme is called progress testing. For example, in the Dutch consortium of medical school, each year, four MCQ tests of 200 items each are sampled from an item bank of over 12,000 items such that content areas from a programme blueprint are represented as agreed upon by the medical schools involved and such that different tests are of very similar difficulty level. Differences in performance between tests are then interpreted in terms of growth, stagnation or decline of knowledge. Given four tests in a year and six years in a medical programme, there are 24 measurements for each student. This method allows us to make all kinds of comparisons of group performance and individual performance over time, consider early intervention and remediation where necessary, consider changes in our item bank, and consider revisions in our programmes where needed, provided that our items are of good quality and we use appropriate analytic tools. This chapter builds forth on an example of progress testing introduced in Chap. 12 and provides a smooth introduction of the time series models presented in Chap. 16.

15.1 Introduction

Progress testing in larger cohorts enables educators, students, and other stakeholders to monitor individual trajectories in performance over time and evaluate these trajectories in the light of cohort tendencies. For example, Fig. 15.1 presents the trajectory of four students from the cohort of $N = 300$ students discussed in Chap. 12, along with the minimum score, maximum score, first quartile, median, and third quartile of the cohort.

J. Leppink, *The Art of Modelling the Learning Process*, Springer Texts in Education,
https://doi.org/10.1007/978-3-030-43082-5_15

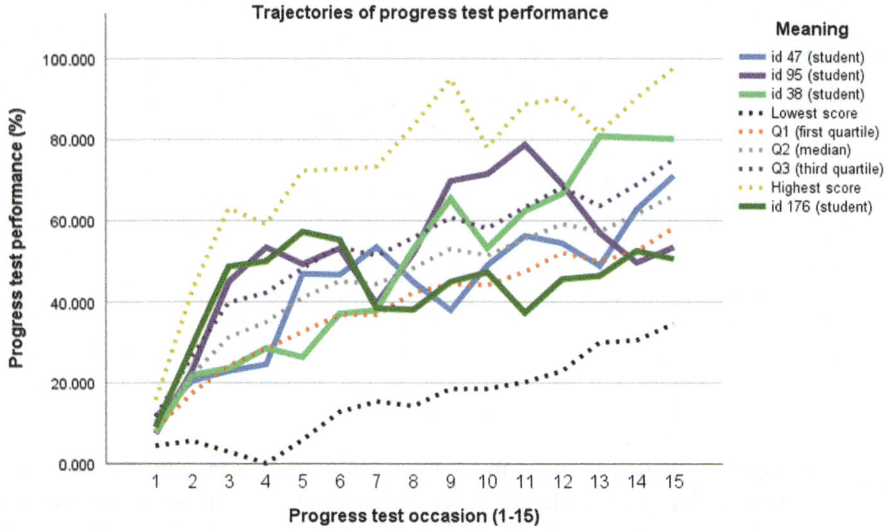

Fig. 15.1 The performance of four students in the light of key statistics from their cohort in fifteen progress tests (SPSS)

Student #176 provides an example of a student who performs relatively well (i.e., scores above or around the third quartile) in the first two years (i.e., first six progress tests) but performs fairly poorly (i.e., scores below or around the first quartile) in the third, fourth, and fifth year. For student #38, the trajectory is more or less the opposite: relative underperformance on the first seven tests (i.e., scores below or around the first quartile) but better performance from the eighth test onward. Student #95 has two clear 'highs' and two clear 'lows', going from relatively good to poorer back to good and back to not so good performance. Finally, Student #47 could be said to fluctuate more or less around median (i.e., second quartile) performance. There may be several reasons for a particular trajectory, and it is important to seek numerical and narrative information from other assessments and perhaps other (i.e., non-assessment) events that may help to for instance explain a dive to poorer performance and seek for ways—with a mentor, tutor or study advisor—to revert that regressive trend. Figure 15.2 presents the boxplots of the fifteen progress tests in this cohort of $N = 300$ students. There are some minor 'outliers' in some of the tests though no signs of extreme cases that would have a major influence on *M*s and *SD*s of some of the tests.

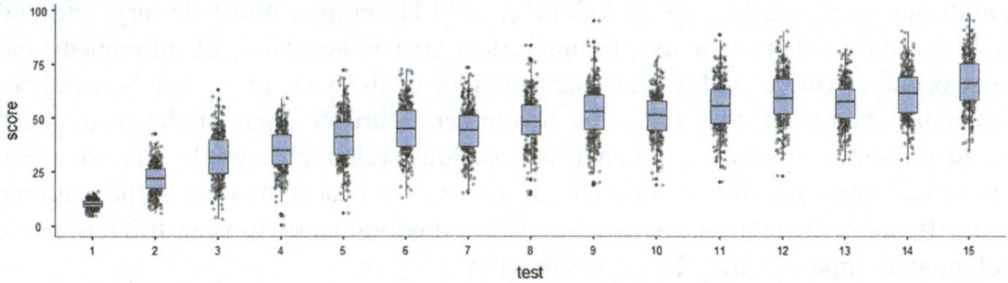

Fig. 15.2 Boxplots of the fifteen progress tests in the cohort (*Jamovi*)

15.2 Residual Covariance Structures

Given a restriction of range in knowledge at the start of the programme, there is relatively little dispersion in performance at the time of the first progress test (*SD* = 2.035) and on the second test as well to some extent (*SD* = 6.828); for the other thirteen tests, *SD* ranges from 9.876 to 12.369. Growth in knowledge is strongest in earlier years, and there is a slight decline in performance from the sixth to the seventh, from the ninth to the tenth, and from the twelfth to the thirteenth test (see also Fig. 12.5) in line with Summer holiday period (July/August). We already learned in Chap. 12 that correlations between subsequent progress tests are strongest between adjacent tests and weakest when the distance between exams is largest (Fig. 12.6). Thus, it is to be expected that we will need a residual covariance structure that accounts for varying V_{RES} and distance-dependent r_{RES}. However, UN is not a sensible option in this case; given 15 tests, we would estimate (15 * 14)/2 = 105 r_{RES}s and 15 V_{RES}s (i.e., *df* = 120 for the random part). If we were dealing with progress test data from several thousands of students, we might consider UN as an option, but with only 300 students this is not a good idea. AR1H and TPH may provide good options when the progress tests are (more or less) equidistant, as in the example at hand (i.e., mid-September, mid-January, and mid-May). Otherwise, AD1 may provide a good alternative, or possibly RI-RS combinations with fewer numbers of RS as discussed in the next section.

15.3 Approaches to Fixed Effects

For the fixed part, we can use test occasion or—if we interested in year differences and/or differences in average performance between progress tests within the same year are very small—year in the programme. Some may opt for a polynomial approach in which for example linear, quadratic, and cubic patterns are considered. While this approach may be defended if the tests are (more or less) equidistant (as in the example at hand), it is problematic when the tests are clearly not equidistant (e.g., yearly tests mid-October, mid-December, mid-February, and end of May), unless there is a specific interest in year rather than test differences and tests occur at (more or less) the same points in the year (e.g., not September–December–March in one year and November–February–June in the next year). Besides, with as many as fifteen test occasions, relatively simple solutions like linear, quadratic or cubic are often too restrictive (as is also the case in the example at hand), although again when the interest lies predominantly in year differences the polynomial approach may be quite attractive.

Another option for the fixed part, if the interest lies in year differences as well as in differences between tests within year (or the latter are of a quite substantial magnitude), is to treat year and season as two-way (i.e., 5 years by 3 seasons). This allows for the estimation of year differences and differences between tests within years and enables us to examine if the pattern of differences between seasons is more or less the same across years. For example, given an academic year starting in September, it is well possible that across years the September test yields the lowest average performance and the May test yields the highest average performance of the three tests. If the pattern of differences in average performance between progress tests varies substantially between years, there is substantial year-by-season interaction, and the two-way model allows for that interaction to be estimated. The fixed part of this two-way model uses as many *df* as the model with test occasion as only fixed effect. In the latter, we use 1 *df* for the intercept and 14 *df* for differences between the fifteen progress tests. In the two-way model, we use 1 *df* for the intercept, 4 *df* for the year main effect, 2 *df* for the season main effect, and 8 *df* for the year-by-season interaction effect. However, if the interaction effect is only small, a main-effects only model may do.

In the two-way approach, an alternative residual covariance structure to be considered is found in the combination of student-level RI and student-level RS for the years or the seasons, although given larger (variation in) differences between years than between seasons within year probably best for the years. Given five years, we would need 4 *df* for RSs; including also the RI and all possible RI-RS and RS-RS covariance terms would mean 4 *df* for RSs, 1 *df* for RI, $(5 * 4)/2 = 10$ *df* for RI-RS and RS-RS covariance terms, and 1 *df* for the remaining V_{RES}, hence $df = 16$ for the random part. This is quite a difference from UN, which would come down to $df = 120$. Finally, if we could leave out the RI component, we would need only 4 *df* for the RSs, 6 *df* for RS-RS covariance terms, and 1 *df* for the remaining V_{RES}, hence $df = 11$ in total.

15.4 Year-by-Season Interaction

Let us take a look at the year-by-season interaction option in more detail. Since we have equidistant progress tests, we can consider AR- and TP-based structures as options. Since we have already done the full exercise of comparisons with simple structures like ID, DI, and CS in previous chapters, and we have seen that for the data at hand we need a structure that enables us to account for both varying V_{RES} and varying r_{RES}, we compare only a smaller number of structures for the data in this chapter (*SPSS*): AR1H (−2RLL = 30,965.915, *df* = 16), TPH (−2RLL = 30,951.150, *df* = 29), AD1 (−2RLL = 30,871.362, *df* = 29), RS for the years and treating the RS terms as uncorrelated (−2RLL = 32,625.078, *df* = 5), RS for the years and RI and treating the RI and RS terms as uncorrelated (−2RLL = 32.495.663, *df* = 6), RS for the years and treating the RS terms as correlated (−2RLL = 32,383.944, *df* = 11), and RS for the years and RI and treating the RI and RS terms as correlated (−2RLL = 32,268.001, *df* = 16). The structure to be preferred is AD1.

Switching to the fixed part (using AD1 as residual covariance structure), we find for the full model: −2LL = 30,873.743, AIC = 30,961.743, and BIC = 31,243.864. For the main effects only model, we find: −2LL = 31,145.647, AIC = 31,217.647, and BIC = 31,448.473. In other words, we have reasons to prefer the full model. Although across years, the September test yields the lowest and the May test yields the highest average performance, the increase in score is most pronounced in the first year: we go from *M* = 10.128 and *SD* = 2.035 on the September test to *M* = 21.889 and *SD* = 6.828 on the January test to *M* = 31.603 and *SD* = 10.782 on the May test. In the other years, the difference between the September and May test in *M* is in the 8–11 points range and *SD*s are larger than in the first year. In other words, we do see a seasonal trend across years, but it is strongest in the first year.

15.5 Within-Student and Between-Students Comparisons

A great advantage of longitudinal data, when collected properly, is that we can separate within-student from between-students variance. Some proponents of progress testing and other longitudinal assessment methods have argued that within-student comparisons are more important than between-students comparisons, that is: that changes in score for a given student from one occasion to the next are more important to focus on than differences in scores between different candidates at a given occasion. Core argument in favour of that view is that assessment is supposed to stimulate learning. While I embrace the latter, for educational and professional practice, *both* types of comparisons are important. Some students may demonstrate some growth in progress test performance across the five-year programme but may still perform in the lowest 25% of the cohort. While above-average progress test performance does not yet make a good doctor, medical knowledge *is* still important, and differences in medical knowledge can to some extent explain differences on clinical skills exams (e.g., moderate correlations between MCQ tests and OSCEs), with high performers on knowledge exams being more likely to be high performers on clinical skills exams compared to average or below-average performers on knowledge exams. Simultaneously, a student who generally performs relatively well on the progress test (e.g., generally above Q3) can have a bad day and relatively underperform (e.g., median performance) on a single test. Punishing that student for not demonstrating growth would not be very appropriate. Having longitudinal data, it would be more appropriate to base decisions regarding performance being 'good enough' on a series of tests rather than on a single test. In other words, while assessment should be about stimulating growth, at some point or another we do need to make judgements about whether a student is 'good enough' to be allowed to enter practice; in a domain like Medicine, abandoning between-students comparisons would likely have grave consequences for patient care.

Unfortunately, longitudinal data is not always treated as is. A common practice in progress testing for example has been to categorise progress test scores into three or four ordinal performance categories (e.g., poor, sufficient, good; or insufficient, sufficient, good, and excellent). The problem with this approach is that it results in a severe loss of information and increases the likelihood of incorrect decisions being made. For instance, a student whose scores fluctuate fairly closely around the poor/sufficient cut-off may receive two 'poor' qualifications and two 'sufficient' qualifications—in a perhaps random order—while the scores indicate sufficient performance across the trajectory as a whole. Another practice which results in an unnecessary loss of information is found in averaging scores from tests within the same year. In the example at hand, this would then result in five aggregated scores for each student, one per year. Looking at Fig. 15.1, it is needless to say that with that approach quite some information about *growth* in performance is lost and this is a pity, because we are (or: should be) interested not only in year-to-year growth but in growth within a year (and possible explanations for that) as well. Categorising and aggregating scores are practices that do no right to the longitudinal nature of data and are, in the light of data-analytic methods available to us, unnecessary.

Another important thing to keep in mind in progress testing, or any other form of longitudinal knowledge assessment for that matter, is that careful sampling of items is crucial. The items in subsequent tests should be of more or less the same content and more or less the same difficulty but should *not* be the same items. The problem with using the same questions is that we cannot tell to what extent increases in scores reflect knowledge growth and to what extent these changes reflect memory effects. In a recent large-scale study involving medical schools across the United Kingdom (Sam et al., 2019), a comparison was made between single-best-answer questions (i.e., MCQs) and so-called 'very-short-answer questions' which are not MCQ but require only a very short response. The very-short-answer questions resulted in lower scores (i.e., poorer performance) than the MCQs and were therefore concluded to appear more authentic and more informative. The problem is that all students in the study were given *the same items* in *the same order* to all students participating in the study, with the very-short-answer questions being presented *before* the MCQs. Of course, with such a setup it is quite normal to expect better performance on the MCQs. A better setup for comparing the two questions would have been a randomised controlled experiment with a different question format for each condition; from the comparison at hand, no conclusions can be drawn with regard to any format being more or less authentic or informative than the other. Equally, in progress testing, we should *not* use the same questions in subsequent tests, but preferably—as for instance done in the Dutch tradition—not reuse items appearing in a particular test for at least three years.

Reference

Sam, A. H., Westacott, R., Gurnell, M., Wilson, R., Meeran, K., & Brown, C. (2019). Comparing single-best-answer and very-short-answer questions for the assessment of applied medical knowledge in 20 UK medical schools: Cross-sectional study. *British Medical Journal Open, 9*, e032550. https://doi.org/10.1136/bmjopen-2019-032550.

Studies with Small Samples or Individuals

16

Abstract

There are settings where students are placed in a particular environment for an extended period, for instance 6 or 12 months, such as internships and longitudinal clerkships. With appropriate and repeated, carefully planned assessments, we can obtain series of measurements of the same performance of interest, which help us to understand how performance changes over time, and how that change over time changes with specific events such as training or difficult situations. Even though numbers of students may be small in such settings, and it may come down to single cases in some settings, with sufficient numbers of carefully placed measurements we can use time series models to understand change. Equally, SCEDs are very popular in some fields where finding participants can be challenging, such as in Special Needs Education. Different types of models for small samples and case studies are discussed in this chapter with their relative pros and cons.

16.1 Introduction

In the practice of Education and educational research, we do not always have (easy) access to large numbers of participants; ethical, financial, and logistic factors may put serious constraints. Besides, in practical settings, our interest often lies in change within the individual learner or in a fairly specific and small group of learners, and time series with sufficient numbers of measurements constitute the most appropriate way to study that change. How to analyse and report on the change of interest depends on what exactly is/are our question/s of interest, how many measurements per individual we have, how these measurements are timed (e.g., equidistant or not), how complex a change pattern studied is, and whether we deal with change in single individuals or in small groups of individuals. However,

J. Leppink, *The Art of Modelling the Learning Process*, Springer Texts in Education,
https://doi.org/10.1007/978-3-030-43082-5_16

generally speaking, where individual change patterns with time are considered, we deal with so-called time series data and therefore need a time series approach (e.g., Box, Jenkins, & Reinsel, 1994; Brockwell & Davis, 2009; Hannan, 1970) to analyse the data and interpret the outcomes.

16.2 Time Series for Education

In fields like econometrics, weather forecasting, earthquake prediction, and astronomy, where it can be relatively easy to have hundreds of measurements in a given time interval, simple and complex time series models are quite common. However, in educational practice and in most research settings (except for perhaps studies in the context of brain research), such large numbers of measurements are rarely available, and measurement is generally much more error prone than measurement in the aforementioned contexts. Consequently, relatively complex models encountered in other fields are rarely usable in Education. For example, in econometrics and weather forecasting, where we have hundreds of observations about prices (in an econometric context) or temperature or rainfall (in a weather context), models that account for seasonal trends are quite common. In educational research, this kind of time series research is rarely if ever feasible and usually not of direct interest either. Therefore, in this chapter, we focus on fairly 'simple', non-seasonal models, that cannot account for eventual seasonal effects but can, as becomes clear throughout this chapter, account for events such as training or treatment.

Another distinction that can be made in time series research is between *analysis* and *forecasting*; while time series forecasting is about using a model based on observed data to predict future outcomes on an outcome variable of interest (e.g., the gold price in a week from now using historic gold price data), time series analysis focusses entirely on estimating meaningful statistics of the data observed. In forecasting, the more accurate or the more forward in future we want to forecast, the more observations we need. Even for fairly simple forecasts for individual change, we may easily need 50 or even 100 observations (Box & Tiao, 1975), and these are numbers we rarely have in education practice or research. However, there are some models we can use, especially where measurements are, as is common in many settings, spaced at equal time intervals (i.e., equidistant).

16.2.1 Common Models

In Chap. 13, ARIMA models are introduced, and especially ARIMA(1,0,0) or AR1, and ARIMA(1,0,1) or ARMA(1,1). In fact, the simplest ARIMA model is ARIMA(0,0,0), which is simply a 'mean model' or model in which scores observed fluctuate around the mean observed score. ARIMA(0,0,1) or the MA1 model adds that the score of individual j at occasion i is not only a function of an overall M but is also a function of the residual around *M* of individual *j* at occasions *i* and '*i* minus 1'. ARIMA(1,0,1) combines the AR1 and MA1 processes into one model. ARIMA(0,0,0) and ARIMA(0,0,1) are sometimes useful when series are *stationary*, that is: it has a constant *M* and a (more or less) constant fluctuation around *M*. Further, all ARIMA models can include a constant, for instance to account for a linear trend over time. In ARIMA(1,0,0), for example, the score of individual *j* at occasion *i* is then a function of the score of individual *j* at occasion '*i* minus 1' plus a constant.

If a series is *not stationary*, the simplest possible model is a so-called *random walk model*: ARIMA(0,1,0). In this model, the score predicted at occasion *i* equals the score predicted at occasion '*i* minus 1' plus the gain (positive or negative) in observed score from occasion '*i* minus 2' to occasion '*i* minus 1', plus a constant to account for an overall gain over time if we add that constant to the model. Other combinations, such as ARIMA(1,1,0) and ARIMA(0,1,1) (with or without constant) are possible but require larger numbers of observations than ARIMA(0,0,0) or ARIMA(0,1,0), and the same holds for extensions like ARIMA(2,0,0) or ARIMA(0,2,1); the more complex our models, the more information (data) we need. Although quite restrictive, an attractive feature of ARIMA(0,1,0) is that it is fairly easy to understand (i.e., fairly easy to compute by hand) and does not require 100 measurements to be used in a meaningful manner. Although as always more observations is better, and there is no magic number for a minimum number of observations that always works, with for example 40 observations ARIMA(0,1,0) may perform fairly well while with fewer than 20 observations ARIMA(0,1,0) some statistics cannot be estimated. In other words, it is safe to say that we should preferably have well over 20 observations—especially if we want to account for events, see next section—and 40 would be better than 30, 50 would be better than 40, et cetera.

An important assumption in time series modelling is that the residuals are *independently and identically distributed* (i.i.d.), which basically means that our model accounts for the pattern in such a way that the *residuals* are uncorrelated and follow a known (e.g., Normal) distribution. Ljung and Box (1978) provided a *Q*-statistic that can test this assumption. In this test, $\boldsymbol{H_0}$ states that the residuals are independently distributed (cf. assumption), while $\boldsymbol{H_1}$ states that the residuals are *not* independently distributed (i.e., there is autocorrelation left to account for). This *Q*-statistic is one of the statistics that cannot computed when the number of observations is smaller than 20 (because $df = 0$) and has limited statistical power when the number of observations barely exceeds 20. The distribution of residuals can be inspected through common graphs such as histograms and boxplots.

Let us have a look at an example of a situation where the random walk model provides a good account of time series data. In a longitudinal clerkship at University X, Year 4 medical students in a five-year programme are placed in a General Practice for 40 weeks. During these 40 weeks, students practice important skills with real patients. At the end of each week, the student's local supervisor rates on a VAS from 0 (minimum) to 100 (maximum) how the student in question has performed on a series of skills, including gathering information from patients,

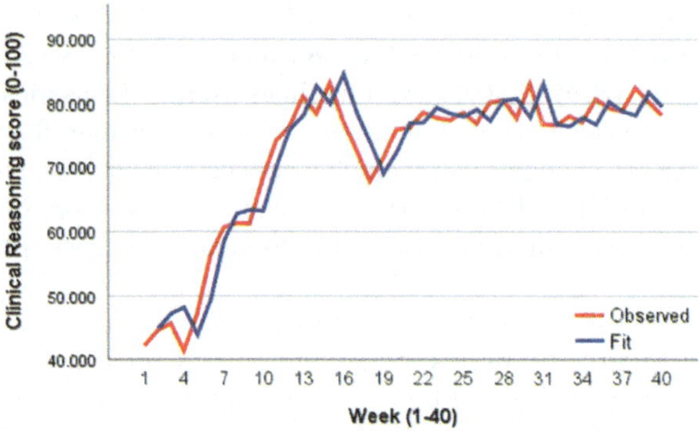

Fig. 16.1 Student #5's weekly clinical reasoning scores provided by General Practitioner (supervisor, red line) and weekly ratings predicted by the random walk model (blue line) (SPSS)

showing empathic behaviour, and clinical reasoning. Let us focus on clinical reasoning for one of these students, Student #5. Figure 16.1 presents the weekly scores provided by the supervisor (red line) and the scores predicted with ARIMA(0,1,0) plus constant (blue line).

As we see, the blue line (predicted scores) is in trajectory very similar to the red line (actual, observed scores), but shifted slightly (i.e., one observation) to the right. Given that the model needs previously predicted and observed scores for the prediction for week i, there is no prediction for the first observation (i.e., the blue line starts only at week 2). Predictions are sometimes higher sometimes lower than the observed scores, though the sign of these differences appears random (i.e., non-systematic). The only predictor in our model is week (i.e., a variable in our data set having values 1–40 cf. the weeks in which we have observed Student #5's clinical reasoning performance). The programme we use, in this case SPSS, generates a number of interesting statistics, one of which is the aforementioned Ljung-Box Q statistic: $Q(18) = 17.844$, $p = 0.466$. In other words, we have insufficient evidence to reject $\boldsymbol{H_0}$ of independent (i.e., non-correlated) residuals. If the Q-statistic generated a statistically significant outcome, we could use (partial) autocorrelation function plots to examine how we could account for the remaining autocorrelation of residuals.

To have a look at the distribution of the residuals, in time series also called *noise residuals*, we can use common graphs like histograms and boxplots. SPSS and other software for time series modelling (e.g., Stata) enable us to *save* these residuals, so we can order the histogram or boxplot for the saved residuals directly. Figure 16.2 presents the boxplot of these residuals for the example at hand, in Jamovi because I like the graphical presentation of boxplots more in Jamovi than in SPSS (though this is a matter of personal preference).

As usual for residuals, $M = 0$. The skewness of the distribution is −0.297, the kurtosis is −0.408, and $SD = 3.543$; residuals range from −7.315 to 6.911, indicating maximum differences between observed and predicted score of about 7

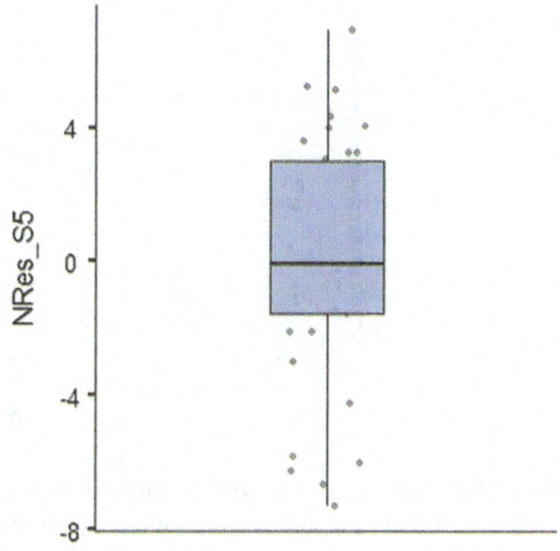

Fig. 16.2 Distribution of (noise) residuals for the time series of Student #5 (*Jamovi*)

points on the 0–100 scale. Figure 16.1 indicates some decline in score from week 15 (about 83 points) to week 18 (about 68 points), and narrative information may help to examine possible reasons for this temporary decline (e.g., difficulty patient encounter[s] or temporary focus on other skills), but this decline is not identified as any kind of outlier in the series. Across the full series, no observations are identified as outliers by *SPSS*. In time series, several types of outliers can be distinguished, but they all have in common that they cause some kind of disruption to a series, either for a short period (i.e., single observation or limited period within the broader series) or for a longer period (e.g., a shift in long-term trend).

16.2.2 Dealing with Events

In educational practice, one source of outliers can be training. In the 40-week longitudinal clerkship period, students may attend training events aimed at specific skills. Regardless of whether the event itself causally influences change (i.e., different factors may contribute to a change), if we see a substantial change in performance during or right after the event, the event may be identified by the software as an outlier. An easy way to deal with such outliers is to add them to the model as predictors. For example, Student #14 takes a two-day training at the beginning of week 15, and the change in score from week 14 to week 15 is substantial, such that when we use the same model as for Student #5, week 15 is identified as an outlier. We then add week 15 as a predictor to our model (i.e., a 0/1 variable called 'week 15' which has '1' in week 15 and '0' in all the other weeks) and obtain statistics for that event. Figure 16.3 demonstrates Student #14's weekly clinical reasoning scores provided by the supervisor (red line) and the model which includes week 15 as predictor (blue line).

Ljung-Box Q-statistic is not statistically significant, $Q(18) = 13.754$, $p = 0.745$, and after accounting for week 15 no other outliers are identified, and the

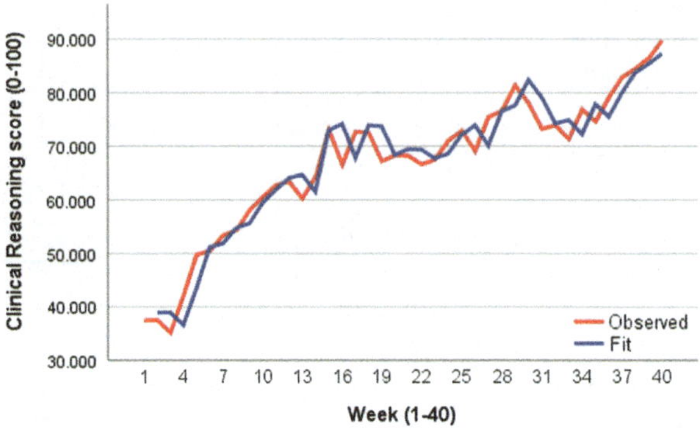

Fig. 16.3 Student #14's weekly clinical reasoning scores provided by General Practitioner (supervisor, red line) and weekly ratings predicted by the random walk model accounting for the two-day training in the first half of week 15 (blue line) (*SPSS*)

distribution of residuals is very similar to what we saw in Fig. 16.2 for Student #5. As we see, Student #14's change in score from week 14 to week 15 is indeed quite substantial (i.e., from about 64 to about 73 points), and for week 15, we find $B = 7.512$, $SE = 3.651$, $t(36) = 2.057$, $p = 0.047$. Note that B is not the same as the actual change from week 14 to week 15 (which is about 9 points), because event statistics are estimated in the light of the broader series.

16.2.3 Individuals and Groups

In settings where it is reasonable to compare individuals, for instance where we have a larger group of students doing the 40-week clerkship under similar conditions (i.e., same skills of focus, same assessment procedures, and same timing of assessments), we have graphical tools at our disposal to look at group-level change and to what extent individual change may differ from that of the group; Figs. 1.1–1.3, 12.5, and 15.1–15.2 provide examples. If we deal with groups of substantial size, such as in Chap. 15 with the progress test, or because a substantial number of students sign up for the integrated clerkship (e.g., 35 students), we can consider some of the mixed-effects models discussed in previous chapters in this book. However, when the numbers of students are small (e.g., only 10–15 students in a longitudinal clerkship), graphs like in Figs. 1.1, 1.3, and 4.1 combined with analyses of individual time series (e.g., cf. for Student #5 and Student #14) provide a more appropriate and more informative approach. With small groups of students, residual covariance structures cannot really be modelled; V_{RES} and r_{RES} tend to be instable, we do not have sufficient information to use a sufficiently complex model, and simple models (e.g., CS or AR1) will not appropriately account for the structure we are dealing with (i.e., likely considerable fluctuation in both V_{RES} and r_{RES} across the series).

16.3 Common Perspectives on Treatment Effects

In educational research, effects of specific treatments on important outcome variables are of interest across the board. While randomised controlled experiments with sufficiently large samples have often been called a 'gold standard', this does not constitute the only method for testing and estimating treatment effects. As mentioned in Chap. 1, whenever the interest lies in treatment effects in individuals or in fairly small populations which may be difficult to study for a variety of reasons, carefully designed SCEDs can provide a good alternative to randomised controlled experiments. For example, if for ethical, financial, or logistic reasons we can include only twelve participants in our study but can take a series of measurements (i.e., time series) for each of the participants, within SCED researchers have a variety of options to design the study, while a randomised controlled experiment where six participants receive treatment and six participants do not receive treatment is unlikely to result in any meaningfully interpretable outcomes. In the world of SCEDs, we have different options for treatment effect statistics (e.g., Michiels, Heyvaert, Meulders, & Onghena, 2017; Parker, Hagan-Burke, & Vannest, 2007; Parker, Vannest, & Davis, 2011), and which ones are most appropriate as usually depends on our research questions, sample size, number of measurements per participant, and the kind of data we end up with.

16.3.1 Parametric Approaches

Where we have sufficiently large numbers of participants, mixed-effects models with effect size estimates like R^2_M can be very useful. However, when we have sufficiently large numbers, we will often opt for a randomised controlled experiment instead for some form of SCED. In practice, SCEDs are often used where the sample size is small. Besides, the numbers of observations are often not that large that we can use time series models discussed earlier in this chapter. In response to these circumstances, researchers often limit themselves to visual (graphical) analysis (Parker et al., 2007, 2011; Tanious, De, & Onghena, 2019)—at group or individual level – or use common parametric methods such as the two-samples t-test and/or Cohen's d or R^2 (Parker et al., 2007; Tanious et al., 2019).

While visual inspection is useful in any statistical analysis, in itself it is rarely sufficient to draw conclusions about treatment effects. Besides, the parametric methods just mentioned have two problems: they assume i.i.d., meaning uncorrelated and preferably approximately normally distributed residuals.

Statistical tests like the t-test rely on an approximately Normal sampling distribution. The sampling distribution follows a Normal distribution whenever the population sampled from follows a Normal distribution. However, in situations where SCEDs are commonly used, such as in Special Needs Education, we often deal with clearly non-normally distributed populations, and in such cases the sampling distribution will approach a Normal distribution only if the sample size is large enough. The numbers of participants in SCEDs commonly encountered—in autism research for instance four to six—usually do not suffice to assume an approximately Normal sampling distribution and make it impossible to meaningfully interpret a distribution of residuals as approximately Normal.

With regard to independence, as we know, residuals in within-subject studies are usually correlated. Thus, parametric procedures such as the two-samples *t*-test and effect size estimates such as Cohen's *d* and R^2 are generally not useful in SCEDs, and for that reason a wide variety of nonparametric statistics have been developed. Given that comprehensive overviews have already been provided by Michiels et al. (2017), Parker et al. (2007, 2011), and Tanious et al. 2019, in the remainder of this chapter we only focus on two commonly encountered and relatively easy-to-use statistics, and look at a third option which is not yet used in this context but comes down to Bayesian Binomial testing.

16.3.2 Nonparametric Approaches Based on Data Overlap

Suppose, we are carrying out a study with $N = 15$ male participants of age 7 years old with autism spectrum disorder, because we want to examine how their performance on an integer metric ranging from 0 (minimum) to 50 (maximum) changes with treatment. For the ease of the example, suppose that we use an AB (i.e., interrupted time series) design, in which for each participant we have 20 measurements *before* treatment (i.e., baseline or A measurements) and 20 measurements *after* treatment (i.e., treatment or B measurements). Figure 16.4 presents the trajectory (i.e., time series) for one of the participants, Participant #1.

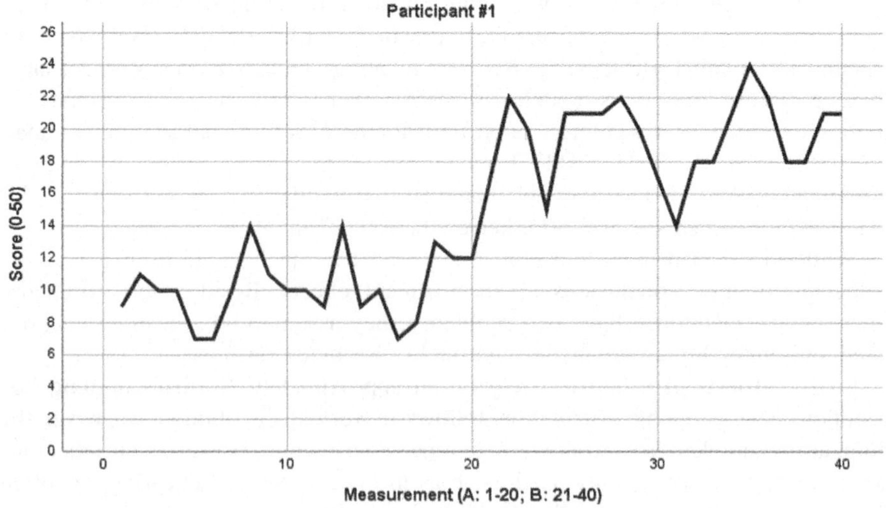

Fig. 16.4 Time series for Participant #1 in autism spectrum disorder study (SPSS)

During baseline (i.e., A), scores range from 7 (observed three times) to 14 (observed two times), whereas the treatment (i.e., B) measurements yield scores ranging from 14 (observed once) to 24 (observed once). An easy nonparametric statistic, which contrary to ARIMA models does not require measurements to be equidistant, is found in the *percentage of non-overlapping data* (PND; Allison & Gorman, 1993, 1994; Parker et al., 2007, 2011; Scruggs & Mastropieri, 1994, 1998, 2001; Scruggs, Mastropieri, & Casto, 1987; White, 1987): the percentage of B measurements that yield better scores than the best score in the A measurements. As a general guideline, PND values above 0.7 are commonly interpreted as effective interventions, PND values in the 0.5–0.7 range reflect questionable effectiveness, and PND values below 0.5 are considered interventions with no observed effect (Parker et al., 2007; Scruggs & Mastropieri, 1994). Within the 0.7–1 range, sometimes a distinction is made between moderately effective (0.7–0.9) and highly effective (0.9–1) interventions.

A second statistic, which is related to PND, is called the percentage of *all* non-overlapping data (PAND; Parker et al., 2007): it is the complement of the lowest possible percentage of measurements from A and/or B measurements that would need to be in the other phase (i.e., in B instead of A, or in A instead of B), or simply removed from the phase they are in, for the highest A score to be lower than the lowest B score (i.e., 100% separation of phases in terms of scores). The addition '*all*' (i.e., the 'A' in PAND) is because contrary to PND, PAND uses *all* measurements instead of the B measurements only. A statistic that uses *all* measurements is generally to be preferred over a statistic that uses only part of the measurements, because we will have more information and more statistical power. For this and other reasons, PAND is generally to be preferred over PND (Parker et al., 2007).

For Participant #1, PND is 0.95 (i.e., 95%), because only 1 of 20 B measurements failed to yield a score higher than the highest A score (i.e., score 14 at measurement 31). For PAND, we use all 40 instead of only 20 measurements, and the minimum possible number of measurements that would need to be transferred or removed to achieve 100% non-overlap is 1 (i.e., measurement 31); 1 out of 40 is 0.025 (2.5%), and thus, PAND = 1 − 0.025 = 0.975.

The fact that PND and PAND yield the a very similar outcome in this example should not be generalised. As Parker et al. (2007) note, PND and PAND tend to yield similar outcomes for effective interventions but can differ substantially for less effective interventions. For instance, Fig. 16.5 presents the trajectory (i.e., time series) for Participant #14.

With participants like Participant #14, it is more difficult to determine PND and PAND from the graph than with participants like Participant #1. Table 16.1 therefore presents the scores for Participant #14 for each of the two phases (A and B).

PND is most straightforward: the highest A score is 21, and 11 of the 20 B measurements yield a score above 21 (i.e., 22–26), hence PND is 0.55. For PAND, the minimum possible number of measurements to be transferred or removed is 3, namely the B measurement that yields score 18, the A measurement that yields

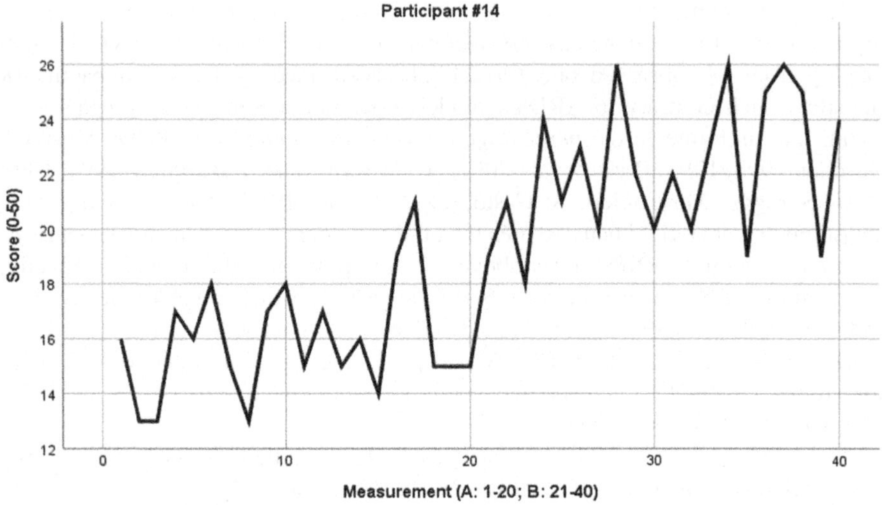

Fig. 16.5 Time series for Participant #14 in autism spectrum disorder study (SPSS)

Table 16.1 Scores and their frequencies for Participant #14 in each of the two phases

Score	Observed frequency	
	Baseline (A)	Treatment (B)
13	3	0
14	1	0
15	6	0
16	3	0
17	3	0
18	2	1
19	1	3
20	0	3
21	1	2
22	0	2
23	0	2
24	0	2
25	0	2
26	0	3

score 19, and the A measurement that yields score 21. Thus, PAND is $1 - (3/40) = 0.925$.

Some may wonder if we should not correct PND and PAND for potential autocorrelation. After all, 40 measurements taken from the same individual likely result in somewhat correlated residuals (i.e., $ICC \neq 0$), and as mentioned in

Chap. 2, the multiplication factor for the required sample size needed (M_N) given *ICC* is:

$$M_N = 1 + [(n - 1) * ICC].$$

However, when dealing with ratios where both numerator and denominator are counts from the same number of measurements from the same individual, both numerator and denominator are corrected by the same factor, and hence for the point estimate of PND and PAND, the outcomes remain the same. Besides, as explained by Parker et al. (2007, p. 196): "*The requirement of serial independence or lack of autocorrelation has little impact on PAND results because the tabled frequency data are unordered.*" This reasoning applies to PND as well. For that reason, Parker et al. 2007) provide an example where for a total of three participants we have a total of 28 measurements, and for each of the participants the minimum number of measurements that would need to be transferred or removed to achieve perfect non-overlap is 2, PAND is 1 − (6/28) ≈ 0.786. They also compute what they call a "*non-overlap beyond chance level*" (Parker et al., 2007, p. 197): 78.6 − 50 = 38.6%, where 50 represents the 50% chance level. The rationale behind the latter is that it will never be needed to remove or transfer *all* measurements; in a situation where exactly half of the measurements are A and half of the measurements are B, the maximum percentage of measurements to be transferred or removed is 50% not 100%. However, when the lengths of A and B are not equal and/or vary across participants, this straightforward 50% correction no longer holds. This is because the maximum possible number of observations needing to be removed or transferred to achieve perfect non-overlap equals the number of observations of the smallest phase; hence, in the case of unequal lengths of A and B, the correction would need to be higher than 50%.

Two limitations of both PND and PAND is that they lack sensitivity for very effective treatments (i.e., PND > 0.9, and PAND easily yielding higher values when —for instance due to a randomised starting point of treatment—one of phases is substantially shorter than the other one) and they do not take into account any potential trend in the baseline period, such as for instance a gradual increase in score which may reflect some kind of learning even before treatment takes place. Therefore, where we have larger numbers of measurements and/or larger numbers of participants, the ARIMA models discussed earlier in this chapter (larger numbers of measurements) and/or group-level mixed-effects models discussed in previous chapters in this book (larger numbers of participants) should be preferred over PAND and PND. Contrary to those statistics estimated with ARIMA or group-level mixed-effects models, PND and PAND have no known sampling distribution, as a result of which *p*-values and CIs cannot be computed and these measures cannot really be interpreted as effect size statistics as for instance Cohen's *d* or coefficient φ. However, PAND can be translated to coefficient φ (Parker et al., 2007), which is a well-established effect size statistic, and this together with PAND using *all* instead of only treatment measurements makes PAND a generally better alternative to PND. Finally, whenever we are in a situation where we cannot use stronger parametric methods in a meaningful manner, the choice seems one between non-parametric alternatives like PAND and φ or presenting graphs only; as would be the case when using parametric methods, reporting both visual and numerical information is generally to be preferred.

16.4 A Bayesian Binomial Treatment Model

PND and PAND are point estimates and there are no CIs around them. From a PND or PAND estimate itself, one cannot tell whether the estimate is based on many or relatively few measurements. A nice feature of CIs is that, keeping other factors constant, they become smaller with more measurements. The Bayesian counterpart of the CI, the CRI, also has this feature; a CRI based on say 35 observations is considerably smaller than a CRI based on only 15 observations. Besides, CRIs allow us to take into account information already available through the specification of the prior distribution and, as demonstrated in the next section, have a fairly important computational benefit over CIs. Finally, as discussed in Chaps. 3 and 14, even where point estimates are not affected by autocorrelation (*ICC*) interval estimations *are* affected by that autocorrelation, and we can correct for that by adjusting our effective sample size (and more specifically: *df*) accordingly. As becomes clear in the final part of this chapter, both PND and PAND can be thought of in terms of two different ways of expressing success/failure rates, and where we talk about successes and failures as the two possible and mutually exclusive options, the Binomial distribution can be used. The Bayesian Binomial model provides a straightforward way to compute success/failure rates for individuals as well as for groups of individuals and can provide meaningful CRIs even where success rates are 0 or 1. Therefore, in the final part of this chapter, I introduce Bayesian alternatives to PND and PAND, henceforth called PND-B and PAND-B (B for Bayes), which can be corrected for correlated residuals to obtain PND-BC and PAND-BC (C for correlation-corrected). Point estimates of these Bayesian alternatives are slightly less extreme (i.e., slightly further away from 0 and 1, meaning a bit closer to 0.5) than PND and PAND, and the 95% CRIs can serve for testing using ROPE.

16.5 Bayesian Binomial Testing and Estimation

To understand the Bayesian Binomial method, let us look at an example of tossing a coin, where Heads stands for success and Tail stands for failure. We want to test $\boldsymbol{H_0}$ that the coin is fair against $\boldsymbol{H_1}$ that the coin is not fair. Based on our experiences with coins, if a coin is fair, the chance of success should equal the chance of failure (i.e., 0.5), but absent data for the coin at hand we should not assume some success probabilities to be more likely than others. This can be translated into a Beta(a,b)

Table 16.2 Prior and posterior distribution for the proportion of success (Heads) for each of ten rounds in the coin tossing study

Prior: Beta(a,b)		Data		Posterior: Beta(a,b)	
a (success)	b (failure)	Successes	Failures	a (success)	b (failure)
1	1	6	4	7	5
7	5	5	5	12	10
12	10	7	3	19	13
19	13	5	5	24	18
24	18	5	5	29	23
29	23	7	3	36	26
36	26	5	5	41	31
41	31	4	6	45	37
45	37	4	6	49	43
49	43	6	4	55	47

distribution that takes the shape of a Uniform distribution ranging from 0 to 1 with *M* and median 0.5 and a 95% CRI of [0.025; 0.975]: Beta(1,1), where the first '1' (a) stands for the number of successes and the second '1' (b) stands for the number of failures.

Suppose, we throw ten times and obtain six successes and four failures. The resulting posterior distribution is Beta(1 + 6,1 + 4) = Beta (7,5). This distribution has a median of 0.588 and a 95% CRI of [0.308; 0.833]. Suppose, we repeat this game nine times, meaning that at the end we have a total of 10 sets of 10 throws. Table 16.2 presents the (simulated) outcomes for each of ten rounds along with the prior and posterior distribution for the different rounds.

As we see, the posterior from one round constitutes the prior for the next round; in the words of Lindley (1972, p. 2), "*today's posterior is tomorrow's prior.*" This is what *Bayesian* (model) *updating* is all about: the prior is *updated* by the *data* as if there had only ever been a single round of tosses. In other words, had we considered the 10 * 10 tosses as one experiment of 100 tosses, we would have obtained the same posterior distribution: a Beta(1,1) prior and 54 successes and 46 failures (data) coming in results in a Beta (55,47) posterior. This posterior distribution has a median of 0.539 and a 95% CRI of [0.442; 0.635]. The median of the posterior is almost equal to the observed proportion of successes (0.54); it is slightly pulled towards 0.5, and more so the more the observed proportion approaches either of the extremes of 0 or 1 but approaches the observed proportion more and more with more observations.

A Beta(55,47) distribution corresponds with $BF_{01} \approx 0.935$ (i.e., around 1) when using a Beta(49,43) prior (i.e., the prior before the start of the tenth round, see Table 16.2) and $BF_{01} \approx 5.854$ when using a Beta(1,1) prior (i.e., the prior before the start of the first round). In other words, there is not much of a shift in likelihood of 0.5 from the end of the ninth round to the end of the tenth round, but there is a clear shift in that likelihood from the start of the first round to the end of the tenth round. We remain open to further data, but the data observed are substantially more likely to have occurred under $\boldsymbol{H_0}$ 'coin is fair' than under $\boldsymbol{H_1}$ 'coin is not fair' ($BF_{01} \approx 5.854$). If the calculations are difficult to follow, JASP enables Bayesian Binomial testing, and in the Summary Statistics module (where you can choose the Bayesian Binomial test) you can fill in the numbers yourself and obtain the outcomes presented here.

16.5.1 Individual Treatment

PND and PAND can be conceptualised in terms of successes and failures. For Participant #1, PND is 0.95 (19/20), which corresponds with 19 successes and 1 failure, and PAND is 0.975 (39/40), which corresponds with 39 successes and 1 failure. For Participant #14, PND is 0.55 (11/20), which corresponds with 11 successes and 9 failures, and PAND is 0.925 (37/40), which corresponds with 37 successes and 3 failures. Doing so, we can apply the same Bayesian Binomial procedure to PND and PAND, using Beta(1,1) as prior.

For Participant #1, we find for PND-B a Beta(20,2) posterior distribution, which is a distribution with a median of 0.921 and 95% CRI of [0.762; 0.988], and for PAND-B we find a Beta(40,2) posterior distribution, which is a distribution with a median of 0.959 and a 95% CRI of [0.871; 0.994]. With fewer observations, the 95% CRIs of PND-B and PAND-B would be wider and the medians would be pulled somewhat more towards 0.5 than is the case with current numbers of observations. The medians of the two distributions provide appropriate estimates of PND-B and PAND-B, because an observed PND of 0.95 based on many observations is more informative and leaves us more confident than an observed PND of 0.95 based on fewer observations. For that same reason, the 95% CRIs provide good intervals for ROPE testing. If for example for PND, we agree that values in the 0–0.5 range reflect ineffective interventions, the ROPE is [0; 0.5], and if we agree that only effective interventions have practical importance, we may want to extend the ROPE to [0; 0.7]. Taking the latter as starting point, we have sufficient evidence in favour of the hypothesis of the intervention being effective whenever the 95% CRI of PND-B has no overlap with ROPE. For Participant #1, the 95% CRI of PND-B does not overlap with ROPE, hence we have sufficient evidence in favour of an effective intervention. For PAND-B, the upper bound of ROPE depends on whether the lengths of A and B are the same or not; when they are the same, PAND ranges from 0.5 to 1 because in the worst-case scenario, half of the observations would need to be transferred or removed to achieve perfect non-overlap. Translating the [0; 0.5] and [0; 0.7] from PND to PAND would then result in ROPEs of [0.5; 0.75] and [0.5; 0.85], respectively. Either way, for Participant #1, the 95% CRI of PAND-B fully excludes ROPE, meaning that we can conclude sufficient evidence in favour of the intervention being effective. That said, when A and B are not of equal length, the lower bound of the PAND range is not 0.5 and a different, case-specific correction needs to be applied.

For Participant #14, the findings are less positive than for Participant #1. For PND-B, we find a Beta(12,10) posterior distribution, which is a distribution with a median of 0.547 and a 95% CRI of [0.340; 0.743]. For PAND-B, we find a Beta (38,4) posterior distribution, which is a distribution with median 0.911 and a 95% CRI of [0.801; 0.973]. If we agree that only effective interventions matter, and we use [0; 0.7] as ROPE for PND-B and [0.5; 0.85] as ROPE for PAND-B, we conclude that there is insufficient evidence to assume the intervention to be effective. As long as a 95% CRI does not fully overlap with the ROPE (which is the case for both CRIs for Participant #14), we cannot conclude sufficient evidence in favour of the hypothesis that the intervention is *not* effective, but as long as there is partial overlap between the 95% CRI and the ROPE we cannot conclude sufficient evidence in favour of the intervention at hand being effective either.

16.5.2 Merging Outcomes from Multiple Individuals

Participant #1 and Participant #14 are only two of the 15 participants in our study. Table 16.3 presents PND, PAND, and the outcomes of PND-B and PAND-B for all fifteen participants in the study.

The 95% CRI for PND-B is fully outside the [0; 0.7] ROPE for Participants #1, #2, #5, and #6, and the 95% CRI for PAND-B is fully outside the [0.5; 0.85] ROPE for Participants #1, #2, #5, #6, and #7. For all other participants, there is at least

Table 16.3 PND, PAND, and the outcomes of PND-B and PAND-B for all participants in the autism spectrum disorder study

Part. #	PND	PAND	PND-B estimates			PAND-B estimates		
			Median	CRI LB	CRI UB	Median	CRI LB	CRI UB
#1	0.950	0.975	0.921	0.762	0.988	0.959	0.871	0.994
#2	1.000	1.000	.968	.839	.999	.983	.914	0.999
#3	0.900	0.950	0.875	0.696	0.970	0.935	0.835	0.985
#4	0.900	0.950	0.875	0.696	0.970	0.935	0.835	0.985
#5	1.000	1.000	0.968	0.839	0.999	0.983	0.914	0.999
#6	1.000	1.000	0.968	0.839	0.999	0.983	0.914	0.999
#7	0.900	0.975	0.875	0.696	0.970	0.959	0.871	0.994
#8	0.900	0.950	0.875	0.696	0.970	0.935	0.835	0.985
#9	0.750	0.900	0.734	0.528	0.887	0.887	0.769	0.959
#10	0.700	0.900	0.687	0.478	0.854	0.887	0.769	0.959
#11	0.800	0.950	0.781	0.581	0.918	0.935	0.835	0.985
#12	0.650	0.900	0.641	0.430	0.819	0.887	0.769	0.959
#13	0.900	0.950	0.875	0.696	0.970	0.935	0.835	0.985
#14	0.550	0.925	0.547	0.340	0.743	0.911	0.801	0.973
#15	0.400	0.850	0.406	0.218	0.616	0.839	0.708	0.928

partial overlap with ROPE, meaning that for those participants we cannot conclude sufficient evidence for the intervention to be effective. For Participant #15, the 95% CRI for PND-B even fully lies within the [0; 0.7] ROPE, meaning that if we were to rely on PND-B as main indicator of intervention effectiveness we would conclude that for Participant #15 we have sufficient in favour of the intervention *not* being effective. That said, even for Participant #15, PAND-B provides a more nuanced picture (i.e., inconclusive, meaning sufficient evidence neither against nor in favour of the intervention to be effective).

Some may wonder if we can use CRIs to conclude about the evidence for the intervention at the level of individual participants. After all, is the goal of research not to establish laws and principles that have a broader use and hence require generalisation from sample to population? Although the answer to this is generally *yes*, in educational practice the interest often lies in individuals as well. While CIs are based on the Frequentist philosophy, which assumes that our samples are *random* from which we can generalise to populations sampled from using SEs, *p*-values and CIs, CRIs are based on a Bayesian philosophy, in which data, once observed, are treated as *fixed*, and update our knowledge of (or belief about) an outcome variable of interest (i.e., from prior to posterior distribution). That process of updating can be done about populations as well as about individuals. Another setting where the individual would be of interest is in knowledge or skill testing, where with every new data point (e.g., a measurement, or a question responded to) we update our knowledge about that individual's knowledge or skill level; CRIs provide a straightforward and intuitive way to quantify our knowledge about that matter at any given point in time.

As long as we are trying to establish evidence for a specific individual patient with regard to the effectiveness of an intervention, we may not want to worry much about autocorrelation in residuals, partly because of the frequency data being unordered (cf. argument by Parker et al., 2007). However, if the goal of research is to *generalise* findings from individuals under study to a broader population, even if that population is small, autocorrelation does become an issue. Whether an outcome variable of interest does or does not take into account the original order of measurements, measurements taken from the same individual tend to yield more similar outcomes than measurements from different randomly sampled individuals, and that creates a situation where $ICC > 0$. A straightforward way to correct the number of observations for $ICC > 0$ is found in:

$$M_N = 1 + [(n - 1) * ICC].$$

In this formula, n is now the number of measurements per individual. In studies where N is large enough, mixed-effects modelling can help us to obtain an accurate ICC estimate. However, in studies where N is limited, for example $N = 15$ in the current study, ICC estimates cannot be trusted and we need a good rule of thumb to apply. For unordered data, ICC values in the [0.01; 0.20] range are very common (e.g., Leppink, 2019), and for dichotomous outcome variables we often find ourselves in the lower part of that range. Therefore, using $ICC = 0.10$ as rule of thumb for sample size correction is decent unless we have sufficiently large numbers of participants to accurately estimate *ICC* using mixed-effects models. Applying this formula to PND and PAND, n corresponds with the number of B measurements in the case of PND and corresponds with the total number of measurements in the case of PAND. In other words, if a participant has 20 B measurements, the correction for PND is a factor 2.9, and if a participant has a total of 40 measurements, the correction for PAND is a factor 4.9. Concretely, this would mean that the effective (i.e., *ICC*-corrected) number of B measurements is $20/2.9 \approx 6.897$, and the effective total number of measurements is $40/4.9 \approx 8.163$. We then correct the number of successes and failures for PND-B and PAND-B accordingly to obtain the distributional outcomes (i.e., median and 95% CRI) for PND-BC and PAND-BC.

For example, for Participant #1, the revised number of successes for PND-BC is 6.552 and the revised number of failures for PND-BC is 0.345. Using the Beta(1,1) prior distribution, this yields a distribution for PND-BC with a median of 0.875 and a 95% CRI of [0.567; 0.990]. For PAND-BC, the revised number of successes is 7.959 and the revised number of failures is 0.204. Using the Beta(1,1) prior distribution, this yields a distribution for PAND-BC with a median of 0.906 and a 95% CRI of [0.635; 0.994]. Given that A and B are of equal length for all participants, the same exercise can be done for the other participants. If the lengths of A and B varied across participants (e.g., a randomised starting point of the treatment), the correction factors would not be 2.9 and 4.9 for all participants but would vary across participants. Table 16.4 presents the outcomes of PND-BC and PAND-BC for all fifteen participants.

Table 16.4 Outcomes of PND-BC and PAND-BC for all participants in the autism spectrum disorder study

Part. #	PND-BC estimates			PAND-BC estimates		
	Median	CRI LB	CRI UB	Median	CRI LB	CRI UB
#1	0.875	0.567	0.990	0.906	0.635	0.994
#2	0.916	0.627	0.997	0.927	0.669	0.997
#3	0.834	0.513	0.980	0.885	0.605	0.990
#4	0.834	0.513	0.980	0.885	0.605	0.990
#5	0.916	0.627	0.997	0.927	0.669	0.997
#6	0.916	0.627	0.997	0.927	0.669	0.997
#7	0.834	0.513	0.980	0.906	0.635	0.994
#8	0.834	0.513	0.980	0.885	0.605	0.990
#9	0.709	0.376	0.931	0.843	0.548	0.979
#10	0.667	0.336	0.909	0.843	0.548	0.979
#11	0.751	0.418	0.950	0.885	0.605	0.990
#12	0.625	0.298	0.885	0.843	0.548	0.979
#13	0.834	0.513	0.980	0.885	0.605	0.990
#14	0.542	0.229	0.832	0.864	0.576	0.985
#15	0.416	0.140	0.738	0.800	0.496	0.964

Since the effective sample size is considerably smaller than the 20 and 40 observations we used before, the 95% CRIs are substantially wider and the medians of the distributions are somewhat more pulled towards 0.5. Even for participants whose PND and PAND is 1, none of the 95% CRIs exclude the ROPE. Some readers may wonder if this does not create problems with the interpretation, but the answer to that is *no*.

Imagine someone telling you in the morning "*I just learned that all inhabitants of York were drunk last night!*", to which you ask "*how did you estimate that?*", and the response is "*well, I asked three people and they all got drunk!*". You would not take that as a serious estimate for all inhabitants of York; instead, you would realise that probably not *all* inhabitants got drunk and that with increasing sample size we would probably also see people who did not get drunk, and we would obtain a more accurate estimate of the proportion of people who got drunk in York last night. A similar reasoning applies to PND and PAND; regardless of what estimates we obtain, when based on many observations we are (or at least should be) more willing to accept them as accurate estimates than when they are based on just a few observations. PND and PAND estimates of 1 should not be understood as an intervention being 100% effective; if we had more measurements, we would likely observe at least one or a few scores that would not indicate success and bring that extreme '1' (100%) estimate down at least slightly. As far as ROPE testing is concerned, the inability to conclude an intervention to be effective and generalise that conclusion to a broader population is not something we should do based on a single participant.

That said, there is an easy way to combine or merge the outcomes of the fifteen individuals into sample-level – and across studies: the level of a meta-analysis – using the Bayesian Binomial approach discussed in this chapter. Not assuming any *ICC*, we have 15 participants * 20 observations for the PND and 15 participants * 40 observations for PAND. For PND, 246 of the 300 observations are successes and the remaining 54 observations are failures; these numbers can be easily recalculated by hand from Table 16.3 (same as for PAND). Using a Beta(1,1) prior distribution (i.e., reasoning cf. the ten rounds vs. one round of coin tossing study), 246 successes and 54 failures yields a Beta(247,55) posterior distribution for PND-B, which is a distribution with a median of 0.819 and a 95% CRI of [0.772; 0.859]. For PAND, 567 of the 600 observations are successes and 33 are failures. Using a Beta(1,1) prior distribution, this means a Beta(568,34) distribution for PAND-B, which is a distribution with a median of 0.944 and a 95% CRI of [0.924; 0.961].

When we correct for autocorrelation (i.e., the *ICC* = 0.1 rule of thumb), using the corrected numbers of successes and failures which result in the outcomes in Table 16.4, the corrected number of successes for PND-BC is about 84.828 and the corrected number of failures for PND-BC is about 18.621. Using a Beta(1,1) prior distribution, this means a Beta(85.828,19.621) distribution for PND-BC, which is a distribution with a median of 0.816 and a 95% CRI of [0.735; 0.882]. For PAND-BC, the corrected number of successes is about 115.714 and the corrected number of failures is about 6.735. Using a Beta(1,1) prior distribution, this means a Beta(116.714,7.735) posterior distribution, which is a distribution with a median of

0.940 and a 95% CRI of [0.889; 0.973]. At group level, the differences in distribution between uncorrected (PND-B and PAND-B) and corrected (PND-BC and PAND-BC) are not as substantial as at the level of the individual, but there are differences nevertheless, and the correction is necessary. While ten rounds of ten random coin tosses may well be counted as 100 independent observations, not correcting for *ICC* when going beyond an individual participant would be like treating 15 participants with 20 or 40 measurements as if they were 15 * 20 or 15 * 40 different participants, hence a form of self-deceit.

For PND-BC, the 95% CRI has no overlap with the [0; 0.7] ROPE, and for PAND-BC, the 95% CRI has no overlap with the [0.5; 0.85] ROPE either, hence this study with fifteen participants appears to provide sufficient evidence to conclude an effective intervention. This does *not* mean that we can now conclude that the intervention is effective for *every* individual; on the contrary, for several individuals we have not acquired sufficient evidence in favour of an effective intervention. However, the findings of all individuals in our study taken together, we conclude that overall there is sufficient evidence in favour of the hypothesis that the intervention is effective.

16.5.3 Other Applications of the Bayesian Binomial Procedure

The Bayesian Binomial procedure discussed in this chapter can also provide a nonparametric alternative in some other situations where mixed-effects models, which are generally much more powerful and much more accurate, cannot be used. Two straightforward examples are the repeated-measures design where the participants are observed twice (e.g., pre-post improvement: yes or no) and matched-pairs design where for instance twins or married couples constitute the pairs. Whether we take pre-post improvement or differences within twins (e.g., random allocation to treatment /control condition) or couples, any difference in a particular, prespecified direction can be conceived as a success while any difference not going in that direction can be conceived as a failure. Another context in which the Bayesian Binomial procedure outline in this chapter (including accounting for *ICC* > 0) can be useful is in using historical performance data on exam items to sample items from a bank such that we compose a new exam of desired level of difficulty and set an acceptable standard (Leppink, 2020).

Absent more informative prior knowledge, the Beta(1,1) constitutes the default prior distribution which can be updated with the numbers of successes and failures observed to obtain a Beta(1 + successes, 1 + failures) posterior distribution. The median provides a good point estimate, and the 95% CRI can be used for estimation and ROPE testing. In these situations, there will be no need to correct for *ICC* (i.e., there is within-measurement-pair correlation, but the pairs can be treated as independent observations) unless the individuals or pairs under study are nested within households or units alike that usually contribute to *ICC*. Absent nesting-related *ICC*, the total number of observations *N* for the Binomial procedure equals the number of pairs, the number of pairs where the change is in the prespecified direction constitutes the number of successes, and the number of pairs where the change is *not* in the prespecified direction constitutes the number of failures.

References

Allison, D. B., & Gorman, B. S. (1993). Calculating effect sizes for meta-analysis: The case of the single case. *Behaviour Research and Therapy, 31*(6), 621–631. https://doi.org/10.1016/0005-7967(93)90115-B.

Allison, D. B., & Gorman, B. S. (1994). Make things as simple as possible, but no simpler: A rejoinder to Scruggs and Mastropieri. *Behaviour Research and Therapy, 32*(8), 885–890. https://doi.org/10.1016/0005-7967(94)90170-8.

Box, G. E. P., Jenkins, G. M., & Reinsel, G. C. (1994). *Time series analysis: Forecasting and control* (3rd ed.). Upper Saddle River, NJ: Prentice Hall.

Box, G. E. P., & Tiao, G. C. (1975). Intervention analysis with applications to economic and environmental problems. *Journal of the American Statistical Association, 70*(349), 70–79. https://doi.org/10.1080/01621459.1975.10480264.

Brockwell, P. J., & Davis, R. A. (2009). *Time series: Theory and methods* (2nd ed.). New York: Springer.

Hannan, E. J. (1970). *Multiple time series*. New York: Wiley.

Leppink, J. (2019). *Statistical methods for experimental research in education and psychology*. Cham: Springer. https://doi.org/10.1007/978-3-030-21241-4.

Leppink, J. (2020). In God we trust, all others bring data: A Bayesian approach to standard setting. *Health Professions Education*, https://doi.org/10.1016/j.hpe.2020.01.003.

Lindley, D. (1972). *Bayesian statistics: A review*. London: SIAM.

Ljung, G., M., & Box, G. E. P. (1978). On a measure of a lack of fit in time series models. *Biometrika, 65*(2), 297–303. https://doi.org/10.1093/biomet/65.2.297.

Michiels, B., Heyvaert, M., Meulders, A., & Onghena, P. (2017). Confidence intervals for single-case effect size measures based on randomization test inversion. *Behavior Research Methods, 49*(1), 363–381. https://doi.org/10.3758/s13428-016-0714-4.

Parker, R. I., Hagan-Burke, S., & Vannest, K. J. (2007). Percentage of all non-overlapping data (PAND): An alternative to PND. *The Journal of Special Education, 40*(4), 194–204. https://doi.org/10.1177/00224669070400040101.

Parker, R. I., Vannest, K. J., & Davis, J. L. (2011). Effect size in single-case research: A review of nine nonoverlap techniques. *Behavior Modification, 35*(4), 303–322. https://doi.org/10.1177/0145445511399147.

Scruggs, T. E., & Mastropieri, M. A. (1994). The utility of the PND statistic: A reply to Allison and Gorman. *Behaviour Research and Therapy, 32*(8), 879–883. https://doi.org/10.1016/0005-7967(94)90169-4.

Scruggs, T. E., & Mastropieri, M. A. (1998). Summarizing single-subject research: Issues and applications. *Behavior Modification, 22*(3), 221–242. https://doi.org/10.1177/01454455980223001.

Scruggs, T. E., & Mastropieri, M. A. (2001). How to summarize single-participant research: Ideas and applications. *Exceptionality, 9*(4), 227–244. https://doi.org/10.1207/S15327035EX0904_5.

Scruggs, T. E., Mastropieri, M. A., & Casto, G. (1987). The quantitative synthesis of single subject research: Methdology and validation. *Remedial and Special Education, 8*(2), 24–33. https://doi.org/10.1177/074193258700800206.

Tanious, R., & De, T, K., & Onghena, P. (2019). A multiple randomization testing procedure for level, trend, variability, overlap, immediacy, and consistency in single-case phase designs. *Behaviour Research and Therapy, 119*, 103414. https://doi.org/10.1016/j.brat.2019.103414.

White, O. R. (1987). Some comments concerning: "The quantitative synthesis of single-subject research". *Remedial and Special Education, 8*(2), 34–39. https://doi.org/10.1177/074193258700800207.

Part V
Conclusion

General Recommendations 17

Abstract

This final chapter provides a synthesis of the other sixteen chapters in this book in the form of a set of general guidelines for educational research and practice: the use of multiple criteria for statistical testing and estimation, ways to deal with different types of data, taking a network perspective on the interdependence of assessments and other measures, and choosing appropriate models for groups and individuals. As such, this chapter provides a concise overview and summary of the other sixteen chapters in this book.

17.1 Introduction

This booked started from the notion that learning is a longitudinal process of change, in expected and unexpected directions, to which a variety of factors may contribute, and that two types of processes are of interest in the context of learning: *within-individual* change and *between-individuals* differences in that change over time. Both types of processes come with their own variances, which can be separated in longitudinal and other repeated-measures research, and both types of processes contribute to an *intercorrelation structure* that defines how repeated measurements with the same method or instrument as well as measurements from different methods or instruments are correlated with one another. Understanding this intercorrelation structure is of paramount importance for understanding learning and for the continuous development of assessments and educational programmes, for early intervention for struggling learners, and for justifying high-stakes decisions which may result in a delay of a learner gaining access to practice or, in some cases, even being denied that access altogether.

J. Leppink, *The Art of Modelling the Learning Process*, Springer Texts in Education,
https://doi.org/10.1007/978-3-030-43082-5_17

Appreciating the longitudinal nature of learning and designing teaching, practice, and assessment accordingly can help us to move from a punishment culture to a growth mindset. Performance of the moment is a fraction of a bigger growth picture. Questions like *what went well*, *what did not go so well*, *what could be done differently next time*, and *what study or practice activities are needed to get there* are key questions for a growth mindset, and accurately modelling *within-individual* change and *between-individuals* differences can greatly facilitate learners' and educators' reflections on these questions.

17.2 Multiple Criteria

As discussed in Part I and Part II of this book, modelling learning processes is about carefully combining a multitude of criteria that need to be evaluated in the light of the (research or practice-driven) questions of interest, the design as well as instruments and procedures used, and the kind of data we end up dealing with. Figure 17.1 presents a line plot with *M* and *SD* test performance in a group of 20 children aged 5–6 years old on 16 training trials for a particular physical exercise.

Statistical analysis should not be restricted to inspecting graphs, and both graphs and numbers must be interpreted in the given context. Questions coming to mind when seeing a graph like the one in Fig. 17.1 include: what was the skill being practised; how were the trials timed; was there any instruction at any point(s) in the trial series; how was performance measured; how was the score composed; what were the theoretical and practical range of the score of interest; did the children have a particular interest in participating; does the nature of the data warrant the use

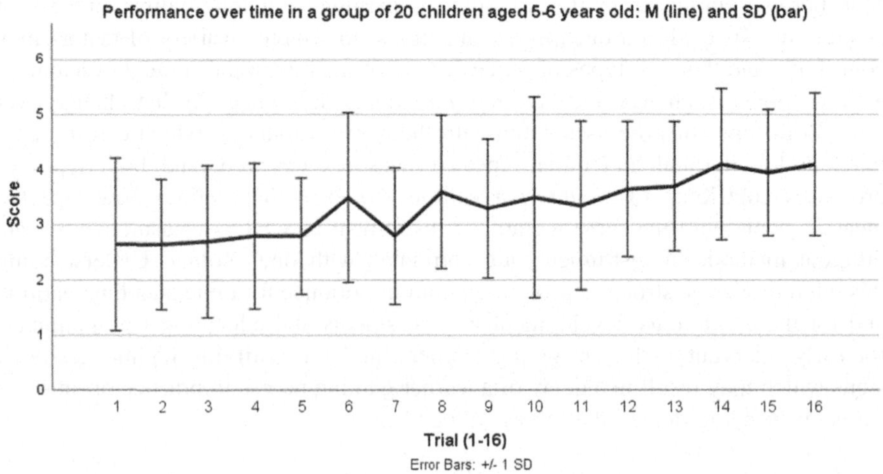

Fig. 17.1 Test performance in a group of 20 children aged 5–6 years old on 16 trials

of *M* and *SD* as key summary statistics of central tendency and dispersion; and, is there considerable variation between individuals in change over time (e.g., Figs. 1.1 and 1.3 as examples of visual inspections of that variation)? These and other questions have implications for our choices regarding which statistical methods and criteria to use for statistical testing and estimation.

A rather forced and unconstructive classification in educational research, which is much less common in other fields (e.g., Forensics), is the *qualitative-quantitative* divide. While the continuation of this divide may be helpful for individuals who want to develop a reputation and career as 'qualitative' or 'quantitative' researcher, in the era of Big Data and AI we have countless examples of why that divide is unrealistic and stands in the way of progress in science. At the end of the day quantitative differences are qualitative differences that have been counted or measured, and qualitative differences are differences that we have not yet managed to quantify in a meaningful manner. In a Forensics context, combining narrative (e.g., the vast body of information from eyewitness testimonies) and numerical (e.g., DNA match and GPS data) to reach informed decisions in a criminal case has been perfectly normal for a long time; why should we pretend that in Education these are separate types of data that cannot be used for the same question of interest? Interviews are commonly labelled as a 'qualitative' and surveys as a 'quantitative' as if one only provides qualitative and the other only provides quantitative data, while even the most 'qualitatively'-oriented interview can yield very useful quantitative information and not so few findings from a survey are hard to interpret as purely 'quantitative'. Classifications like 'quantitative' needing software and 'qualitative' requiring coding 'by hand' may have been natural in former times, but recent examples of advances in Machine Learning, such as the ones in Chap. 3 on the classification of materials as 'thermoelectric' and Facebook processing billions of messages and other communication on a daily basis, demonstrate that such dichotomies are no longer useful. It is time for us to embrace the reality that 'qualitative' and 'quantitative' are not two entirely different spaces separated by a thick wall but are *one* and should be treated as such in both research and everyday educational practice. Even where narrative information cannot be quantified, coded data may perfectly lend themselves for several of the methods discussed in Chap. 5 (dichotomous data), Chap. 6 (multicategory data with no evident order), and Chap. 7 (multicategory data with evident order). Simultaneously, whether we deal with categorical or noncategorical data, some of the assumptions made in the models we use are assessed in a rather 'qualitative' manner. For instance, there are no absolute rules with regard to some threshold for a distribution deviating 'too much' from an assumed ideal (e.g., Normal, or proportional odds); a multitude of criteria are to be taken into account and explained.

Estimations of and decisions on relations and differences of interest are also to be based on a variety of criteria. While we appear to slowly have left behind an era where the *p*-value had an almost 'holy' status (e.g., decisions about whether something 'works' used to be made largely and often entirely based on *p*-values), moving to a single alternative (e.g., BF) would not be a route to be recommended. All criteria have their strengths and weaknesses (e.g., BFs provide a straightforward way to compare different models but can be quite sensitive to different choices in prior distribution), and more informed decisions usually come from combinations of criteria. CIs and CRIs provide testing intervals that can help us to establish evidence against or in favour of relative equivalence of conditions, groups, or repeated measurements under comparison (i.e., TOST, ROPE, and FOST introduced in Chap. 3).

17.3 A Network Perspective

As demonstrated in Part III of this book, network analysis can serve many purposes. To start, it provides a useful emerging tool along with established methods like factor analysis, IRT, latent profile analysis, and latent class analysis to study the psychometric structure of the instruments we use (Chap. 9). While like its more established alternatives network analysis puts considerable demands on the sample size, especially when more complex structures are considered, network plots provide powerful visuals of which items may be grouped together, which items might also relate substantially to items outside that item grouping, and how item interrelations might vary across groups, conditions, or occasions (Chaps. 9 and 11). When the sample size allows for it, these network plots also help us to understand how scales from different instruments are related (Chaps. 10 and 12). As demonstrated in Chap. 12, a network perspective on our educational programmes can help us to understand for instance how different assessments in our programmes are related. Even though different types of assessments usually measure somewhat different types of knowledge or skills, they do tend to have some explanatory power for each other.

17.4 Change Models for Groups and Individuals

In Part IV of this book, we encounter different options for studying change in groups (Chaps. 13–16) as well as in individuals (Chap. 16). Where the sample size is sufficient, randomised controlled experiments (Chap. 13) continue to provide a strong approach to a wide variety of research questions involving condition-by-time interactions. Special attention is needed for so-called *baseline measurements*, which are measurements occurring *before treatment*: as long as treatment is absent, participants randomly allocated to different conditions are to be treated as coming from the same population, which implies regression to a *common M* instead of to different *M*s.

Since much of our learning takes place through interaction with others, and advancements in technology increasingly enable us to monitor such interactions, social network analysis is an indispensable part of our statistical toolbox that can provide powerful visuals of how different actors in a network are interrelated and that can provide a variety of statistics that can be used for explanatory and predictive modelling, sometimes through fairly basic methods like single-level linear regression and sometimes using mixed-effects modelling (Chap. 14).

In some fields of Education, well-established practices of longitudinal assessment can already be encountered. For example, in some medical schools, progress testing has provided an important method to monitor growth in knowledge at individual and group level across years in a medical programme (Chap. 15). Likewise, in other fields of Education, studies involving a multitude of repeated measurements of the same outcome variable(s) of interest are already common practice (Chap. 16). For instance, in Special Needs Education, where for a variety of reasons researchers often do not have the luxury to sample numbers of participants suitable for a meaningful randomised controlled experiment, and besides, the interest often lies in whether an intervention is effective for specific individuals, SCEDs involving relatively long series of measurements are much more common than randomised controlled experiments. Chaps. 15 and 16 provide graphical and numerical options for the study of change in longer series of measurements at individual and group level. Given the limitations we may encounter in some settings, especially where only few individuals are involved and the number of measurements is not very large, both parametric and nonparametric options are discussed. While the parametric options are generally to be preferred over the nonparametric ones when there are no stringent limitations that invalidate the parametric outcomes, the Bayesian Binomial treatment model discussed in Chap. 16 provides a straightforward nonparametric approach that overcomes some of the limitations of nonparametric methods commonly used in SCEDs in some settings (e.g., PND and PAND) and is also applicable to other types of studies where the interest lies in a change in a particular direction (e.g., pre-post and matched-pairs designs) but where sample size and/or data limitations do not reasonably allow for the generally more powerful and more accurate parametric solutions.

17.5 To Conclude

The practice of statistics is not limited to linear relations in 'large' samples; it encompasses all kinds of patterns from highly complex to very basic, and can be use when dealing with data from entire populations, for samples large and small, as well as for making informed decisions about specific individual cases. In educational research, the interest usually lies in generalising findings obtained from a sample to a larger population. However, in everyday educational practice, questions concerning individual progress and the effectiveness of interventions for particular individuals are quite common. Either way, we have statistical solutions available, and new statistical solutions are being developed on an ongoing basis. Whether we deal with research data or data from a setting in educational practice, different people looking at the same data will likely make different choices and end up with somewhat different outcomes. Whether we are trying to contribute to the research literature in our field or we are dealing with assessments of knowledge or skill in an educational programme or exit/entrance exam, transparency is key; it is our ethical and moral obligation to document steps, choices, findings, and conclusions such that they make sense to our audience. It is therefore important that we carefully document every step taken, every choice made, and explain how we have come to our findings and conclusions. When we document things with that accuracy, the audience can decide for themselves if our conclusions make sense or they might draw somewhat different conclusions.

The manufacturer's authorised representative in the EU is Springer Nature Customer Service Centre GmbH, Europaplatz 3, 69115 Heidelberg, Germany. If you have any concerns regarding our products, please contact ProductSafety@springernature.com

Printed and bound by CPI Group (UK) Ltd, Croydon, CR0 4YY
30/09/2026
02225643-0008